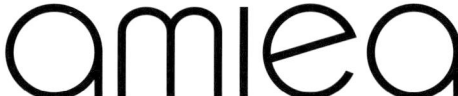

PERMANENT MAKEUP

The essential steps to become an artist

Toni Belfatto in cooperation with Elena Nikora, Olga Kravchenko and Sara Lopez

INDEX

PERMANENT MAKEUP. THE ESSENTIAL STEPS TO BECOME AN ARTIST. was written to answer the needs of dermopigmentation professionals, supporting them with research, knowledge, and very detailed step-by-step instructions. We will describe different application techniques for eyebrows, eyes, and lips, with relative levels of difficulty: different types of training and level of expertise will determine the best choice.

DIFFICULTY LEVEL

The icons describe the procedures that are best suited for BEGINNERS (LOW), ADVANCED PROFESSIONALS (MEDIUM), AND EXPERT PROFESSIONALS (HIGH).

= LOW, recommended for beginners

= MEDIUM, recommended for advanced professionals

= HIGH, recommended for expert professionals

SPECIALIZATIONS

The following icons indicate the 4 areas of specialization within dermopigmentation, and are found throughout the book alongside the descriptions of needles and of the fields of application.

= PERMANENT MAKEUP

= PARAMEDICAL TATTOOING

= SCALP PIGMENTATION

= BODY TATTOO

PARAMETERS

The icons below indicate the parameters necessary for performing the procedure correctly and safely. The many different movements, hand speed, and the different angles of the handpiece will be described, as well as the frequency at which to set the device, and the needles and pigments to be used in each step.

- ➡ = Movement
- ✋ = Hand speed
- ◢ = Angle
- ± = Frequency
- 🌡 = Needle
- 💧 = Pigment

....

PROCEDURES

These icons indicate the different procedures for eyebrows, lips, and eyes.

- 👁 = Eyebrows
- 👄 = Lips
- 👁 = Eyes

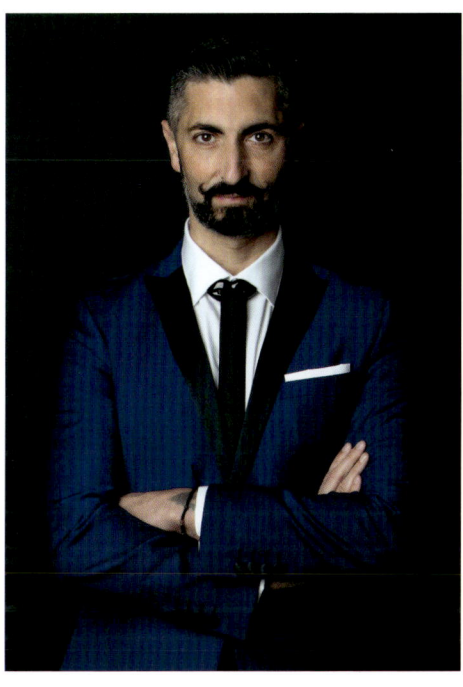

In 1998 Toni Belfatto took his first steps in the world of dermopigmentation, moving from body tattoos to dedicating himself to permanent make-up. Years of study, research, and experimentation, combined with a strong passion for aesthetics and beauty made him a committed dermopigmentation professional and teacher.

In 2007, he patented Scalp Pigmentation ®, a completely innovative specialization that totally revolutionizes the world of dermopigmentation. The same year, he became CEO of Orsini & Belfatto, a business that sells products and equipment for dermopigmentation, as well as being a training center with over 5,000 graduates.

In 2008, he participated in a global project for creating a book on visagism-based dermopigmentation, translated into five languages, in collaboration with specialists in infectious diseases, microbiology, and dermatology. He became president of AIDER (Italian Dermopigmentation Association).

Since 2010, he has been a jury member at several permanent makeup championships, a speaker at more than 100 medical and dermopigmentation conferences, and he has collaborated with one of the most famous and renowned surgeons in the world. Some publications have called him, "the guru to the VIP". He has received several awards from institutional authorities like the Abruzzo Region, the Province of Chieti, and other national industry associations.

From 2014 to 2015 he wrote his first two books: "Secrets to Hyper-Realistic Male and Female Eyebrows", and "Scalp Pigmentation, the Original", translated into 6 languages. These two manuals, together with forthcoming books, will form the "Encyclopedia of Dermopigmentation".

Belfatto Lab is Toni Belfatto's latest creation. He is the visionary and soul behind this project, which was conceived to overcome professional boundaries by opening several dermopigmentation centers throughout Italy and the world. It is a truly innovative project, which has been supported by a group of highly qualified dermopigmentation specialists who share his passion. The centers are aimed at answering a growing demand from clients, who see these procedures as a definitive solution to their problems.

In 2017, he launched Tricorigen, a line of therapeutic hair products. This innovative system effectively and safely controls hair loss without side effects.

....

These days, talking about beauty seems to imply a narrow focus on the importance of appearance. But I don't believe that the means should ever be sacrificed in favor of the ends, so I am fighting to turn the spotlight back onto an approach that is based on common sense. An approach which (apparently) has long been replaced by the more sales-oriented motto of "at any cost". I can't accept the loss of the ideal of authentic beauty: that is why, through my work, I insist on recovering the ethics of beauty before even beginning to discuss aesthetics. Our field should be populated by professionals with steadfast and incorruptible guidelines, who do not share the ease with which other sectors pursue profit above all else. What makes us different, and maybe what also makes us unique, is our ability to understand people's needs. Helping those who come to us to solve an aesthetic concern doesn't mean enabling every outlandish request, but rather maintaining our own sense of moral rigor and holding firm to a recognized aesthetic ideal. The goal shouldn't be to disrupt harmony, but to restore it; an astonishing final result becomes an end in itself if it is not underpinned by order and balanced proportions. Nothing should seem fake: anything that looks right aesthetically can only be so because it is already ethically sound.

But what is beauty, then?

An object, a landscape, a work of art, or a person is "beautiful" because we feel an attraction to it, even if it is difficult for us to explain this "feeling". We can start to define beauty more successfully by bringing together Apollo, the god of harmony, music, and the sun, with Dionysus, the god of drunkenness, of pleasure, of life: beauty is created when it meets life.

Beauty, deeply understood, really can promise happiness and can certainly be a harbinger of something that, with time, can come true.

People place their hopes for happiness in the hands of professionals who can restore balance when it becomes lost, whether due to an accident, or simply through the loss of certainties.

The profession I've chosen is based on human contact, experience developed over time, innovation, and ideas that are ready to become practical actions. Through experimentation, I am able to transform ability into experience. I can't stand by and watch the commodification of beauty, I can't stand still with my hands in my pockets when I see these continued attempts to abuse beauty.

My story is that of a thirst for knowledge, passion, and confidence in what can still be done. Gathering the fruits of my labor, in my case, isn't a question of celebrating goals reached, but of looking forwards to the next victory. My work has allowed the very concept of tattooing to evolve, cross over into different fields, and reach the greatest number of people. Because an idea can't be withheld or worn out until it becomes useless; it should be transformed. I've brought together body tattooing and permanent makeup to create physical harmony and order. The happiness I promise comes from the fields of dermopigmentation and permanent makeup The effort, perseverance, and continuously updated preparations, the frantic need to keep improving, always and anywhere, lend authenticity and pragmatism to my invitation to follow in my footsteps.

What drives me to write for those who want to join my field is similar to the desire to provide an effective tool to complete and enrich professional training courses; it's my way of applying the philosophy behind an ancient Chinese proverb: give a man a fish and you feed him for a day, teach him how to fish and you feed him for a lifetime.

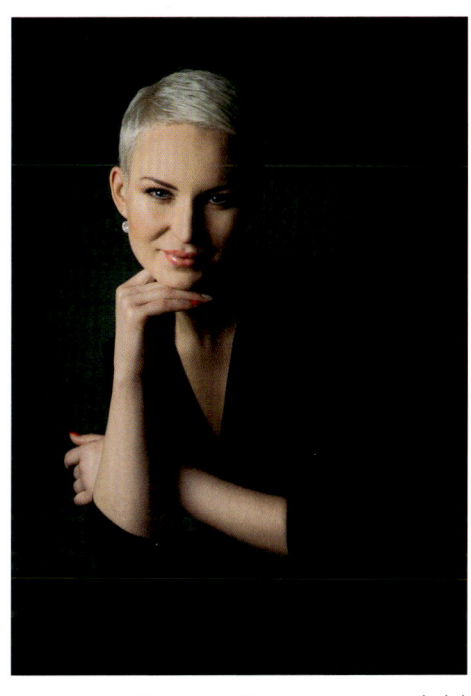

My name is Elena Nikora, amiea international master trainer. I originally come from Russia, but my career path led me to my current residence in Berlin, Germany, where I work as Head of Training for amiea.

My personal love story for this profession began with my first professional steps in 2008. I lived in the south of Russia with my husband and little son in a small town called Stavropol, where I was born.

After obtaining a master's degree in tourism, my dream was not only to travel, but also to express myself in an artistic way. Since I was a child, I have enjoyed creating small detailed drawings. I could sit for hours observing how beauty was manifested after each step of creation.

One day I came across a professional website about permanent makeup and I immediately fell completely in love. I very quickly made the decision to get a loan from the bank, and I went to Moscow for a basic course in permanent makeup. I chose the school that trained with German equipment and pigments by Medium-Tech (the former name of the MT.DERM company).

One of the reasons behind my choice was a desire to learn from the best artists and with products of the highest quality and safety standards. This is why I preferred to start my career with products "made in Germany" instead of cheap devices, although my budget was very limited. My first device was a tiny and simple "Symphony I" and I dove deep into practical work with my first clients while trying to improve my techniques. After one year, one of my colleagues who believed in my competence suggested that I participate in an international permanent makeup championship in Moscow. I was very proud to make it to the final competition and to be among the top three winners.

A few more competitions followed, and at one of them in 2010, Jörn Kluge, the amiea company owner, distinguished my work with the special prize: an amiea Linelle Supreme device, which I'm still using. Also, the official distributor of the amiea brand in Russia "Soling company" offered me a trainer-representative position in Moscow.

This achievement was more than just one victory in the competition. It was a turning point in my whole life. That is how I became a new member of the amiea family and moved to Moscow to teach permanent makeup. One of my dreams came true!

Since then, I have never stopped learning and developing my skills, participating in workshops and conferences with the best trainers worldwide. At the same time I have tried to develop my own personal micropigmentation style. I always wanted my work to look flawless, natural, almost invisible, stylish, and unique.

In 2012, I completed a "Train the Trainer" course by amiea in Berlin, and I was invited to lecture in the first edition of the Permanent International Congress in the same city. Both experiences were very exciting and opened the international stage to me. I became one of the international amiea faces and started educational activities all over the world, spreading natural-looking micropigmentation techniques across more than 27 countries, where I was lecturing and performing master classes in the framework of international conferences or as a jury member at championships.

Several of my professional articles about different micropigmentation techniques have been published in various international magazines.

At the end of 2016, amiea offered me a position as Head of Training and I did not think twice: I moved to Berlin in order to support the amiea team by developing new products and creating new working techniques and teaching materials.

....

The book you are holding in your hands now is a result of gathering our educational experience in all countries where the amiea brand is present. We have tried to put together the most essential materials and to answer all questions that arise during the learning process of this very complex but very interesting profession of micropigmentation.

I am eternally grateful for my professional and life path and for the opportunity to share my knowledge with students and to see them grow. Use this book as a guide for your first steps and hopefully it will help you find your own way and personal style in this wonderful profession.

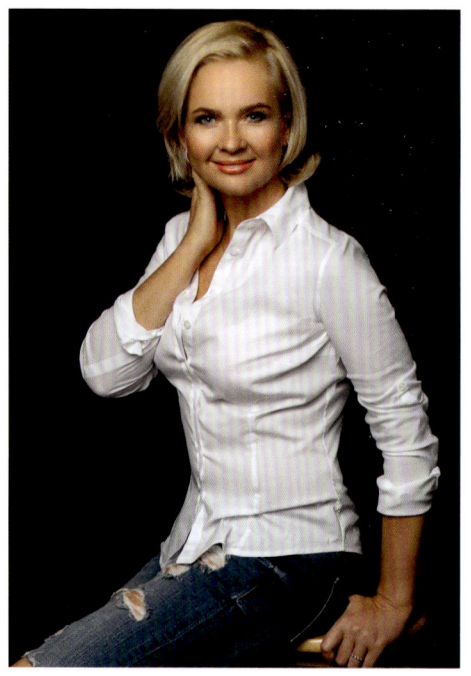

My name is Olga Kravchenko, amiea international master trainer. I am the director of the OK PMU CENTER Academy in Tallinn, the capital of Estonia, and it is a great honor for me and my team to be an educational partner of the amiea brand.

My creative history and professional path to permanent makeup were not simple. A lot of effort, work and material costs were necessary to get to the point where I could open my own training academy. However, it was worth it!

I began my career in Riga (Latvia) in 2008 after completing basic training in the best school at that time, Long Time Liner. Then I boldly plunged into the interesting world of beauty and the magic of permanent makeup.

At first it was not easy, but the basic knowledge I received helped me to avoid mistakes and laid the foundation for further growth. Of course, I continued studying both at conferences and at individual master classes from the best masters in the world. I am convinced that we must improve our expertise all the time – never stopping the progress of our professional development.

A few years later I realized that I wanted something technologically more perfect. At that time in my country, I heard about a new, young, and very promising brand – amiea. It sounded like it could secure my future happiness!

Having worked with the equipment from this brand for about two years (by that time I already had my first students), I decided to open a studio to teach permanent makeup.

I attended a "train the trainer" course in Berlin, where I got a trainer's certificate, and after working together for a few years, amiea offered me the opportunity to represent the brand on the world stage. Further developments in our professional field in recent years have been dizzying. The equipment has become more complex, the number of masters has increased incredibly, and my knowledge and skills have been required in different countries.

I traveled the world speaking at conferences and teaching master classes, and discovered what a huge responsibility and pride it is to share my knowledge and see how my students grow.

Today, I run the Academy in addition to working on my own clients, and my wonderful team helps me with the daily work. I also develop my own techniques and our OK PMU CENTER permanent makeup textbook. I have been asked to publish several articles in professional beauty and PMU magazines.

....

I am proud to be able to participate in the publication of the first book on the basic techniques of permanent makeup, which you're holding in your hands, I am grateful to my partners and friends and would like to extend my thanks to all my colleagues and partners who have helped me become the person and professional I am today!

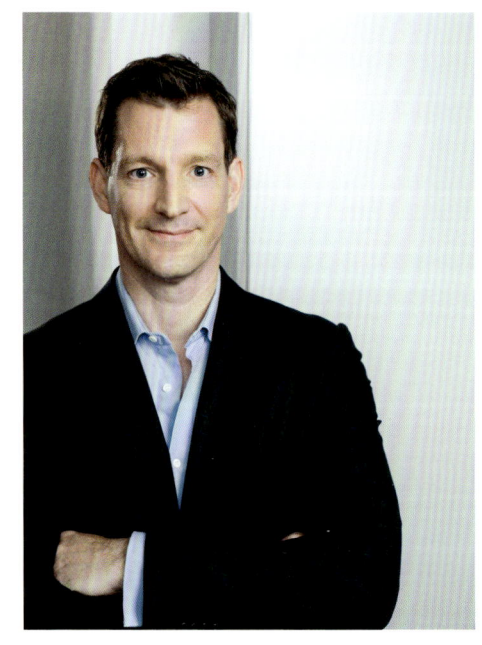

MADE IN GERMANY –
MADE FOR THE WORLD

German quality is a philosophy.
Inspired by technology and our artists.

Jörn Kluge – CEO MT.DERM

EXCLUSIVE BEGINNERS' TRAINING BOOK

You have decided to take the first step to becoming a permanent makeup professional by choosing this beginners' book.

The globally renowned micropigmentation artist Toni Belfatto, together with the international amiea Master Trainers Elena Nikora and Olga Kravchenko have compiled all the information, techniques, and insider know-how you will need to start your PMU artist career with the best possible knowledge. We wish you success in your business and a lot of fun while reading this book.

AMIEA – PROFESSION. PERMANENT. PASSION.

In the last 10 years, amiea has become the world leader in micropigmentation. Through innovation and the highest quality, amiea is continuously setting standards in the permanent makeup industry and micropigmentation. Our devices, cartridges, and pigments are developed, engineered, and produced in Germany.

MT.DERM, the parent company, is a pioneer in the field of injecting colors and substances into the skin. For 20 years, we have been investing continuously in research and development to turn current trends into long-lasting, high-quality reality. We hold a medical certification ISO 13485. Our numerous international patents are instrumental to our ongoing success story.

MICROPIGMENTATION

Professional permanent makeup accentuates natural beauty by introducing color pigments into the skin to perfect facial contours. With high-precision devices and needle systems, we provide subtle highlights and nuanced shades of color, which work together to complement individual personalities. Our procedures enhance facial expressions and provide the perfect base for daily makeup routines.

amiea's cosmetic micropigmentation achieves perfect eyebrow definition, subtle eyeliner, and soft lip contours – bringing out your true radiance.

Highest Quality – Made in Germany. amiea strives for perfection. Our systems are easy and convenient to use.

The most important components of our success are our products. They are made in Germany, and through our ambitious R&D department, we strive for quality, safety, and innovation. Quality is a must in our company, therefore we are an ISO 13485 certified company with an in-house quality management team that assures that we are always in compliance with European law. amiea places great value on knowledge and training. That is why we cooperate with micropigmentation experts, training academies, and distributors around the world (in more than 50 countries).

MT.DERM is a global leader in the field of transdermal delivery of substances into the skin. In addition to cosmetic applications and tattoo equipment, the company is also active in the medical field. We are an ISO 13485 certified company.

We provide all required (and additional) certifications and independent tests for the products. We strive for perfection. Our systems are easy and convenient to use. Highest Quality – Made in Germany. This claim ensures a long product life cycle as well as unmatched precision. As a trendsetter, MT.DERM can bring together the best in science, technology, business, and people to help solve challenges in micropigmentation and microneedling.

SAFETY & CERTIFICATION

The reward of our efforts is ISO 13485: the medical standard for quality management systems. Our devices comply with all relevant guidelines.

We recruit great minds. Our team consists of ingenious people who relentlessly strive for engineering innovation.

In order to recruit the best professionals, we collaborate with leading universities like the TU Berlin. We love to invite people with more than just a passion for disruptive ideas and the courage to bring them to life. Working collaboratively and acting as if MT.DERM were their own company is all part of our ownership culture. As a technology innovation driver, we own numerous patents and invest a significant amount in R&D. We constantly rework our portfolio and adjust it to current standards and legal requirements.

The health-care and cosmetic industries keep evolving at a fast pace and are now on the verge of a new era: digitalization. With our headquarters, R&D, and production site in Germany, we develop individual solutions together with customers to ensure that processes and products satisfy both current and future requirements.

Permanent makeup (PMU) is a method of implanting pigments into your skin to create a lasting cosmetic effect. Micropigmentation can be used to achieve soft and natural results and restore confidence in your overall appearance. It can be applied with good effect to the eyebrows, eye lines, and lips. We understand professional needs and have devoted ourselves to technical innovation and safety since 1998. Besides devices, handpieces, and sterile modules we also develop and produce the most advanced and highly graded cosmetic enhancement pigments that are used to carry out permanent makeup procedures.

PERMANENT MAKEUP DEVICES

Our equipment for permanent makeup consists of certified high-tech products reflecting the highest standards in technology and design. With high standards of medical hygiene, the greatest possible precision, and user-friendless, this equipment is a must for every cosmetic studio or medical spa.

OPTIMAL CONTROL DEVICE

Only high-quality electronic components are used in all our equipment. To ensure faultless results, control occurs via digital microprocessor. This ensures uniform needle operation – the guaranteed best possible prerequisite for high color injection. The upper surface of every piece of equipment comes fitted with an easy-to-clean surface.

....

UNIQUE ADVANTAGES

- Rapid change of needle combination
- High precision
- No handling of bare needles
- Simple setting of puncture depth
- Hygienic operation
- Ergonomic handling
- Quiet running
- Made to last
- Certified to EN ISO 13485 and CE standards

....

CARTRIDGE SYSTEM

MT.DERM developed the first cartridge system that offers the client absolute safety as far as sterile conditions are concerned. The needles and the needle nozzles are integrated into a disposable hygienic cartridge. This cartridge is sealed at the rear by a membrane, thus preventing the tool from being soiled by contaminating liquids.

HIGHLIGHTS OF THE MT.DERM CARTRIDGE

- Wide choice of needle configurations
- Quick switching of color and needle array
- Optimized needle capacity
- Precision needle deployment
- Sterilized disposable material
- Packed in clean rooms with batch traceability
- Safe for the client, safe for the professionals

BROAD COLOR SPECTRUM OF PIGMENTS

As regards the dyes used for pigmentation, the highest standards of quality and safety are called for. The dyes are prepared in our own in-house laboratory.

Only pigments of class I, as laid down in the directive EEC 76/768/EED-I, are employed. Use tested for biological and dermatological safety at an independent laboratory (Dermatest®).

1

DERMOPIGMENTATION

1.1. FIELDS OF APPLICATION

Dermopigmentation is a practice that regulates the injection of pigment into the skin, using non-hollow needles.
There are many different fields of application for dermopigmentation,
each of which has its own particularities and uses different techniques and knowledge.

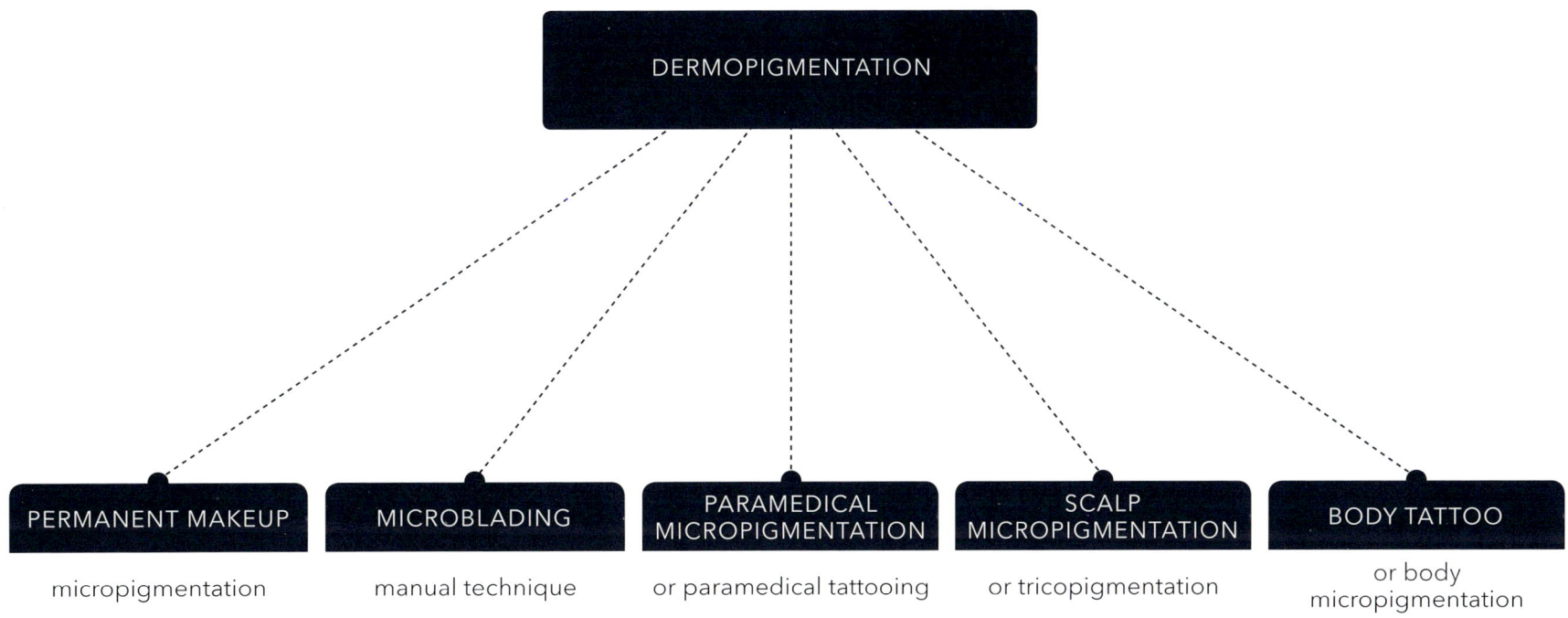

WHAT ARE THE MAIN DIFFERENCES BETWEEN THE SECTORS?

Before getting into the details of the major differences between the sectors listed above, it is important to specify that the boundaries between them are defined by the client's motives in seeking out a particular aesthetic procedure. From a more technical perspective, although the action of applying pigment may be the same in all of these sectors, there are significant differences both in terms of the equipment and pigments used and in terms of the specific technical knowledge which each area requires.

PERMANENT MAKEUP

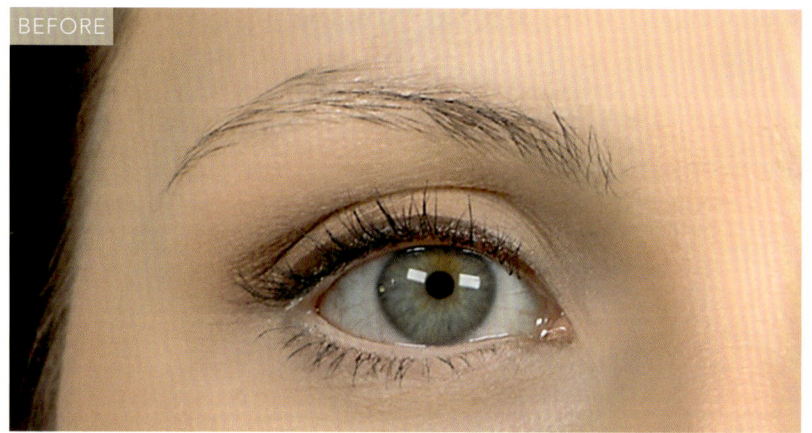

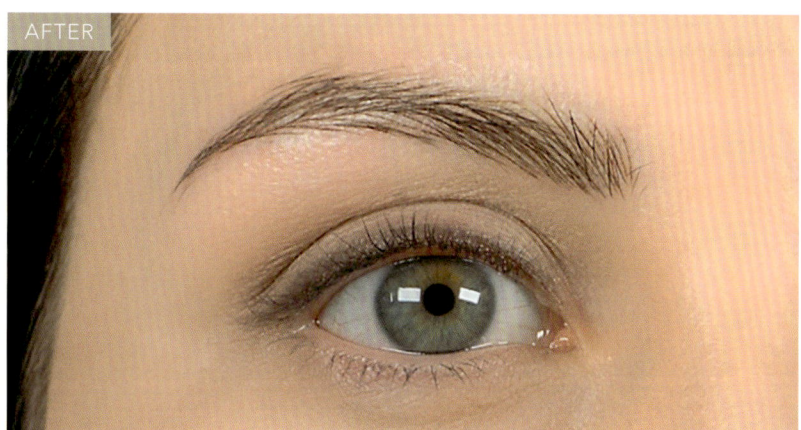

This sector concerns the face, intervening on the eyebrows, lips, and eyes. The goal is to restore harmony and balance, making the look and the lips more attractive and defined. The client's motives for seeking this procedure can vary: correcting asymmetries, defining shapes, emphasizing parts of the face, or simply for the day-to-day convenience of replacing regular makeup routines or looking put together during athletic activities.

PARAMEDICAL TATTOOING

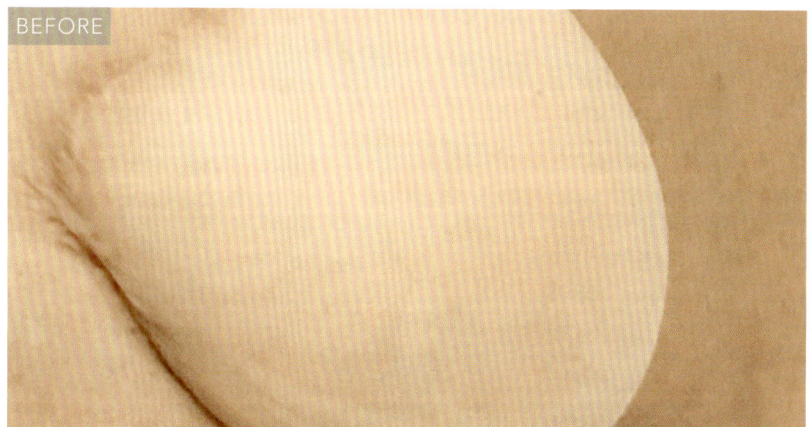

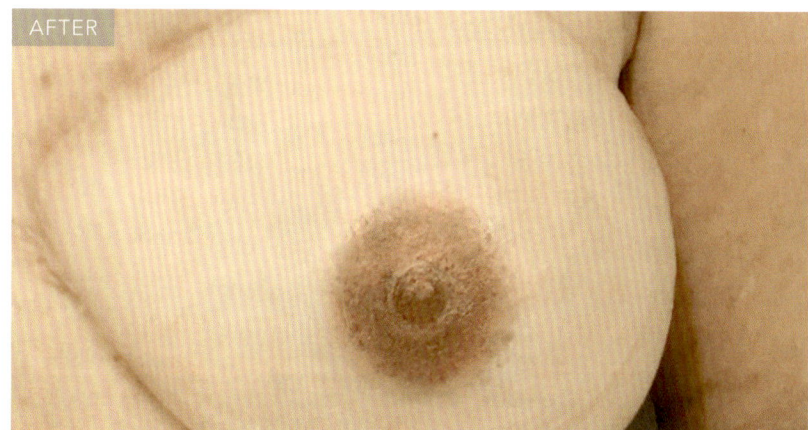

This activity complements cosmetic surgery and aims to resolve cosmetic defects caused by surgical operations or diseases.

This includes reconstructing areolae, covering scars around the areola resulting from breast surgery or breast lifts, covering general scars, re-pigmenting hypopigmentation or hyperpigmentation patches, or correcting vitiligo and stretch marks.

SCALP PIGMENTATION

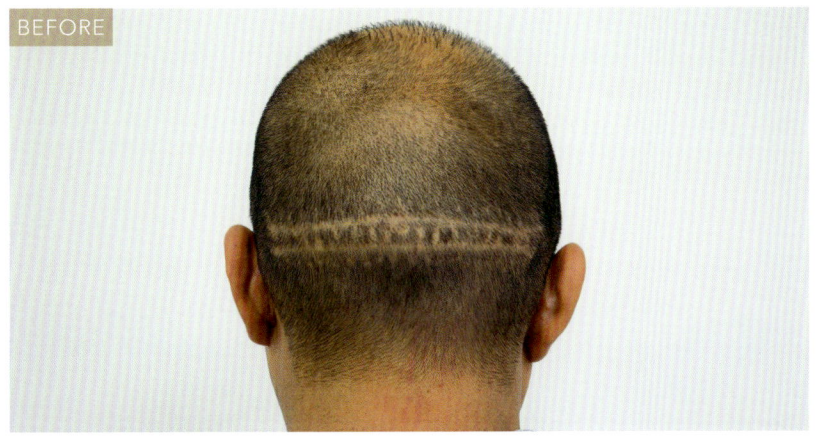

BEFORE

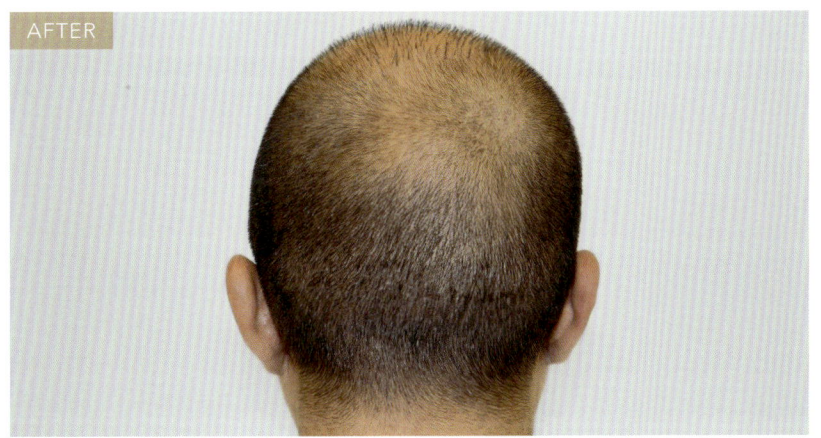

AFTER

This is the most innovative specialization to come out of Toni Belfatto's research. After a lengthy, ten-year period of experimentation, he registered a patent for it in 2007 under the name tricopigmentazione (scalp pigmentation). Aimed at treating baldness and scarring from hair transplants, this specialization is the most commom entry point into the world of dermopigmentation for men. This practice is often done to complete hair transplant surgery, and different techniques may be used to create a shaved look, the appearance of short hairs, or a more dense appearance.

BODY TATTOO

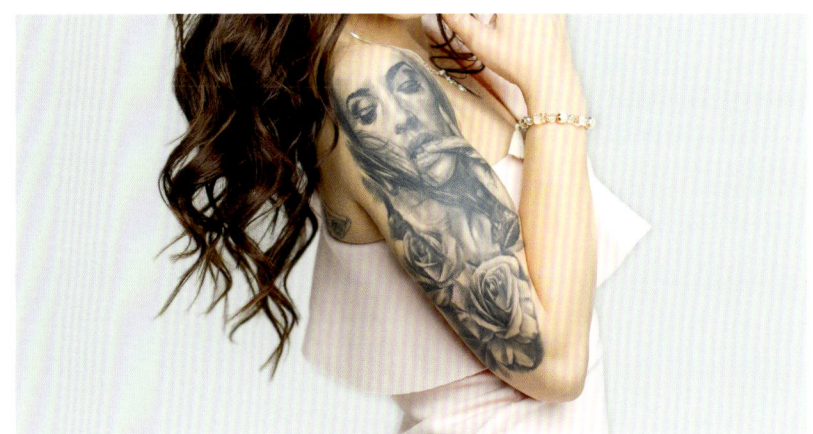

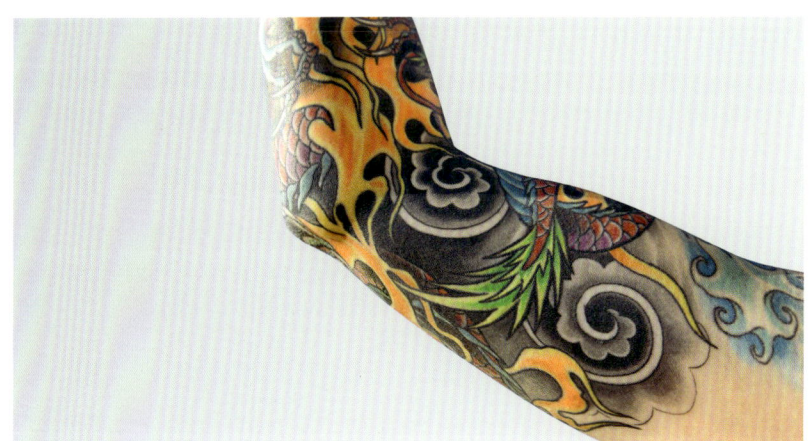

Artists express themselves on the skin, turning their client's emotions into a drawing. Tattoos are chosen to commemorate important events in one's life, to remember a loved one, to decorate one's body, or in recent years, to display a famous artist's work on one's own skin. Although this practice shares certain fundamentals with the other sectors, its techniques, equipment, and the pigments used are different.

THE DIFFERENCE BETWEEN PERMANENT MAKEUP AND BODY TATTOOS

In many cases, clients considering dermopigmentation are exposed to false information, which often results in confusion and ambiguity. Among other aspects, this includes misinformation about the difference between body tattoos and permanent makeup, especially with regards to their duration and the techniques used. People often think that tattoos are for life while permanent makeup is temporary because of how deeply the pigment is inserted; the pigment being injected much more deeply for tattoos than for permanent makeup. This is not true. Inserting pigment too deep in the dermis can lead the color to migrate and sometimes cause hypertrophy in the area.

This results in pseudo-scars which cause the tattoo to be raised. The only difference is in the type of pigment used, which will be discussed in detail in the following pages. Clearly, there are big differences between these two worlds, from the motivations that lead clients to consider these practices, to the equipment used. Body tattoo equipment, for example, is much noisier and more powerful, because it needs to push very large needles into the body, including magnums of up to 40 needles at a time.

The equipment used for permanent makeup is made with more focus on style and has greater precision. They also vibrate less, since vibrations could cause unacceptable technical results when used on the face. Let's learn more about the equipment and pigments used in both practices.

1.2. DIFFERENCES: EQUIPMENT AND PIGMENTS

Applying permanent makeup starts with the handpiece, a sophisticated, extremely innovative piece of equipment. The handpiece is dynamic and silent, with controlled pulsations and relatively small needles, making it very lightweight. Its slim, ergonomic shape allows the professional to apply pigment precisely and safely.

LINELLE SUPREME

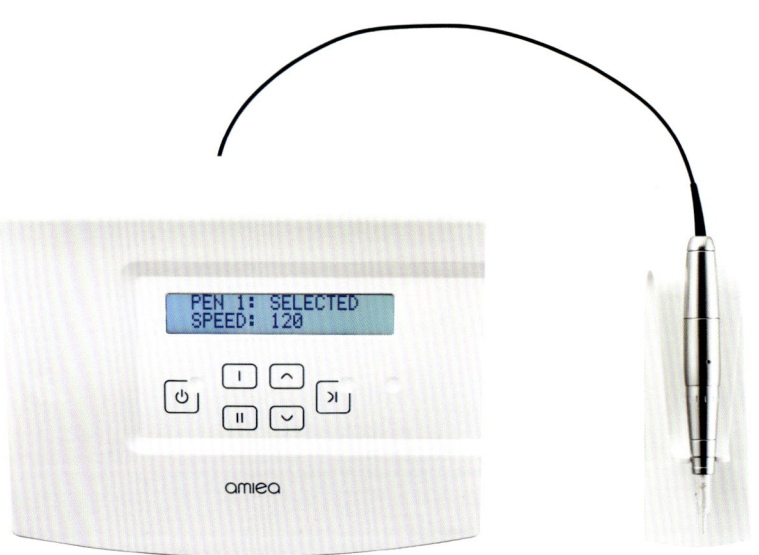

NO. 1 IN SALES WORLDWIDE

The sleek intuitive control unit is digitally controlled. It ensures top precision results, which allows you to focus fully on your work. The amiea Linelle Supreme operates with minimal noise and vibration.

FEATURE & BENEFITS

Adjustable needle speed:

- high power
- perfect pain management
- minimal downtime
- 50 – 150 pps

ADJUSTABLE NEEDLE LENGTH

- appropriate needle length for each area of application
- range of depth 0.02 – 0.14 inches / 0.5 – 3.5 mm

Precision and power:

- low epidermal trauma
- low noise and vibration
- superior results

Values:

- German technology
- R&D and production in Berlin
- two-year warranty

OPERATING CONDITIONS

- Ambient temperature: 59° to 77°F / 15° to 25°C
- Relative humidity: 30% to 75%
- Width x height x depth:
  10.28 x 3.50 x 8.62 inches
  26.1 x 8.9 x 21.9 cm
- Weight of handpiece: 3.53 oz / 80 g
- Total weight: 1.98 lbs / 31.75 oz / 900 g
- Manufactured in: Germany according to quality standard ISO 13485

TECHNICAL PARAMETERS

- Type: DA30310US
- Rated voltage: 15 V – (DC)
- Power input: 7 V A max
- Working frequency: Selectable from 50 to 150 hits per second
- Drive: Precision: DC motor
- Operating mode: Continuous operation

PATENTS

- US 6,505,530; US 6,345,553; US 8,029,527; US 9,504,814 EP 1 495 782; EP 1 618 915; EP 1 958 659; EP 2 462 979
- Additional patents pending

BODY TATTOOING EQUIPMENT

Tattoo machines are mechanical devices with rotary mechanism coils, making them significantly heavier and more aggressive.
They have a more powerful rhythm since more needles are pushed into the skin at one time. The equipment used in permanent makeup is often also used for paramedical tattooing: more powerful equipment is needed to work on scar tissue, since it is thicker and harder than healthy tissue.

ATTENTION ⚠

Scalp pigmentation is done using specific equipment with a different duty cycle and much thinner needles compared to traditional needles to safely work on the scalp. Using regular permanent makeup needles would cause color to migrate and form mega dots (dots that are too big).

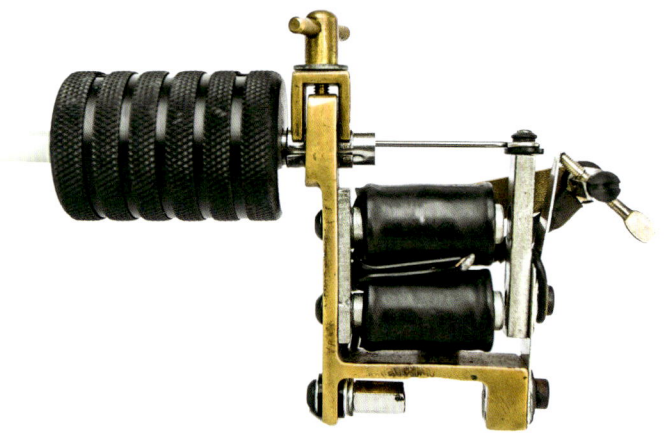

SKILLS: Each of these specializations requires advanced knowledge in order to guarantee quality and reduce technical and histological risks as much as possible. Studying anatomy, specifically that of the skin, is helpful for all dermopigmentation practices since this is the organ into which we insert the pigment. No student should approach permanent makeup without a basic understanding of visagism. To be able to tattoo, professionals must be familiar with art movements and have an inclination for drawing. Paramedical tattooing requires specific knowledge about medical and scientific aspects, and delegation by a qualified doctor is also desirable. Scalp pigmentation requires knowledge about the scalp, hair transplant surgery, as well as a very skilled hand, since it requires performing an enormous quantity of dots of the same width, color, and density.

EVERYTHING ABOUT PIGMENTS FOR PERMANENT MAKEUP, SCALP MICROPIGMENTATION AND PARAMEDICAL TATTOOING

Tattoo pigments and PMU pigments are partly eliminated by macrophages. Both types could be resorbable or non resorbable.

The pigments used in permanent makeup are predominantly non resorbable, and partly the same as those used in tattoo. In tattoo inks, organic pigments are used because of their intense color shades, such as carbon black.

The pigments used in permanent makeup are predominantly non resorbable. Generally, iron oxide pigments are used because of their natural colors. But there are many PMU colors on the market, which are based on organic pigments or mixed with organic and inorganic pigments with intense color shades.

In general, the most widely used pigments in micropigmentation are made up of:
• the functional principle or coloring agent
• solvent
• binding agent

The functional principle refers to the coloring substance, a precise mix of mineral powders. The liquid excipient is made up of glycerin, water, and isopropyl alcohol. Glycerin allows the pigment to more easily penetrate the skin and prevents it from drying out: it is crucial for ensuring that the color is viscous, thick, and substantial. The water makes the color more liquid and fluid.

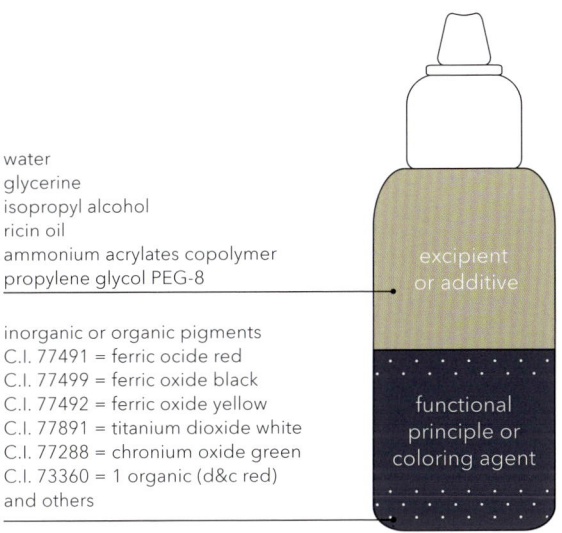

COMPOSITION OF BODY TATTOOING PIGMENTS

water
glycerine
isopropyl alcohol
ricin oil
ammonium acrylates copolymer
propylene glycol PEG-8

excipient or additive

inorganic or organic pigments
C.I. 77491 = ferric ocide red
C.I. 77499 = ferric oxide black
C.I. 77492 = ferric oxide yellow
C.I. 77891 = titanium dioxide white
C.I. 77288 = chronium oxide green
C.I. 73360 = 1 organic (d&c red)
and others

functional principle or coloring agent

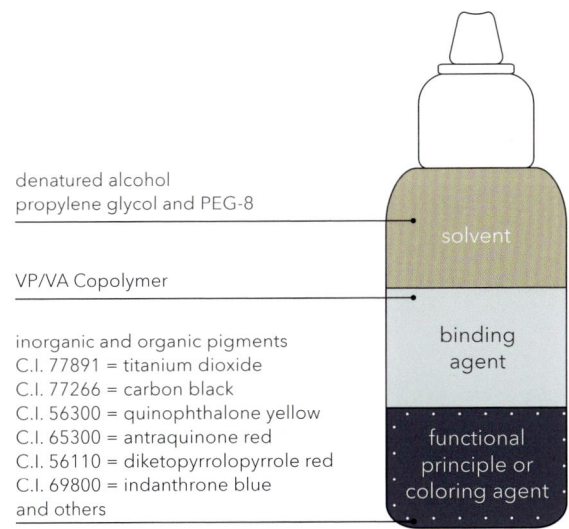

COMPOSITION OF PERMANENT MAKEUP PIGMENTS

denatured alcohol
propylene glycol and PEG-8

solvent

VP/VA Copolymer

binding agent

inorganic and organic pigments
C.I. 77891 = titanium dioxide
C.I. 77266 = carbon black
C.I. 56300 = quinophthalone yellow
C.I. 65300 = antraquinone red
C.I. 56110 = diketopyrrolopyrrole red
C.I. 69800 = indanthrone blue
and others

functional principle or coloring agent

The isopropyl alcohol keeps the color sterile and prevents the proliferation of bacteria during the procedure, and also serves as a preservative and anti-foam agent.

The color and the size of the molecules (generally below 12 microns) determine how long the pigment lasts inside the skin. The size of the molecule impacts the duration of the procedure's results, but not their irreversibility.

The skin contains macrophages which can choose, swallow, and then digest all of the molecules present (this is called the phagocytosis process). Imagine a little Pacman that can ingest pigments and eliminate them through the lymph nodes, sweat, and urine.

It is recommended not to mix body tattoing and permanent makeup pigments because of the different composition. Mixing different solvents might lead to bad pigment retention or even undesired reactions in the skin.

The goals of body tattooing are different from those of permanent makeup and scalp pigmentation. Therefore, the consistency and composition of tattoo and permanent makeup pigments is different. Tattoo pigments are more liquid, so the pigment concentration is lower and more additives are used.

Tattoo pigments should be avoided for scalp pigmentation because they can undergo problematic color changes following sun exposure, which tends to oxidate the pigments and result in undesirable colors. The same choice should be made as for permanent makeup.

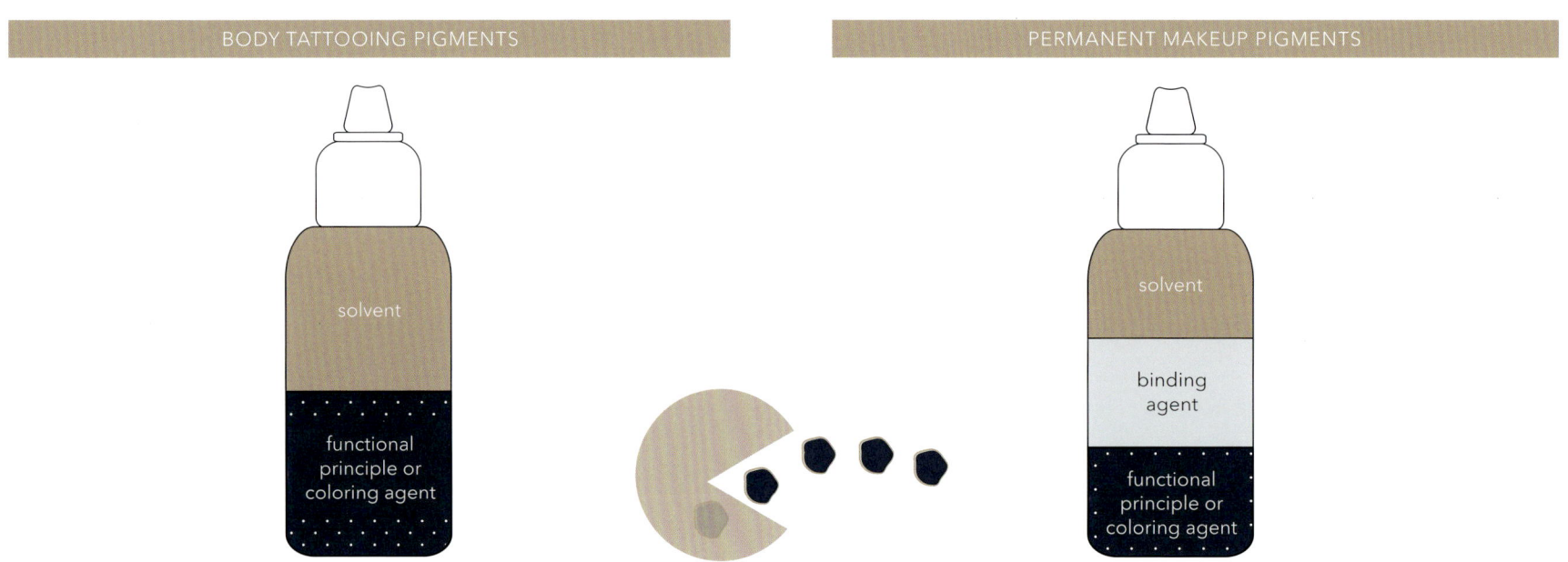

BODY TATTOOING PIGMENTS

solvent

functional principle or coloring agent

PERMANENT MAKEUP PIGMENTS

solvent

binding agent

functional principle or coloring agent

THE DIFFERENCES BETWEEN PERMANENT MAKEUP AND MANUAL MICROBLADING

Microblading (or eyebrow embroidery) is a relatively new manual method.

It is considered to be semi-permanent, as compared to the traditional permanent makeup hairstroke technique. It is based on the oldest technique of tattooing called "tebori" in Japan.

It is performed with manual tools and blades, which create fine incisions or micro-cuts in the skin. The results are natural looking lines, hair-like strokes. Different factors affect the procedure results and determine how long pigments last in the skin. Results can last from 1 up to 10 months depending on the conditions below:
- SKIN TYPE
- SKIN CONDITIONS
- SKIN STRUCTURE (bleeding, swollen, immediate reaction)

LIMITATIONS OF MICROBLADING

- The microblading technique can be used for creating eyebrow hairstrokes. However it is hazardous to use for lips, eyes and paramedical pigmentation. It is also very limited regarding shading techniques for eyebrows.
- The microblading technique does not last as long as PMU (short-term treatment).
- Microblading procedure is not suitable for all clients and skin types. Only recommended for young to medium age normal skin types or thick skin types as for example, asian skin. Not suitable for mature clients with thin, sensitive, or dry skin, for example.

POSSIBLE COMPLICATIONS

- Higher trauma level in comparison to micropigmentation. More bleeding and swelling during the procedure. Healing process takes longer than with permanent makeup.
- Difficult to control needle depth. In case microblading treatment is performed too deep, color healing will turn too cool, or gray.
- Scars, even hypertrophic scars, might appear. In this case, neither laser removal treatment nor micropigmentation can be applied on the area.
- Not long lasting. Results can last from 1 up to 10 months.

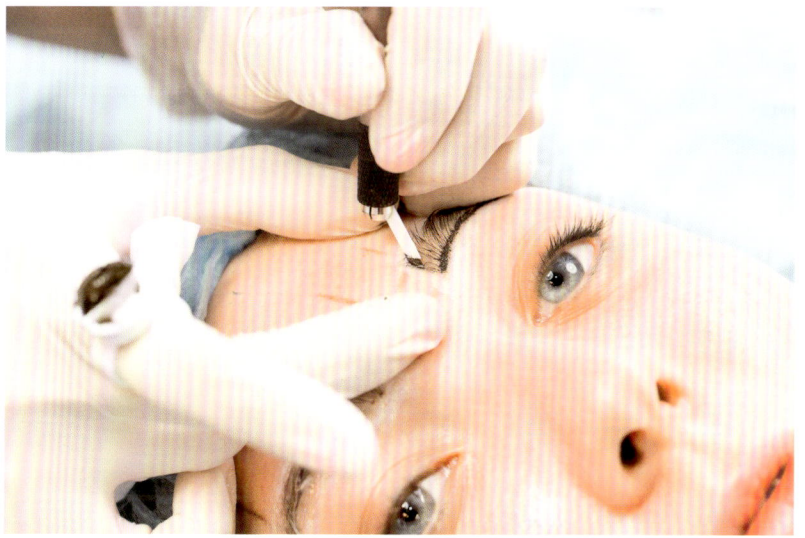

2

THE SKIN

2.1. THE SKIN FOR DERMOPIGMENTATION PROFESSIONALS. BY DR. SILVIO SCIARRETTA

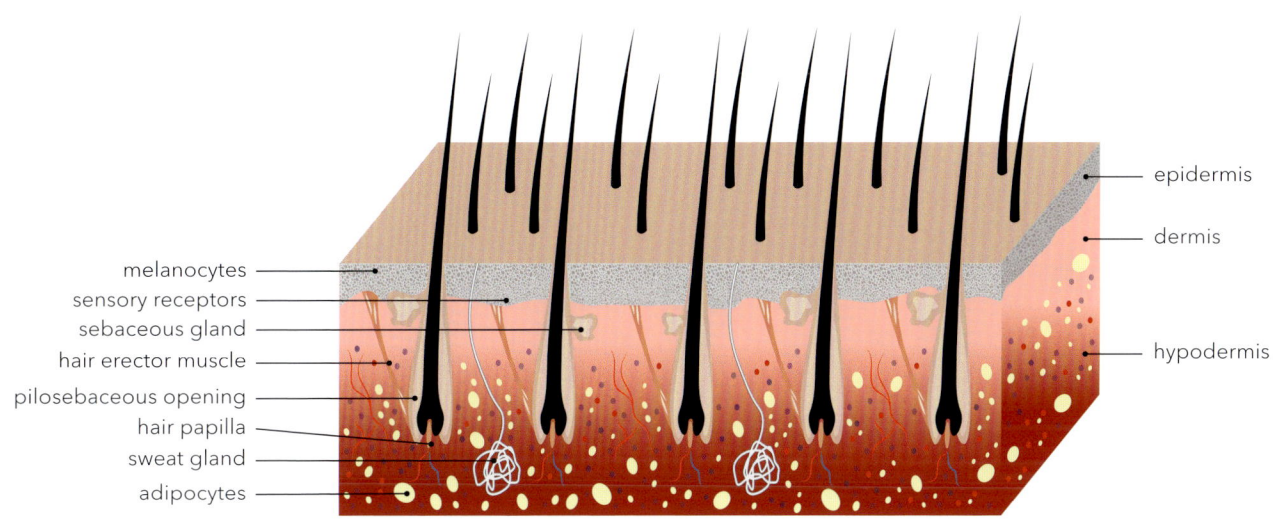

epidermis

dermis

hypodermis

melanocytes
sensory receptors
sebaceous gland
hair erector muscle
pilosebaceous opening
hair papilla
sweat gland
adipocytes

Individual well-being includes healthy skin. Taking care of one's skin, and potentially deciding to correct blemishes arising from the most disparate causes, is a means of finding balance and feeling good about oneself.

Our skin's appearance and health strongly and inevitably impacts our daily life. But it is best to learn more about the skin when considering potential procedures.

In all anatomical and histological texts, the skin is described as an organ made up of several layers: the epidermis, the dermis, and the hypodermis. It is extremely important for a dermopigmentation professional to understand the skin from a histological perspective, and to be able to analyze its physiology in order to predict normal reactions to micropigmentation procedures and to understand that perfect results depend on various factors (color, depth, part of the body, blood flow, etc.). The basic concepts we will discuss make up the fundamental knowledge that every dermopigmentation professional needs.

A — Distinguishing the skin's cellular components and their different functions

B — Describing the skin's structure

C — Understanding the skin's functions

D — Identifying the various colors that skin can have, and knowing how to choose the most appropriate materials

E — Understanding how skin reacts when color is introduced (pain, bleeding, scarring, cell turnover, sweat, macrophage reactions, etc.).

F — Studying how anesthetics work and their use.

Dermopigmentation professionals should analyze the skin from a two-dimensional perspective, which takes into account breadth and depth, rather than seeing it as a simple envelope that covers muscle and bone (a one-dimensional perspective), especially since the skin's depth has a significant impact on achieving perfect results.

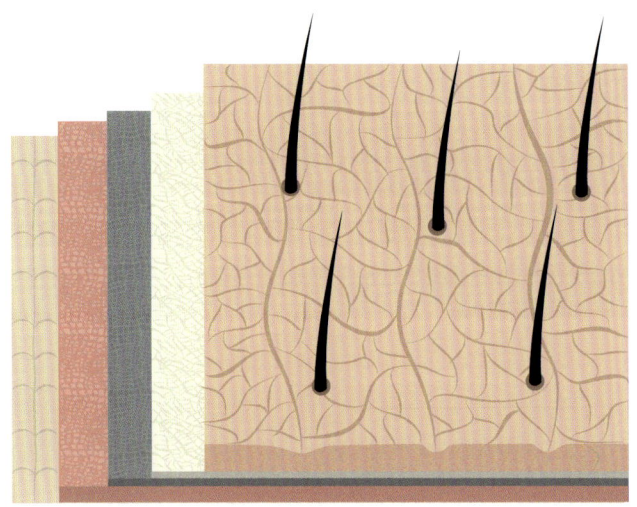

ONE-DIMENSIONAL PERSPECTIVE TWO-DIMENSIONAL PERSPECTIVE

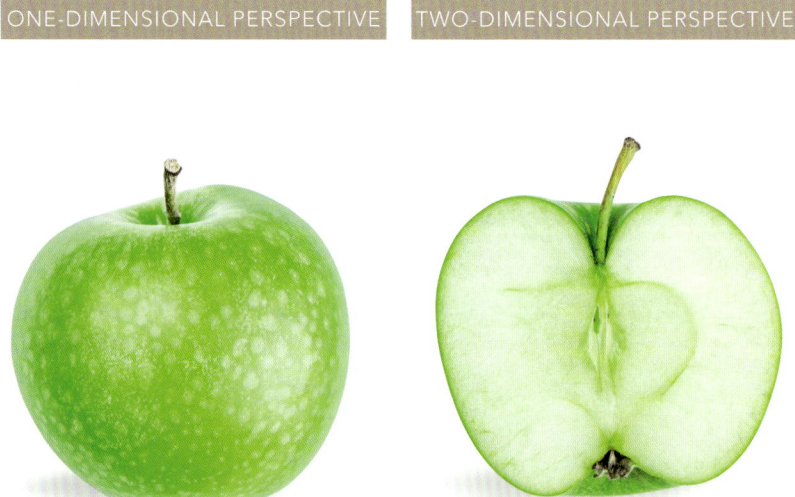

2.2. FAQ: QUESTIONS AND ANSWERS

Below, are practical tips and concrete answers to questions that may arise before, during, and after performing a procedure.

WHY, WHEN USING THE SAME TECHNIQUE, MAY THE ACHIEVED RESULTS BE DIFFERENT?

Usually, any technician will offer one of two answers to this kind of problem: "I must have done something wrong" or "There's something wrong with the skin." In reality, things are not always that simple. The skin's different macroscopic textures (dry, oily, dehydrated, buffed, smooth, wrinkled, etc.) can cause different results, even if the technique used is the same.

The skin is a dynamic organ, and its appearance is caused by different factors, whether they are endogenous (genetic) or exogenous (environmental). These factors, individually or in combination with each other, can cause the skin's structure to change over the course of a person's life. Young skin is more compact and even. The different layers of the epidermis are organized neatly, and there is intense cellular activity. The underlying dermis is characterized by a more compact, fibrous structure, and the way the elastic fibers are organized ensures strength and elasticity. The ability to bind with water makes skin hydrated and luminous, while intense cell turnover allows the skin to repair itself remarkably.

Less youthful skin is characterized by slower metabolic processes, and consequently will always appear less elastic and more dehydrated. Nutrients are absorbed more slowly, resulting in the skin becoming progressively thinner and subsequently less compact. If reduced blood flow is added to the mix, the skin will seem duller and not very luminous.

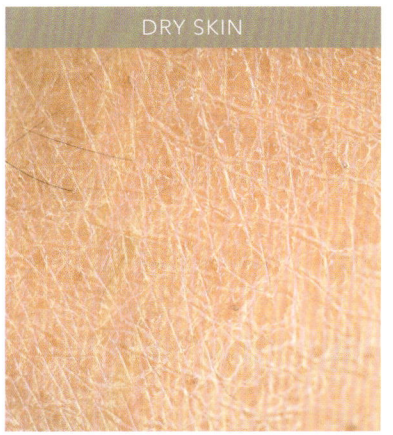
DRY SKIN

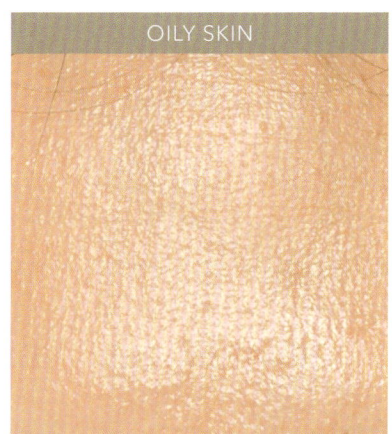
OILY SKIN

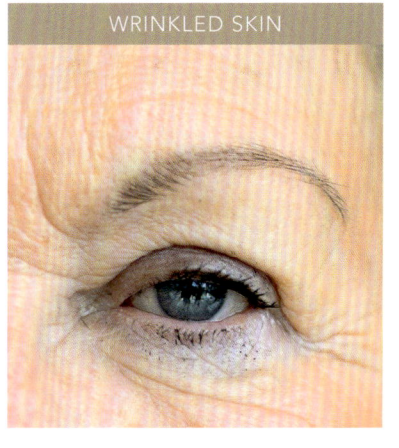
WRINKLED SKIN

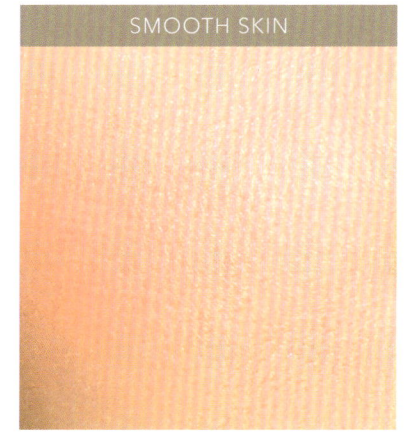
SMOOTH SKIN

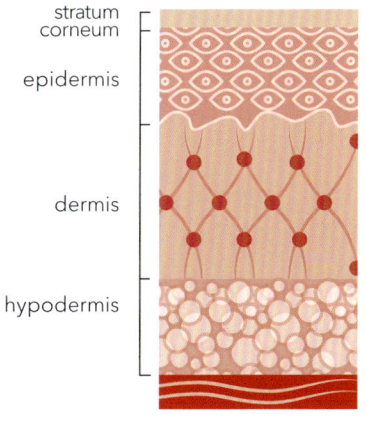

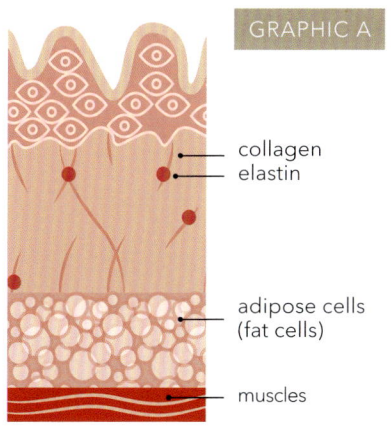

GRAPHIC A

stratum corneum

epidermis

dermis

hypodermis

collagen
elastin

adipose cells
(fat cells)

muscles

WHERE AND HOW DEEP SHOULD I PLACE PIGMENT IN THE SKIN?

The skin can be divided into two main regions: the epidermis and the dermis, plus an underlying region called the hypodermis. The epidermis and the dermis, with their structural characteristics, are the most relevant areas when applying permanent makeup and they are both involved in obtaining perfect results. First of all, the dermis is where the pigment is deposited. To obtain even results, it is important to evaluate which technique to use and above all, to carefully analyze the macroscopic and microscopic aspects of each client's skin (Graphic A).

WHY IS THE EPIDERMIS INVOLVED IN THE FINAL RESULT?

Let's start by considering how the epidermis is structured. The epidermis is characterized by the presence of different cellular elements, laid out in different layers, with different functions. Keratinocytes (keratos = keratin, cyte = cell, meaning the cell that produces keratin) are the most numerous cells in the skin (about 90% of skin cells). They are continuously renewed, and undergo a process of keratinization, in which they are transformed into corneocytes, cells that have no nucleus which belong to the outermost layer of skin (Graphic B).

Melanocytes (from melas = black) (1%) are cells that synthesize melanin, the brown-black pigment that causes the various light or dark skin colors of different skin types. These cells have a branched morphology and are distributed among the keratinocytes in the epidermis. They disperse melanin granules from their extremities. Below, we'll take a moment to analyze the physiological role of this pigment and its impact on the choice of colors and a procedure's final results (Graphic C).

Merkel cells are not particularly numerous, and are defined as tactile cells, since they are responsible for tactile sensitivity.

Langerhans cells (2-7%) trigger the body's immune defenses and serve as the sentinels who alert the body to the presence of viruses, bacteria, and toxins which could penetrate the skin.

As we'll see below, the cell turnover process, characterized by the movement of keratinocytes, could determine the transfer of pigment from the deeper layers to the outermost layers of the skin. Relatively darker complexions, the result of intense melanin production, could alter the final color results. It is important to emphasize that the professional should consider the dermis as the only area of intervention. Because of the intense cell turnover and the possibility of pigment being transported, avoid tattooing only in the epidermis. It is extremely important to perfectly

GRAPHIC B

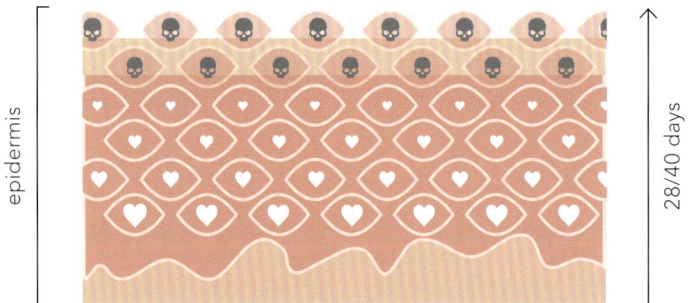

epidermis

28/40 days

GRAPHIC C

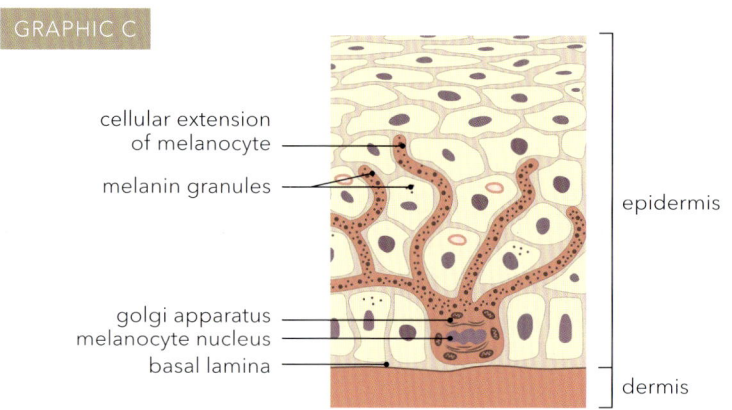

cellular extension of melanocyte

melanin granules

golgi apparatus
melanocyte nucleus
basal lamina

epidermis

dermis

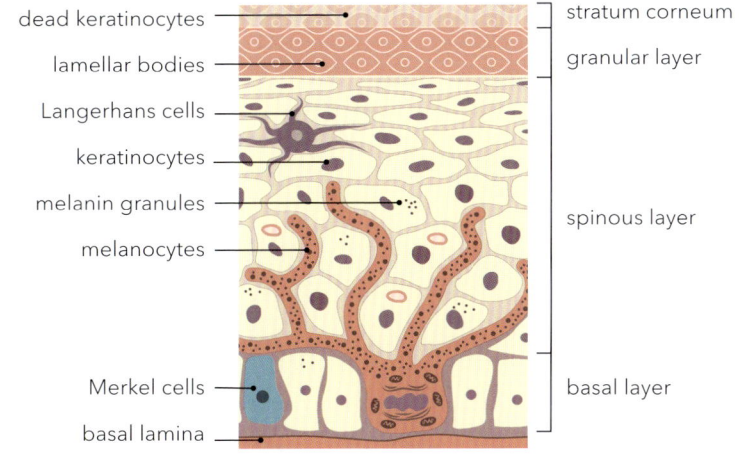

dead keratinocytes — stratum corneum
lamellar bodies — granular layer
Langerhans cells —
keratinocytes —
melanin granules — spinous layer
melanocytes —
Merkel cells — basal layer
basal lamina —

The presence of these elements throughout the dermis, with their own morphological and functional characteristics, can alter the aesthetic results of the procedure.

understand the structural characteristics of the epidermis to plan for the physiological response to the process of inserting the needle and releasing color into the skin (Graphic D).

WHY DO THE RESULTS FADE AFTER A FEW WEEKS?

The epidermis has the extraordinary ability to regenerate continuously. A substance injected at both the dermic and epidermic level is deposited inside the cells' cytoplasma and the transformation process causes the color to lighten in tone.

Over time, the amount of pigment present in the dermis remains unchanged, while the color in the epidermis is eliminated through the process of cell turnover (exfoliation).

As the color-filled corneocytes migrate from the deeper epidermis towards the outer layer, they tend to take color granules with them. Once they have been transformed into small, enucleated lamellae, they will disintegrate completely before being shed from the skin's surface. The lost cells are quickly replaced by new cells thanks to the activity of the keratinocytes, which are responsible for the cellular division process known as mitosis.

The nutrients and oxygen which are necessary for cell multiplication are provided by the blood vessels in the underlying dermis. The cell turnover cycle takes approximately 28–40 days, from the birth of a new keratinocyte to its exfoliation through the shedding of squamous lamella.

Before beginning any dermopigmentation procedure, the professional should therefore pay particular attention to three aspects:
- cell turnover;
- the person's age;
- the season during which the procedure is performed.

Color-filled keratinocytes will actually migrate more quickly in younger people, and more slowly in older people, and will also accelerate during the summer, due to stimulus from sunlight, compared to the winter.

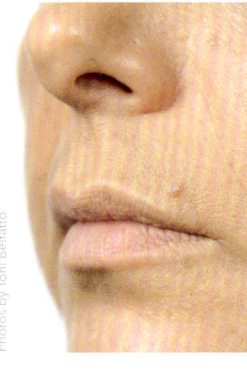
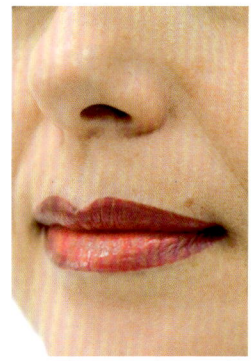
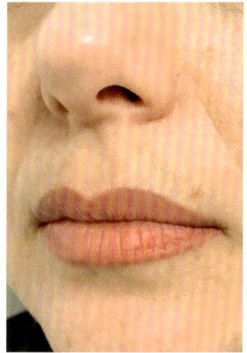

Photos by Toni Belfatto

WHICH ASPECTS OF THE SKIN SHOULD BE EVALUATED BEFORE BEGINNING THE PROCEDURE?

To create the best conditions for the procedure and obtain the desired result, it is good practice to perform an in-depth aesthetic diagnosis of the client's skin.

Here are the aspects which the micropigmentation professional should pay attention to from the start:
- the layer of skin
- its color
- the presence or lack of wrinkles, opening, and folds

Normal skin is smooth, elastic, and luminous. Good blood flow ensures that the skin receives the correct nutrients. Skin color depends on a number of variables: skin type, the number of melanocytes, the part of the body, age, and the presence of diseases. In the Caucasian skin type, skin appears pinkish-white in newborns, then darkens among adults, and appears yellowish among seniors.

It is said that the color of the skin depends on the presence of melanin (the pigment produced by melanocytes) and the level of blood flow, and it can change based on age, skin type, different parts of the body, and different exposure to ultraviolet (UV) rays.

People basically have the same amount of melanocytes regardless of their skin color, but in those with a darker complexion, the melanocytes are more active and therefore produce more melanin. In people with lighter skin tones, the melanin is concentrated near the nuclei of the keratinocytes, and therefore, the cells have less color.

In the end, we can affirm that the skin's pink color is the result of a mix of colors:
- brown tones from melanin
- red from the oxyhemoglobin found in the oxygenated blood that flows through the arteries
- yellow from carotenoids and pro vitamin A
- gray tones created in the superficial stratum corneum

Two types of melanin are present in humans:
- eumelanin, which imparts a brown-black color
- pheomelanin, which imparts a yellow-red color containing sulfur pigments.

STAGES OF SKIN AGING

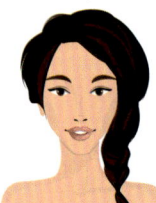

AT 25 YEARS:
- smooth and elastic skin
- luminous skin
- defined face contours

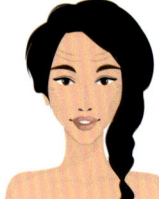

FROM 26 TO 35 YEARS:
- wrinkles around the eyes
- wrinkles on the forehead

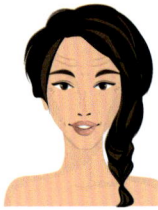

FROM 36 TO 50 YEARS:
- wrinkles on the forehead increase
- wrinkles around the eyes increase
- wrinkles around the mouth

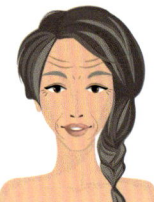

AFTER 50 YEARS:
- wrinkles on the forehead increase
- wrinkles around the eyes increase
- wrinkles around the mouth increase

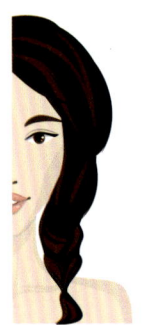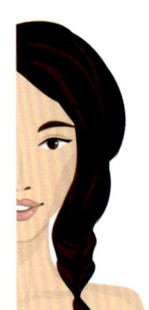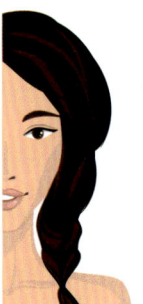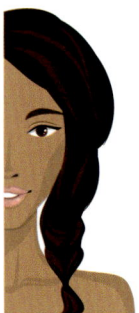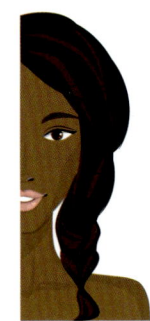

HOW SHOULD THE LEVEL OF PIGMENT IN THE SKIN BE ASSESSED?

Skin color is mainly the result of two factors:

- genetic predisposition
- greater or lesser intensity of pigmentation based on sun exposure, use of pharmaceuticals, or hormonal influence

Humans are subdivided into three skin types, each with their own peculiarities:

- Caucasian
- Asian
- Dark

The main differences in the colors of the different skin types are not due to the number of melanocytes, but to their different levels of activity.

Different pigmentation between members of the same skin type can be due both to more intense synthesis of melanin by the melanocytes due to a particular environmental stimulus, or to melanocytes that are larger or have more branches due to some genetic predisposition.

Seasons are a determining factor in evaluating skin color.

Sun exposure, which stimulates both the synthesis and oxidation of melanin, and consequently causes the skin to tan, is one of the external factors with the most influence on skin pigmentation, and therefore on the results of the procedure.

Without continued stimulus, a tan fades over time as the melanin granules in older keratinocytes break down, and as we've learned, these cells are progressively eliminated through exfoliation, which occurs more quickly due to sun exposure. Therefore, different results are to be expected for procedures done in the summer compared to those done in the fall or winter.

The process of melanogenesis, in addition to making people more aesthetically attractive, is the most important protective mechanism against UVA and UVB rays. When performing a comprehensive assessment of the work to be done, the substantial differences between different parts of the body should not be overlooked, since the amount of melanin varies from one area to another.

Freckles, moles, the backs of the hands and feet, nipples, areolae, and genitals have higher concentrations of melanin than other body parts.

Hemoglobin and carotenoids also cause skin color to vary.

Hemoglobin, the red pigment found in blood, imparts the reddish-pink color of blood vessels that are visible through the skin. Therefore, the skin looks more red in areas like the lips, where capillaries are closer to the surface.

Carotene is a yellow pigment which the body mostly obtains from food. A person's diet determine the concentration of this pigment. Carotene is found, for example, in subcutaneous tissue and in the thicker stratum corneum like the skin of the heels or in foot calluses. Last but not least, professionals should ask their clients if they are undergoing, or planning to undergo, pharmaceutical or hormonal procedures, since these substances can notably influence levels of pigmentation in the tissues.

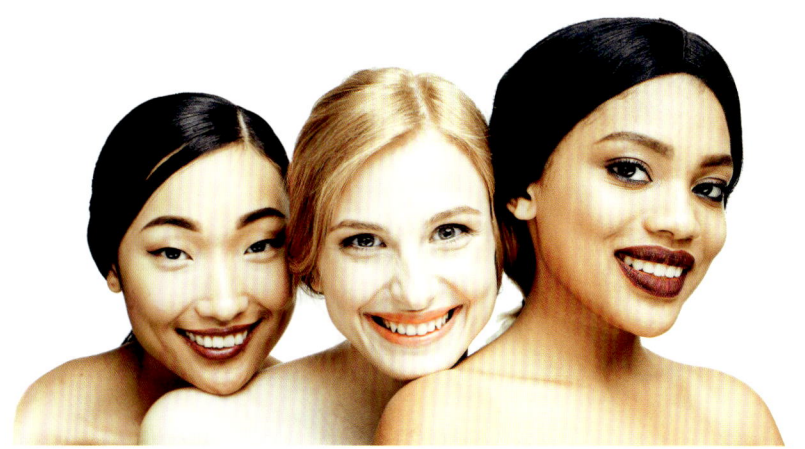

SKIN VASCULARIZATION

Wounds bleed, which is another crucial factor to carefully consider during the dermopigmentation procedure.

The elements of a perfect procedure are:
- minimal bleeding (regarding the abundantly vascularized dermis, compared to the epidermis, which has no blood vessels);
- the sound exam;
- no perceivable alterations in the vibration;
- constant flow from the needle.

Although they function as a whole, it is good to understand which parts of the body are the most vascularized, and therefore pose the most risk of bleeding. This helps reduce bleeding, and therefore reduce the risk of bacterial, viral, or chemical contamination. Vascular networks made up of arteries and veins run through the dermis, parallel to the skin's surface. The arteries and veins that run perpendicular to the surface originate from these vessels, enabling the skin to carry out all of its most important functions. A dense web of capillaries originates from the arteries found in the subcutaneous tissue. These capillaries extend up to the dermis, guaranteeing circulation and distributing nutrients to the epidermis, which otherwise has no blood vessels. Capillary veins then take over from the capillary arteries, draining all of the skin cells' waste substances into the body's veins.

The circulatory system's main functions are:
- providing the skin with nutrients through substances which are dissolved in arterial blood;
- supporting the skin's metabolism, and therefore cellular turnover;
- regulating body temperature through vasoconstriction and vasodilation mechanisms. Variations in climate conditions allow the body to reduce or increase how much heat it disperses: in the summer, abundant vasodilation causes the skin to appear flushed and hot as heat is dispersed outwards, while in the winter, the opposite mechanism, which is vasoconstriction, makes the skin appear paler as it retains heat and limits its outwards dispersion;
- eliminating toxins and waste products from cellular metabolism through the dense vascular network, lymphatic vessels, or transdermal routes.

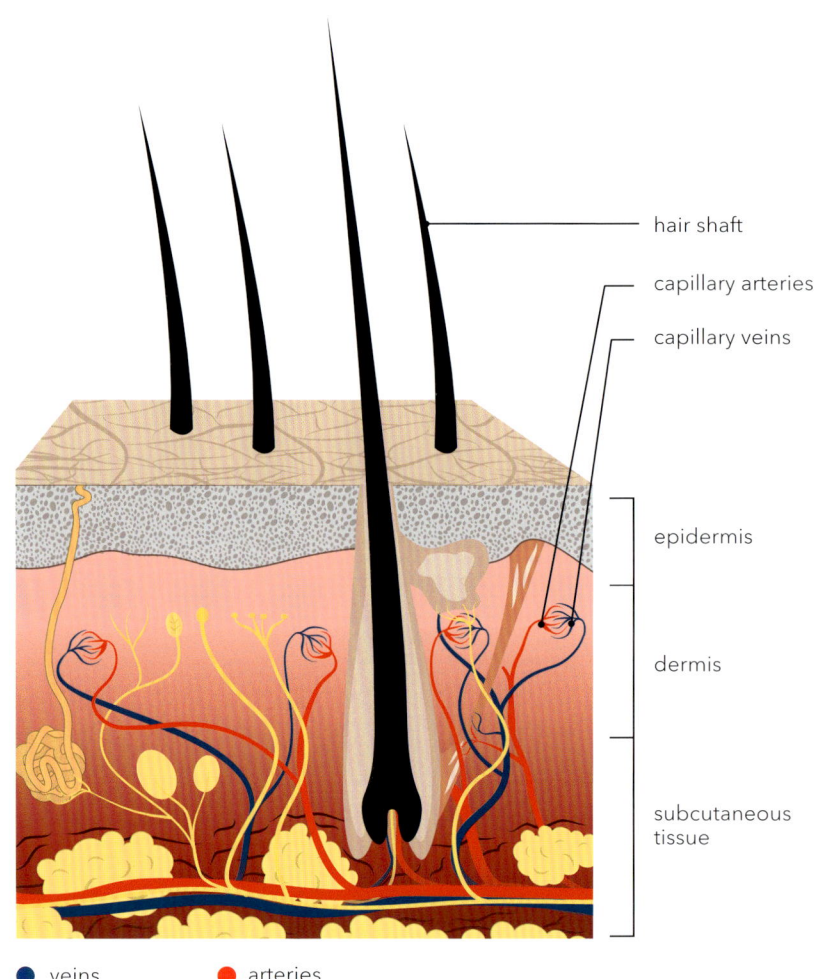

hair shaft

capillary arteries

capillary veins

epidermis

dermis

subcutaneous tissue

● veins   ● arteries

It is important to note that both the circulatory and lymphatic systems are the natural means through which fragments of the pigment introduced by micropigmentation are eliminated.

Before being carried into blood stream, the pigment fragments are absorbed by the white blood cells, like neutrophil granulocytes and macrophages (sometimes called the body's "street sweepers"), which are blood cells that specialize in destroying and eliminating foreign elements from the body. In the dermis, the normal process through which pigment is destroyed can cause noticeable color fading after the procedure is completed.

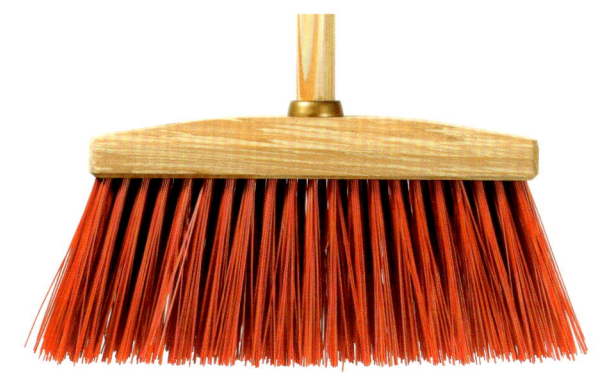

THE SKIN AS AN ORGAN OF PAIN AND PLEASURE

The presence of nerve endings, which are distributed differently throughout the various layers, makes the skin a true sensory organ. The sensory receptors can receive, elaborate, and transmit different kinds of stimuli from the body's surface (the outermost layer of skin) to the central nervous system. Some receptors are made of simple nerve endings such as those for pain and temperature, while others are more complex.

The following receptors are distributed throughout different parts of the skin:

- nociceptors: pain receptors that are activated when tissue is wounded. These are the most common nerve endings in the skin and mucous membranes;
- thermoreceptors: nerve endings that can distinguish between hot and cold;
- mechanoreceptors: activate in response to vibrations, pressure, or pulling of the skin. Among these, we also find Merkel "hair disks", which are located in the basal layers of the epidermis. Hair receptors respond to vibrations transmitted through the hair. Meissner tactile corpuscles are located in the dermis and are responsible for tactile sensitivity. They are concentrated in particularly sensitive areas like the fingertips, eyelids, palms,

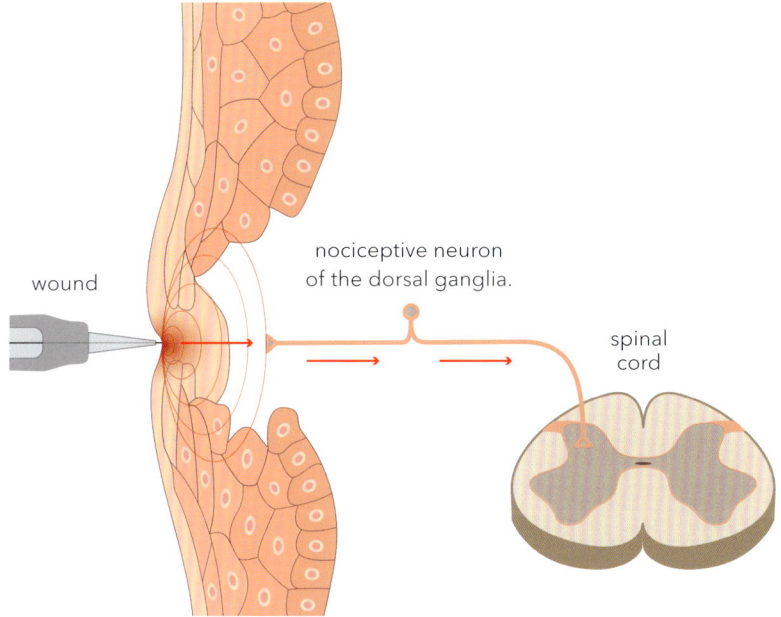

wound

nociceptive neuron of the dorsal ganglia.

spinal cord

nipples, lips, and genital areas. Pacini corpuscles, which are sensitive to vibrations and tickling, are concentrated in the deep dermis of the hands, feet, breasts, and genitals.

WHY ARE SOME AREAS MORE SENSITIVE THAN OTHERS?

Pain is not always a negative thing: in some situations, it serves to protect the body. The pain we feel when we touch a burning object, for example, triggers a nervous reflex that in turn stimulates the muscles and allows us to move away from the object. It should be noted that every stimulus, regardless of its nature (mechanical, thermal, etc.) can turn into a sensation of pain once the threshold level is exceeded. This can occur during a dermopigmentation procedure because of the involvement of certain receptors present in notoriously sensitive areas (e.g. lips, eyelids, limb extremities, genitals, etc.).

Pain receptors are distributed differently throughout the body's surface. Their nerve fibers run through the gaps between the keratinocytes and the granular layer. Every single nerve ending can cover an area of skin measuring around 7cm in diameter.

For example, consider the skin on the back: if the skin in this area of the body is stimulated using two needles placed at points 7cm apart, the puncture is only felt in a single point. That's because the back, like other areas of the body, does not need to be able to make such accurate distinctions. On the other hand, there are parts of the body (fingertips, lips, eyelids, genitals) in which each nerve ending covers an area of skin with a diameter of less than one millimeter, and with a much higher density of fibers. That means that in these areas, if two points even just 2 mm apart are stimulated at the same time, they will be perceived as separate and distinct. The pain that is felt when specific parts of the body are stimulated depends on the type of nerve endings, their organization and density, and the type of stimulus applied.

SCARRING OF SKIN WOUNDS

Micropigmentation can cause tiny lesions, which compromise the skin's integrity and trigger a series of pathophysiological mechanisms which aim to repair injured tissue. The tiny lesions trigger a series of events which causes the wounds to scar, and therefore heal. These can be superficial (epithelial) or also involve the dermis, but regardless of the type of wound, healing takes place through three phases that overlap as time goes by. Scarring is the end result of the tissue repair process. Micropigmentation causes tiny wounds, which do not require the scarring and healing process needed by larger wounds. However, we still think it is useful to provide a general overview of the three most important phases in the healing process, whose extent depends on the depth or seriousness of the wound itself.

1. Inflammatory phase (0 to 4 days)
2. Proliferation phase, with formation of granular tissue. (4 to 20 days)
3. Tissue remodeling phase (6 to 10 days to 12 to 20 months)

The true inflammatory phase is preceded by a hemostatic (coagulatory) phase which lasts around 10 minutes. It is crucial for avoiding excessive blood loss, and prevents platelets from

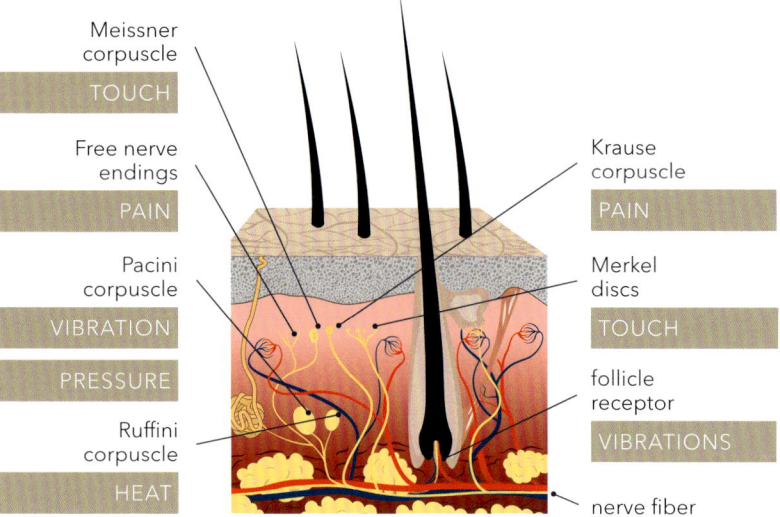

Meissner corpuscle
TOUCH

Free nerve endings
PAIN

Pacini corpuscle
VIBRATION
PRESSURE

Ruffini corpuscle
HEAT

Krause corpuscle
PAIN

Merkel discs
TOUCH

follicle receptor
VIBRATIONS

nerve fiber

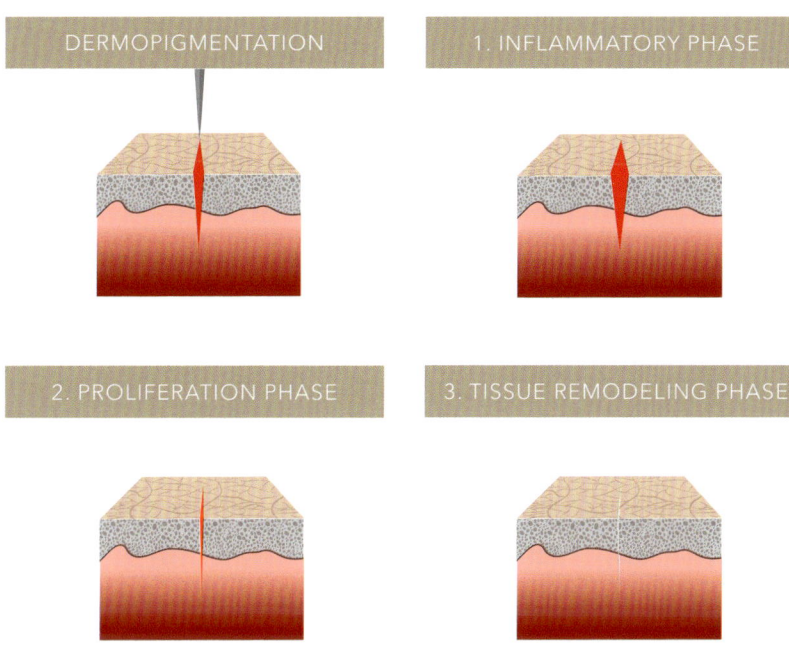

| DERMOPIGMENTATION | 1. INFLAMMATORY PHASE |
| 2. PROLIFERATION PHASE | 3. TISSUE REMODELING PHASE |

getting involved. At first, rapid vasoconstriction (a few seconds) can be seen, which is triggered by vasoactive substances in the wounded cells. Vasodilation follows, then platelets form a cap over the lesion. This coagulation solidifies and creates a scab around the wound in order to occlude it from the external environment and defend it from bacterial infection.

After hemostasis and coagulation, the real inflammatory phase begins. Following vasodilation and the subsequent increase in blood flow, the wound may appear red. The wound is painful because nerve endings are exposed, and a bruise may form because liquid and cells leak from the capillaries.

The blood cells that are called to intervene after the platelets are the neutrophin granules (2-4 hours after the wound): their job is to clean the wound of foreign particles like the ink used for the pigmentation procedure), and to destroy any bacteria present by ingesting them. Around 24 hours after the granulocytes

intervene, monocytes arrive, and become active macrophages inside the lesion. Their job is to ingest microorganisms, eliminate dead neutrophins, and remove both waste and the coagulation. Macrophages play an essential role in the transition from the inflammatory phase to wound repair: they release chemical messengers and trigger the start of the proliferation phase.

Creation of granulation tissue. About 24 hours after the wound, a new epithelial tissue begins to form on the surface, followed by granulation tissue deeper in the skin. The latter will form new blood vessels and new collagen fibers. In this phase, new keratinocytes from the epidermis migrate along the margins of the wound, stacking themselves from the edges of the wound inwards under the scab. They remove the coagulated blood, the damaged tissue, and any residuals (such as color particles) from the wound. Remodellng phase. This is the longest phase in the wound healing process. It can last from a few weeks to several months. Through a phenomenon in which the vascular network (capillaries) is reduced, the previously formed granulation tissue turns into a fibrous mass, which is known as a scar.

Although scars are essentially made of collagen, elastin, and other structural elements with a similar composition as dermal connective tissue, there are substantial differences in both the type of collagen fibers and their architecture.

This different organization is the reason for some of the physical properties of scar tissues, including less elasticity and resistance to stretching than normal skin. This is where the normal tissue repair process comes to an end. Of course, all of the phases of wound repair can be more or less pronounced depending on the wound's seriousness. When micropigmentation is done well, some of the phases may blur together with much quicker repair and healing processes.

LOCAL ANESTHETICS: WHEN AND WHY THEY SHOULD BE USED

In certain situations, depending on the area of the body being treated, but always with the prior approval of a qualified medical professional, these procedures can require the use of topical local anesthetics. These products are available in the form of creams or gels and are used to anesthetize the part of the body receiving the micropigmentation procedure. The use of local anesthetics should always be targeted and limited, given the possibly toxic effects they can cause in the central nervous system and to the heart. Even with topical use, the possibility of systemic absorption should not be excluded, since the area of application, quantity of product used, and the presence of potentially vasoconstrictive substances like adrenaline can all have substantial impact Applying topical anesthetics to abundantly vascularized parts of the body causes more absorption than their use in parts of the body with little vascularization.

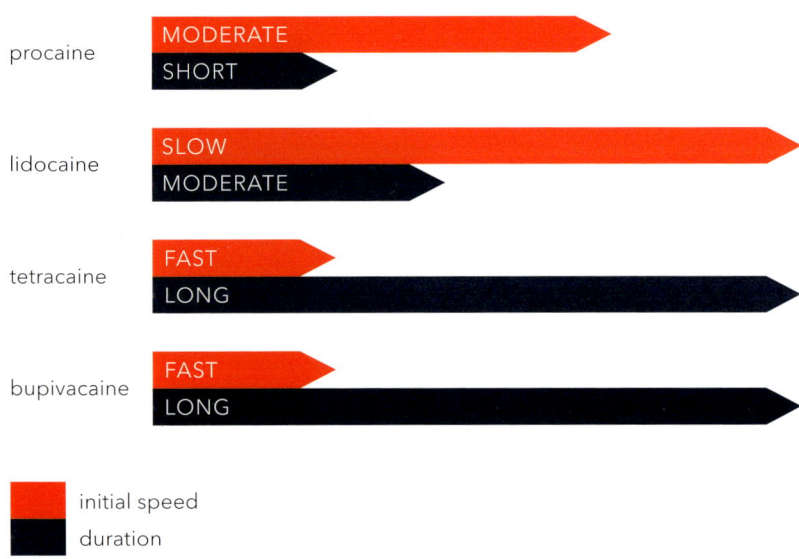

procaine
MODERATE
SHORT

lidocaine
SLOW
MODERATE

tetracaine
FAST
LONG

bupivacaine
FAST
LONG

■ initial speed
■ duration

But how do anesthetics work? These substances are absorbed by the dermis and prevent the sensory receptors from transmitting pain signals along the skin's nerve fibers. Determining which local anesthetic to use depends mostly on the length of the procedure. Starting with short-acting anesthetics like procaine, to those with intermediate durations like lidocaine and mepivacaine, to tetracaine and bupivacaine which have long-lasting effects.

There are two ways to extend the effects of moderate- or intermediate-lasting products: either by increasing the dosage, or by adding vasoconstriction substances like adrenaline, which slows the rate at which the anesthetic leaves the area of application, reducing the amount of product absorbed into the bloodstream and therefore the risk of toxicity. Vasoconstriction also reduces the risk of bleeding in the area of application, creating better conditions for the procedure. As mentioned, local anesthetics, if absorbed into the bloodstream at high levels, can cause severe toxic reactions in the cardiovascular and central nervous systems. Adverse reactions in the heart may lead to severe cardiac arrhythmias and heart failure.

As for the central nervous system, the most frequent symptoms include restlessness, drowsiness, changes in sensory perceptions such as visual or auditory disturbances, and convulsions.

Anesthetics may also cause local allergic reactions, from small skin rashes to anaphylactic shock. Keep in mind that technically, anesthetics actually harden tissues, thus making it harder to insert the pigments into the dermis.

3

HEALTH AND HYGIENE

3.1. CROSS-INFECTIONS

Infections occur when microorganisms (viruses, bacteria, fungi, protozoa, etc.) invade the body. There are two basic types of infection: symptomatic and asymptomatic.

When preparing the room for a procedure, don't overlook the aspects of health and hygiene, which are of primary importance in this work. Before even thinking about how to set up an operating room, we must underscore the risks of contracting infections that may arise within it.

As discussed previously, performing a dermopigmentation procedure may lead to bleeding. The professional will inevitably touch the blood with disposable gloves, and transfer it onto all the objects handled with those gloves.

Unless all the contaminated areas are disinfected with appropriate products and methods at the end of the procedure, the next client could be infected by a virus from the previous client (here, viruses may also be used to refer to bacteria, algae, fungi, AIDS or hepatitis).

Infectious diseases are caused by a wide range of microorganisms: prions, lipid and non-lipid viruses, bacteria with spores and without spores, micro-bacteria, and fungi.

Prions are abnormal among infectious agents because they lack nucleic acid and are resistant to disinfectants and boiling. Non-lipid viruses are more resistant than those with a lipid lining, and microbacteria are more resistant than bacteria.

Bacterial spores are resistant to all disinfectants as well as boiling.

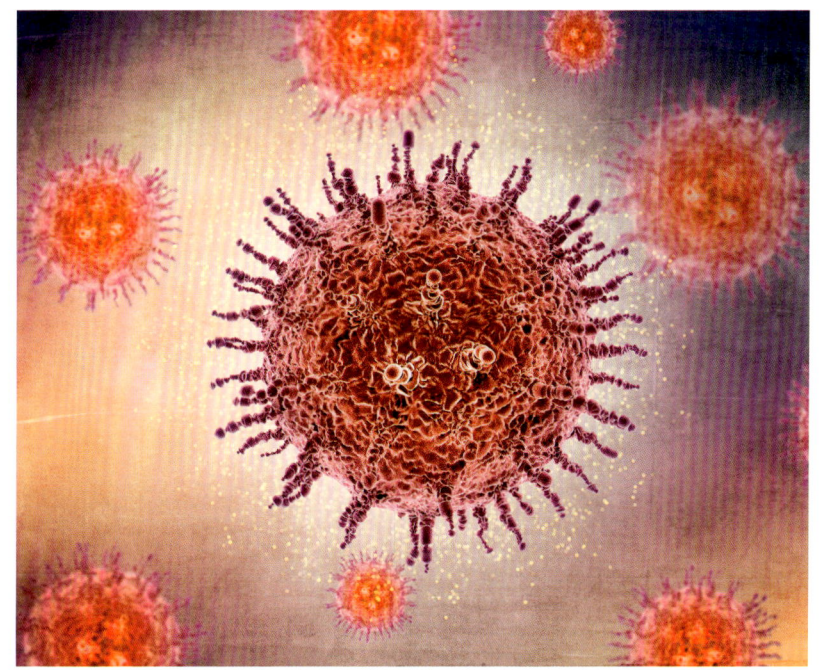

3.2. GENERAL PRINCIPLES OF INFECTIOUS DISEASES

Germs, upon penetrating the organism, colonize the target area and then, moving deeper, induce an inflammatory and immune reaction, successively provoking generalized and symptomatic manifestations.

Infections can be transmitted in two ways:

- directly: through blood, mucous membranes, or inhalation;
- indirectly: through needles or instruments, hands, insects, objects, clothing, or food.

Often, infections are immediately counteracted by immune defenses, through the combined actions of white blood cells, gamma globulin antibodies, competition with non-pathogenic bacteria such as saprophytes and many other substances (interferons, cytokines, lysozyme, complement, etc). Of course, the best defense is the specific protection obtained from vaccines. Vaccines are a legal requirement for those working in the health care sector, and dermopigmentation professionals cannot and should not forgo them. Health care workers are considered at-risk personnel because of their frequent contact with patients and potentially infectious materials: that is why undergoing the relevant vaccinations is crucial.

An adequate immunization process of health care workers is fundamental for preventing and controlling infections. Well-implemented vaccination programs may in fact substantially reduce the number of susceptible workers and the resulting risks, either of acquiring dangerous occupational infections, or of transmitting preventable pathogens by vaccinating patients or other workers. The legal basis for vaccinating health care workers is Legislative Decree of April 9, 2008, n.81, in which article 279 states: "Workers carrying out activities whose risk evaluation has identified a health risk are subject to health surveillance."

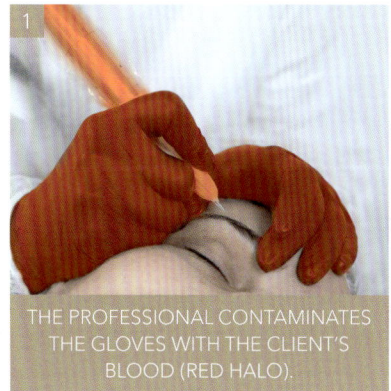

THE PROFESSIONAL CONTAMINATES THE GLOVES WITH THE CLIENT'S BLOOD (RED HALO).

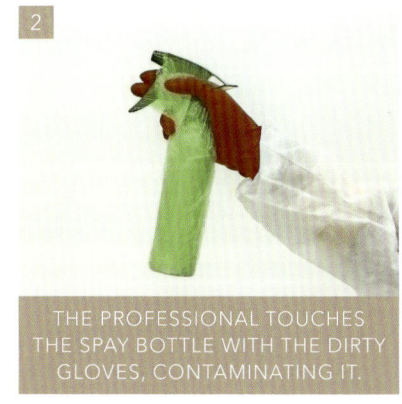

THE PROFESSIONAL TOUCHES THE SPAY BOTTLE WITH THE DIRTY GLOVES, CONTAMINATING IT.

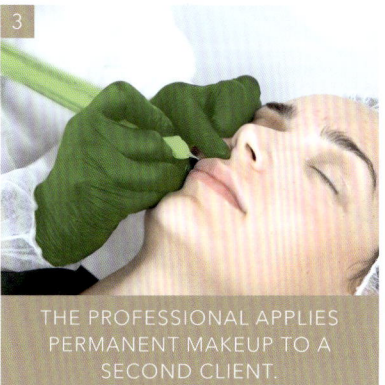

THE PROFESSIONAL APPLIES PERMANENT MAKEUP TO A SECOND CLIENT.

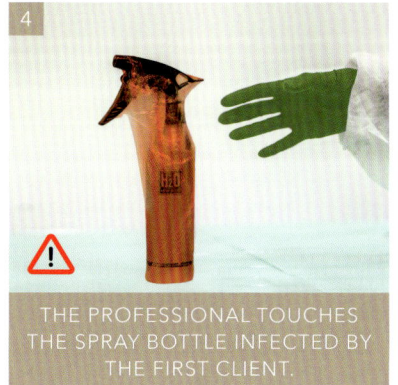

THE PROFESSIONAL TOUCHES THE SPRAY BOTTLE INFECTED BY THE FIRST CLIENT.

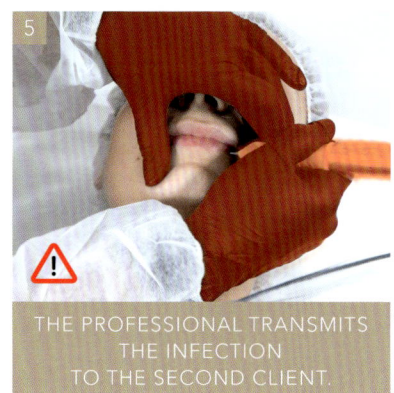

THE PROFESSIONAL TRANSMITS THE INFECTION TO THE SECOND CLIENT.

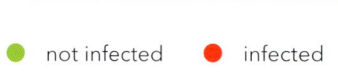

● not infected   ● infected

3.3. VACCINATIONS

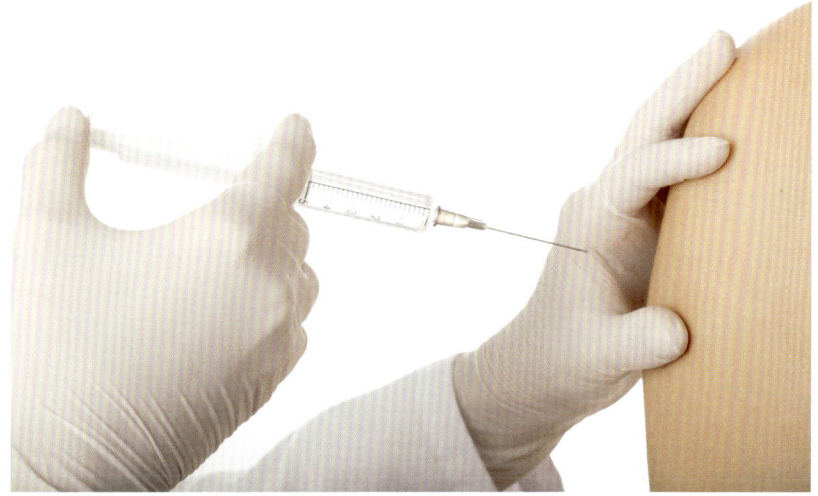

The employer, in consultation with the treating physician, must implement protective measures for those workers who need special protection measures, including for individual reasons. The company's treating physician is therefore responsible for identifying or performing the vaccinations required by the health workers.

In other cases (like with anti-influenza vaccinations) active immunization not only protects the individual professional, but above all protects the patients to whom the professional could transmit the infection, causing significant damage.

For these reasons, the following vaccinations are strongly recommended for all health workers, health care students, and dermopigmentation professionals:

HEPATITIS B VACCINE

Hepatitis B represents the biggest risk of infection for health professionals, and it is therefore essential that they all be vaccinated, if possible before starting any risky activity.

The vaccine is administered in three doses, 0, 1, and 6-12 months apart. However, for those exposed to an immediate risk of infection, the vaccine can be administered on an accelerated schedule in 4 doses (0, 1, 2, 12 months), which guarantees higher chances of protection after just the first 3 doses.

Serum conversion (presence of anti-HBs antibodies) should be verified one month after the last dose (according to the Ministerial Decree of 20 November 2000, art.4), to ensure that immunological memory has been established.

Students in the health care area and health professionals born after 1980 are presumed to have been vaccinated against hepatitis B at the age of 12, but the test is still recommended in order to verify the level of anti-HBs before beginning risky activities. A positive result means there is immunological memory, and no further intervention is needed.

However, it is recommended that subjects with negative test results receive a single dose of the vaccine and are checked for antibodies again one month later.

Positive anti-HB results indicate the presence of immunological memory, while continued negative results indicate the vaccination cycle must be completed with the next two doses, followed by a new serum test one month later.

For subjects who do not respond to the vaccination cycle, up to 3 additional doses (0, 1, and 6 months apart) can be administered to attempt to protect the professional. Recently, a new system of vaccines was proposed for those who don't respond, which includes simultaneously administering 2 doses into the deltoid muscles, followed by analogous administration 2 months later and serum tests to check for serum conversion (anti-HBs ≥10 mUI/ml) two more months later.

FLU VACCINE

This vaccination, in addition to protecting the professional, has the dual purpose of protecting the patients with whom they may come into contact and to whom they can transmit infections. This prevents the overloading of essential assistance services, in case of a flu epidemic.

For these reasons, every health care company must actively promote all initiatives deemed appropriate in order to encourage their professionals and students to get vaccinated during the annual autumn vaccination campaign.

TETANUS VACCINE

This vaccine protects against tetanus, a disease that affects the body's muscles and nerves. It is a serious disease, which usually occurs when a wound in the skin is contaminated by a bacteria that is fairly common in the ground, Clostridium tetani. After entering the body, the bacteria produces a neurotoxin called tetanospasmina, which can spread throughout the entire organism through the blood stream and lymphatic system and interfere with nerve function, causing muscle spasms.

If not treated in time, tetanus can be fatal. Death can occur through cardiopulmonary failure, due to contraction or paralysis of the muscles. The first symptom of tetanus often includes muscle spasms in the jaw, which may be accompanied by difficulty swallowing. Spasms in other muscles may follow, from the head down to the neck, shoulders, back, and limbs, until the subject curls up on themselves.

Symptoms can occur any time between a few days to a few months after coming into contact with the bacteria. Its incubation period actually lasts between two days and two months, and in most cases, the disease manifests within 14 days.

Anti-tetanus prophylaxis includes getting the vaccine even after an accident that results in a wound or lesion, since the objective is always preventing any infection from occurring in the first place.

The infections we aim to prevent include those transmitted through the blood, like prions and the hepatitis B and C viruses, as well as HIV (the virus that causes AIDs), non-blood infections like tetanus, and bacterial infections in the wound like staphylococcus and streptococcus. A good way to avoid any kind of infection is to sterilize tools in an autoclave and to hygienically prepare both the professional and the client.

Not all objects, however, can be sterilized in an autoclave. That is why often, different hygienic methods are used (plastic wrap being the most common) to avoid continued contaminations on different kinds of objects.

3.4. PPE (PERSONAL PROTECTIVE EQUIPMENT)

Because the professional is at risk of infection, they must put on the appropriate personal protective equipment before entering the treatment room and beginning to set up the materials. PPE refers to any equipment intended to be worn by professionals to protect themselves against the many risks of their work environment. In reality, there is a proper order for putting on and taking off this equipment before and after every procedure.

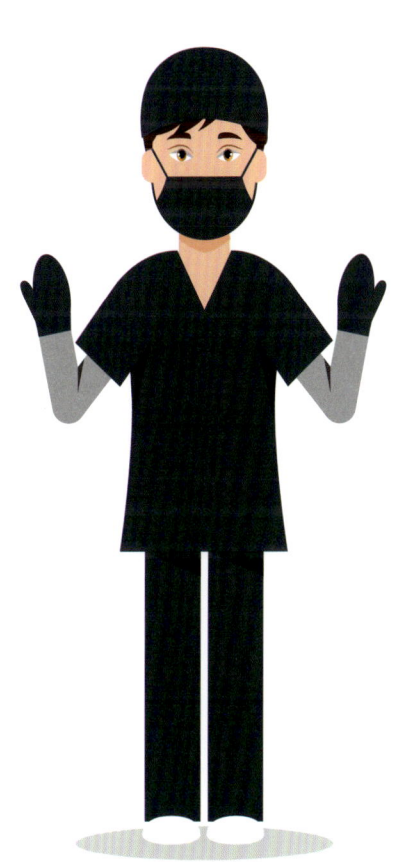

STEPS FOR PUTTING ON PPE

gloves	1
visor	2
mask	3
cap	4
shirt	5
leg coverings	6
change gloves	7

STEPS FOR TAKING OFF PPE

1	leg coverings
2	change gloves
3	shirt
4	cap
5	masks
6	visor
7	gloves

3.5. INFECTION RISK FACTORS FOR THE PROFESSIONAL

Professionals, aestheticians, tattoo artists, and body piercers can risk infection (biohazard) through accidental transmission by any infected clients. Biological agents can include bacteria (such as tetanus, staphylococci, streptococci, pseudomonas, etc.), viruses (hepatitis, AIDS, cytomegaly, mononucleosis, herpes, etc.), fungi (candida, pityriasis, etc.), and parasites (scabies, fleas, etc).

There are also "good" germs however: our skin and mucous membranes are covered with bacteria that prevent "bad" germs from gaining a foothold. Intestinal bacteria produce a lot of vitamins; many bacteria help us create food such as sourdough bread, wine, beer, certain cheeses, cured meats, and yogurt.

The skin and mucous membranes, together with our immune system, provide defenses that in most cases protect us from infection.

But if any infectious agent pass through these natural barriers, or if they are particularly aggressive or unusually numerous,
or if our immune defenses are temporarily weakened, these biological agents can win the upper hand and find a place to reproduce, colonize, and infect.

Parenteral infections are transmitted through cuts and punctures by infected tools or exposure of the mucous membranes to infected blood.

This could include pricking oneself with a needle used on an infected client, or injuring oneself with a tool contaminated with someone else's blood, or contaminating one's mucous membranes (eyes, nose, mouth) with these fluids. AIDS and hepatitis B, C, and D are some examples diseases that are transmitted this way.

Direct contact is another, equally important way through which herpes viruses, bacteria, fungi, and mites can spread. Some infections are airborne, including the influenza and tuberculosis viruses, and respiratory bacteria.

3.6. PREPARING THE TREATMENT ROOM

After donning the PPE, it is time to prepare the operating area: all of the surfaces with which the client and professional come into contact must be prepared with specific hygienic modules or plastic film. Lay a sterile, single-use towelette on the work table, onto which the single-use containers of color, disinfectant soap, sterile drawing instruments, and the properly covered machine will be placed.

The following is a list of the main protective materials for the equipment: plastic casing to cover the console and the handpiece, an envelope that covers the entire cord of the handpiece and the handpiece itself; latex sheaths to protect the handpiece and seal the envelope that surrounds it.

For the furniture:
the treatment chair must be carefully sealed using plastic film, then place paper where the client will be positioned. The professional's chair and backrest should also be covered with plastic film. If the treatment chair is electronically operated, seal the controller. If it is manually operated, seal the lever. Also seal the handles of the cart, the dispenser, and any other items that may be used during the procedure.

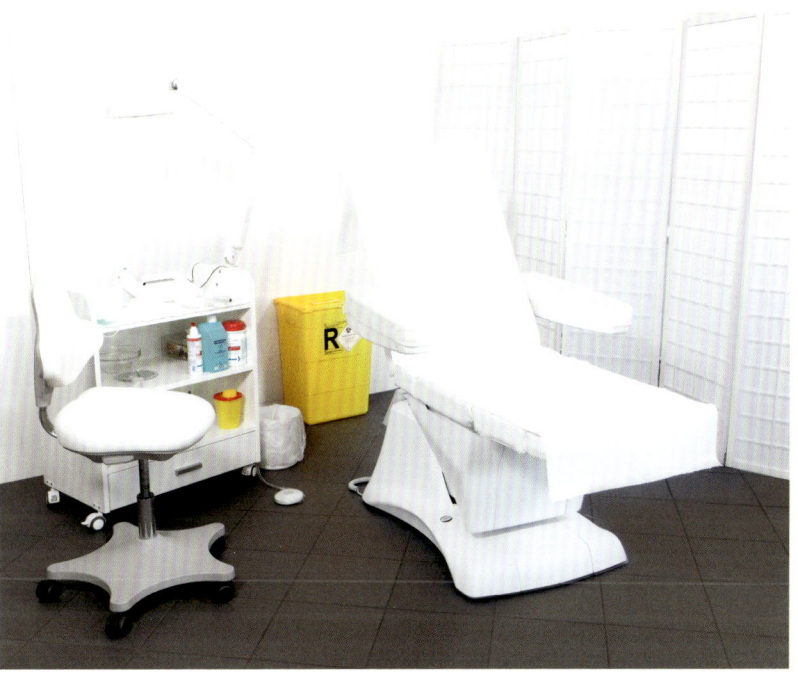

3.7. MAINTAINING HYGIENIC TOOLS

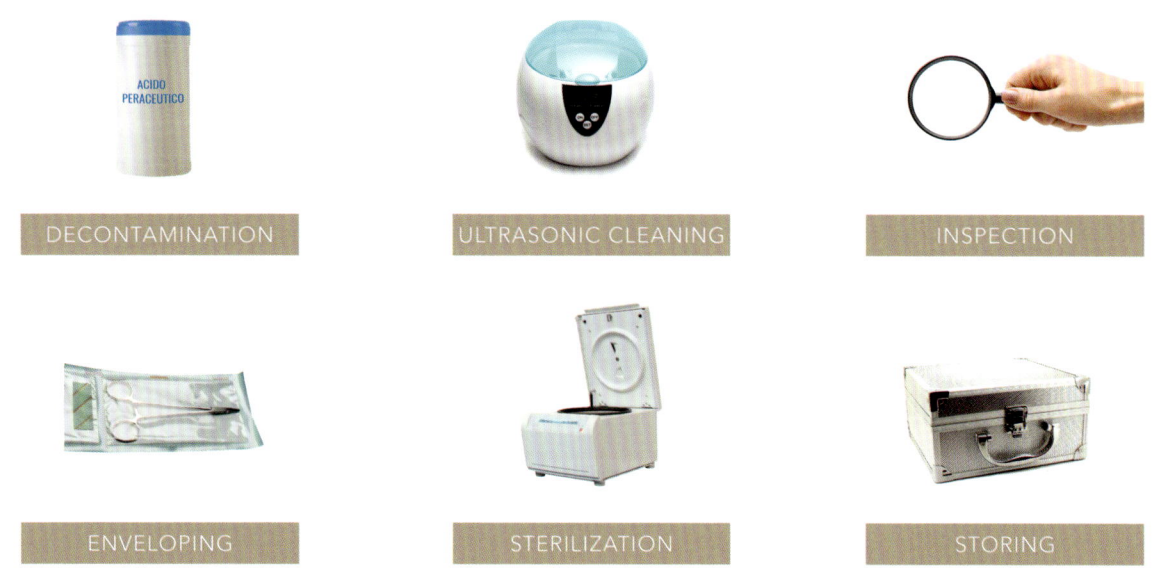

| DECONTAMINATION | ULTRASONIC CLEANING | INSPECTION |

| ENVELOPING | STERILIZATION | STORING |

Although the majority of tools used for dermopigmentation procedures are entirely single-use (needles, needle holders, and pigment containers), some items like the tweezers for removing eyebrow hairs, or different grips for microblading, need to be sterilized before being re-used.

Therefore it is worth going over the 6 phases and methods to follow to make sure that the tools used during dermopigmentation remain safe and reliable.

DECONTAMINATION

The first phase is decontamination, to prevent any microorganisms from spreading from the object into the surroundings. To do this, immerse the tool into a container of peracetic acid or glutaraldehyde immediately after use. To accelerate the activation process for the peracetic acid, we recommend immersing the container in hot water. This product is time-sensitive: it loses its effectiveness completely within 24 hours. Glutaraldehyde requires a fume hood because it is toxic and corrosive. It should be disposed of with special waste liquids.

CLEANING

The second phase in maintaining hygienic tools is cleaning, in which objects are washed to remove any residues from pigment, blood, or skin cells. This is generally done using an ultrasonic tool, which is an electric appliance that emits vibrations thanks to water contained inside it. A single-use, autoclavable plastic cup is placed inside the ultrasound, filled with enzymatic liquid to make the cleaning process even more effective.

INSPECTION
Next, a visual inspection determines whether the tool is damaged, corroded, or dirty, and if necessary the cleaning process is repeated.

ENVELOPING
In the fourth phase, the cleaned tool is placed inside specific envelopes before being sterilized.
Two kinds of envelopes are used here:
• self-sealing envelopes are closed on one side, and the object is inserted in the other;
• heat sealed: a heat sealer closes them using heat.

STERILIZATION
In this fifth phase, the envelope is placed in the autoclave, taking care to position it with the paper side facing up so that the steam can enter more easily without being obstructed by the tray. Sterilization removes any form of life (including spores) from a contaminated object, with a 98% success rate.

There are 3 kinds of autoclaves:
N: sterilize objects that are not hollow, and not placed in an envelope
S: sterilize objects that are not hollow, but are placed in an envelope
B: sterilize objects that are hollow and placed in an envelope thanks to a feature called fractional vacuum, which allows vapor to enter the object's cavity.

Unlike many other sterilization systems, the autoclave uses heat and pressure because it works with the physical constants of pressure (2.5 atmosphere), heat (134 °C) and time (30 minutes).

By law, autoclaves must pass three types of tests:
• physical test: a sensor inside the autoclave confirms that the three physical constants are functioning;
• chemical test: verifies the pressure using litmus papers;
• microbiological test or spore test: performed once a month by an external professional to verify that bacteria, viruses, and spores are eliminated correctly.

Each time an object is sterilized in the autoclave, its sterilization must be recorded and suitably dated in the sterilization log, within a maximum of 15 days from use.
In general, the autoclave used in the field of dermopigmentation is regulated by the class B norms of the ASL.

STORING
Once sterilized, the object must be placed inside a hermetically sealed container in order to keep it sterile.

3.8. HYGIENICALLY PREPARING THE CLIENT

Permanent makeup procedures or general dermopigmentation are not high-risk procedures if all of the hygienic and health procedures described above are followed. However, like in the medical field, it is extremely important to discuss the declaration of consent, which is an agreement and disclosure between the client and the professional which protects both parties and most importantly, informs the client of all the procedures they will undergo, together with their benefits and risks.

RISK FACTORS RELATING TO THE CLIENT'S STATE OF HEALTH

The client's risk of contracting an infection is mainly related to whether they are under conditions of immunodepression: as is the case for example with AIDS patients, people who have undergone a transplant, people undergoing cancer therapy or cortisone therapy, "biological" therapies, radiotherapy or dialysis. Clients should also be evaluated on a case-by-case basis to determine if they are at risk because of severe debilitation or malnutrition, or if they suffer from chronic illnesses or congenital or acquired defects.

Contraindications may also include pregnant and breastfeeding women as well as a wide variety of allergies, skin diseases, congenital and / or acquired coagulation disorders, seizures, or the presence of moles or pre-cancerous lesions. It is also best to avoid any procedure if the client plans to donate blood or organs within the next 6 months, or if the client regularly uses alcohol or drugs, vasodilators, anti-coagulants, or anti-platelet medication. The client has to be an adult according to national legislation; treatment of minors is not allowed. The specific age may differ from country to country. To protect the practice, it is best to require a declaration of consent, including for the risk of any post-procedural infections that arise because the client does not follow the professional's hygienic advice.

HAIR REMOVAL

There are many ways to remove body hair: wax, depilatory creams, electric razors, disposable razors, or tweezers. The safest hair removal is always the one carried out by the professional right before the procedure using the classic eyebrow tweezers or a razor for paramedical procedures on the body.

This ensures better control of the area to be depilated, and reduces the risk of germs entering the skin through the tiny cuts left behind by less adept use of the razor. Studies on surgical depilation show that the longer the interval between shaving and the procedure, the more the probability of infection in the wound increases. Wax is definitely not recommended because of the micro-traumas it causes on the local level.

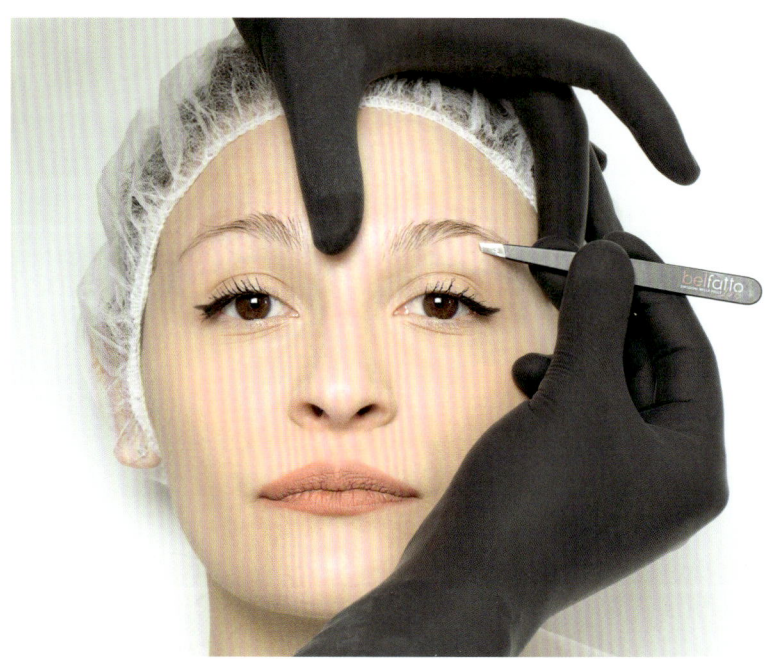

DRESSING THE CLIENT

After the disclosure, the client should be prepared for entering the operating room.

It is good practice for the client to be hygienically prepared, like the professional: clothing should be clean (arriving at the practice for procedure in work clothes is contraindicated) to reduce the presence of bacteria (Fig. A).

Nobody else should accompany the client into the treatment rooms, since they could be vehicles for infection or become exposed to infection. If the client insists on having their companion with them, this person must wear all of the materials included in the personal protective equipment.

To avoid hypoglycemia or fainting, the client should not undergo the procedure after fasting, nor immediately after a meal. The soap used does not necessarily have to be disinfecting. The most important thing is that the client, in the days following the intervention, scrupulously self-medicates, follows rigorous hygienic norms, always washes their hands before and after medicating their permanent makeup, cleanses or disinfects the wound, applies the appropriate ointment recommended by the professional, does not expose the wound to dust or polluted water, and does not visit unsanitary areas.

DISMISSAL

Before the client leaves, it is best to have them wait until their immediate reactions to the procedure can be observed, and the professional can confirm that the client is generally in good condition. When the appointment is over, it is important to remind the client to follow hygienic rules and to give them written reminders in accordance with the type of procedures they underwent (Fig. B).

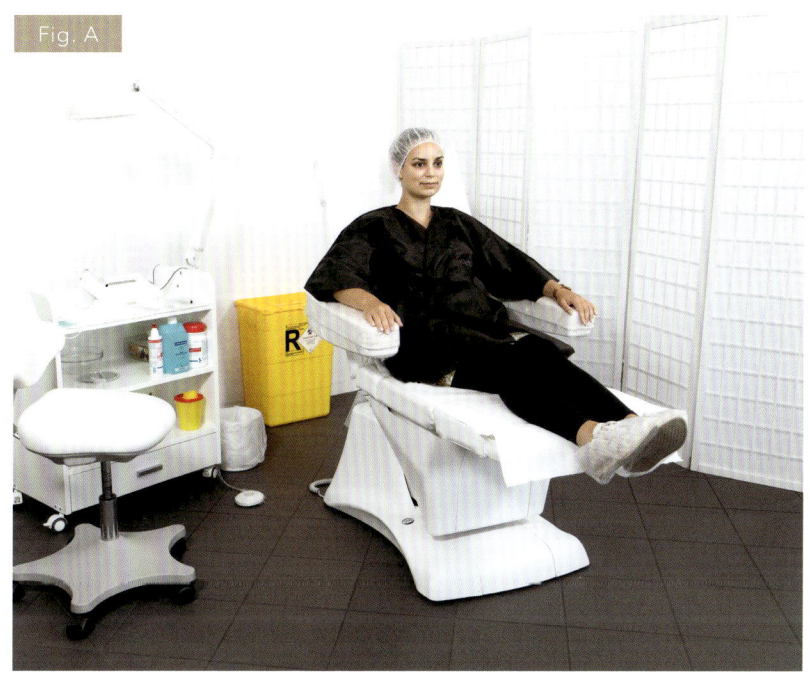

Fig. A

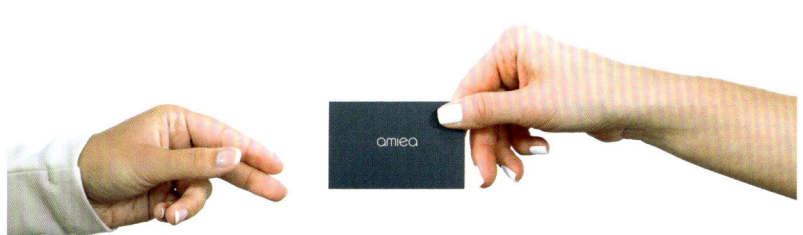

Fig. B

3.9. WHEN TO AVOID DERMOPIGMENTATION

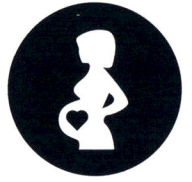

PREGNANCY AND BREASTFEEDING

MINORS UNDER 18 YEARS

BLOOD CLOTTING DISORDERS
(e.g. haemophilia)

UNCONTROLLED DIABETES MELLITUS

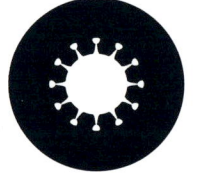

SYSTEMIC INFECTIONS OR INFECTIOUS DISEASES (HIV, HEPATITIS A, B, C, D, E OR F)

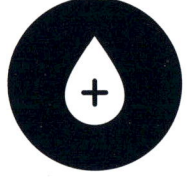

ANTICOAGULANT THERAPY

ECZEMA/EXANTHEMA/ OPEN WOUND

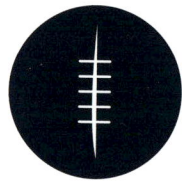

SCARS NOT OLDER THAN 6 MONTHS

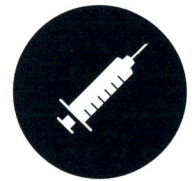

FILLER INJECTIONS IN THE PAST 6 MONTHS

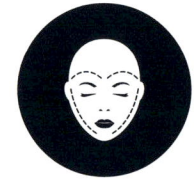

PLASTIC SURGERY IN THE PAST 12 MONTHS

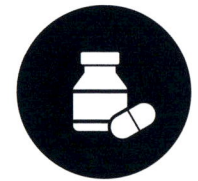

ALLERGIC REACTIONS TO TOPICAL AND LOCAL ANESTHETICS

PREGNANCY AND BREASTFEEDING

It is always advisable to wait until after pregnancy and breastfeeding before undergoing invasive aesthetic procedures.

Pregnancy lowers the woman's immune defenses, making her more vulnerable to local infections, or worse, more severe infectious diseases. During pregnancy the skin becomes more sensitive and is more prone to allergic reactions or to rejecting the pigments.

MINORS

Proceed only with prior consent from both parents or, if the parents are separated, from the parent with custody.

DISEASES

Avoid performing dermatological procedures on people with hemocoagulatory diseases (including diabetes in certain circumstances) or heart diseases. People with verified autoimmune disorders should also abstain from these procedures.

MOLES AND SCARS

Never apply pigment to moles. It is always best to work at a cautionary distance of at least one centimeter since moles have deep roots that are not visible on the surface of the skin. Hypertrophic scars and keloid scars cannot be treated. Hypertrophic scars are caused by an excess of scar tissue (connective tissue, collagen, and fibroblasts). Keloids become larger and are more invasive and problematic. Unlike hypertrophic scars, keloids may appear even months after the lesion.

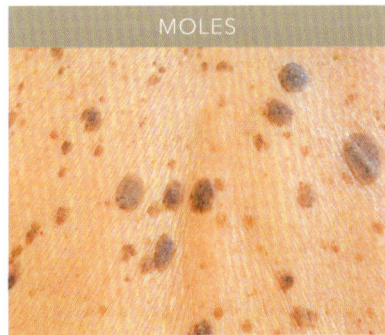

MOLES

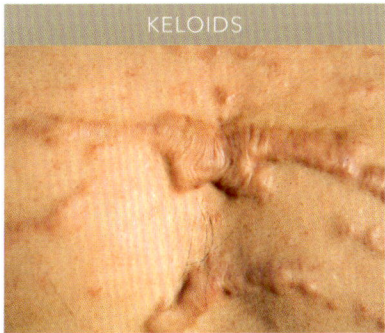

KELOIDS

4

LEGAL MATTERS

In the last few years, the growing popularity of tattoos and permanent makeup has been proven both by the exponential increase of people with tattoos and PMU, as well as by the wide availability of specialty products made available online.

The resulting proliferation of unsuitable dermopigmentation centers, with improvised and unqualified staff and products without guarantees, has created a need for ad hoc regulations to provide legal protection and standards of reference.

Despite the Regulatory Authorities' attempts to issue a uniform legal framework, the regulations that oversee the tattoo and PMU industry and products are still constantly evolving.

4.1. LEGAL REFERENCES

EUROPEAN REGULATIONS

The European legislation on cosmetics (Directive 1223/2009) has banned the use of many dangerous substances in cosmetic products, but tattoos and PMUs are not covered by this ban. As of today, the European Union (EU) has not issued any specific regulation regarding products for tattoos and PMU. These products are among those regulated by the General Product Safety Directive 2001/95 / EC (GPSD) which mandates that only safe products can be placed on the market.

In 2003 the European Commission, through the Scientific Center (JRC), began a research project to collect and evaluate all the available data needed to undertake a possible coordinated European initiative on tattoo and PMU pigments and processes. The European Commission's work is summarized in the publication: "Recommendations for European Union (EU) regulatory action on the safety of tattoos, body piercing and related practices in the EU" Also in 2003, in response to the growing popularity of tattoos and PMU, the Council of Europe (CoE) published a

non-binding resolution, the CoE ResAP, on the requirements and criteria for tattoos and PMU safety.

RESAP(2003)2

ResAP(2003)2 was an initial attempt to create a European standard for legislation concerning the safety of tattoo and PMU products.

The European Council's motives in creating these regulations include:

- the growing popularity of tattoos and permanent makeup;
- the health risks arising from potential microbiological contamination, the presence of dangerous chemical substances in the inks, and unfit hygienic conditions;
- the lack of national legislation in many EU countries regarding the use of products and practices for tattoos and permanent makeup;
- the safety advantages resulting from a unified perspective for solving potential problems.

For many European nations, ResAP(2003)2 provided fundamental guidelines for the formulation of their own national laws. In the following years, the European Commission deemed it necessary to revise the previous resolution by publishing ResAP(2008)1.

RESAP(2008)1

In February 2008, the geopolitical panorama changed with the entry of new nations into the EU, the acquisition of new scientific data regarding products for tattoos and permanent makeup, and a more definite understanding of consumer health risks, leading the Counsel of Europe to revise its previous resolution ResAP(2003)2.

Below are the requirements of the new regulation:

1. Risks should be evaluated correctly before products are placed on the market;
2. Chemical requirements and lists of chemicals that should not be present in tattoo and permanent makeup inks (negative lists);
3. Hygiene and packaging requirements;
4. Proper consumer information regarding potential health risks caused by tattoos and permanent makeup;
5. Labeling requirements for products intended for use in tattoos and permanent makeup.

The main characteristics and differences can be found in the table.

Banned chemical substances:

1. 27 aromatic amines or amines released from azo dyes (Annex 1, table 1);
2. Carcinogenic, mutagenic, reprotoxic, or sensitizing pigments (Annex 1, table 2);
3. Maximum concentrations of impurities (Annex 1, table 3);
4. Ingredients banned in cosmetics (EC Regulation n. 1223/2009
5. Colorants specified in (EC) regulation no.1223/2009, Annex IV, column g, (Annex I, table 4);
6. Carcinogens, mutagens and reprotoxic substances (CMR) of category 1A, 1B and 2 classified according to (EC) regulation n. 1272/2008 (CLP), Part 3 of Annex VI, Table 3.1

Satisfy the minimum requirements for further organic impurities in colorants used for food and cosmetics products.

Labeling:

1. The name and address of the manufacturer or the person responsible for placing the product on the market;
2. The minimum shelf life;

MAIN DIFFERENCES BETWEEN COE RESOLUTIONS (2003)2 AND (2008)1.

		COE RAOAP(2003)2	COE REAAP(2008)1
1. Risk evaluation	safety assessment	done by manufactures or importers/ distributors	manufactures: Prove composition of products and toxicology of substance (using existing guidelines if any). Authorities: Take steps to replace negative lists with positive lists of safe substances.
2. Chemical requirements	aromatic amines negative list	26 aromatic amines in Table 1	paraphenylen diamine added to Table 1
			concentrations should be determined by test methods to be harmonized
	purity criteria	none	maximum allowed concentrations of metal and polycyclic aromatic hydrocarbon (PAH) impurities (Table 3)
			minimum requirements of organic colorant impurities for colorants used in foodstuffs and cosmetic products (Directive 95/45/ECC)
	preservative	should not be used	only to ensure preservation after opening, not as purity correction nor inadequate hygiene
			only after safety assessment and in the lowest effective concentration
3. Hygienic and packaging requirements	container size	Single use recommended	if multi-use containers, designed to avoid contamination durig use
4. Public information	risk	risks including potential sensitation	added: aftercare, removals, physician consultation if medical complications

68

3. Usage conditions and warnings;
4. The batch number or other manufacturer's reference for identifying the batch;
5. The list of ingredients based on their IUPAC nomenclature, CAS (Chemical Abstract Service of the American Chemical Society) number, or color code (color index-CI);
6. Guarantee that the contents are sterile.

Risk assessment:
The manufacturer or person responsible for the commercialization must perform a risk assessment based on data and toxicological information using a digital document that is easily accessible by the relevant authorities.

Application conditions:
Tattoo and permanent makeup products must be sterile and supplied in a container that preserves sterility until the time of application, ideally single-use. Non-contamination during use must be guaranteed. It is of crucial importance to follow specific hygienic norms established by national public health services.

Information:
Tattoo artists should always provide the clients with complete, reliable, and understandable information regarding the risks arising from such practices (raising awareness about the necessary procedures following the application of a tattoo, about the reversibility and removal of tattoos, and about the need to consult a doctor in case of complications).
All potential clients should receive reliable and verified information regarding the risks posed by tattoos and permanent makeup through all appropriate means, for example through mass information campaigns or via the internet.

Legislative framework in EU countries, EFTA (European Free Trade Association) and other jurisdictions.

In 2014, the change in Europe's political geography following the entry of new countries into the European Union, each with their own legal framework, led to a new revision of the JRC's 2003 guidelines. The "Safety of tattoos and permanent makeup: Final report" of the Joint Research Centre (JRC) of the European Commission intends to provide the scientific evidence required to decide if the European Union should adopt further, specific restrictive measures to ensure the safety of the inks and processes used in tattoos and makeup. The report presents an updated overview of legislative reference framework in the various

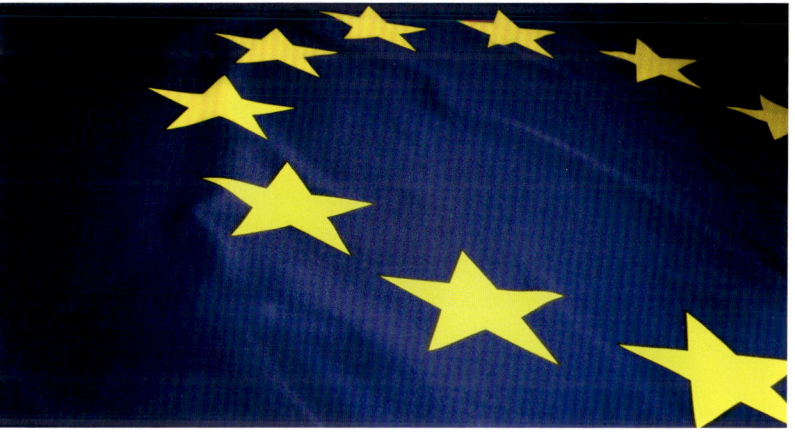

member states (EU) and EFTA countries (Iceland, Liechtenstein, Norway, and Switzerland), the ingredients of the inks used, and the description of the negative health effects reported, as well as new data on analytical methods, statistics, market oversight, risk perception, and communication with consumers.

EU/EFTA COUNTRIES

The situation varies widely between countries. Within EU and EFTA countries, ten countries (Belgium, France, Germany, Liechtenstein, Norway, the Netherlands, Slovenia, Spain, Sweden, Switzerland) have integrated the two ResAP 2003 and 2008 resolutions' recommendations regarding tattoos and permanent makeup products into their own national legislations.
Furthermore, Austria, Denmark, and Latvia have aligned their own national legislation with the ResAP 2008(2008)1.

....

The Czech Republic, Finland, Italy, Malta, Romania and Slovakia have adopted consumer health and safety measures by regulating tattoo artists' activities, including thorough hygienic requirements for tattoo studios. In addition, thorough RAPEX notifications, the Italian and Slovenian health ministries have implemented oversight of tattoo and permanent makeup pigments with reference to the list of dangerous chemicals found in ResAP(2008)1.

....

Bulgaria, Croatia, Cyprus, Estonia, Greece, Ireland, Luxembourg, Poland, and Portugal have not yet established a legislative framework specifically for tattoos and permanent makeup, although like all member countries, they should take safety measures for consumer products and follow the REACH and CLP legislation on chemicals.
No information is available for the United Kingdom, Hungary, Iceland, or Lithuania.

....

The EU/EFTA countries that follow the ResAP recommendations include a series of specific provisions in their own legal framework which concern both the materials and procedures used in tattoos and permanent makeup.

For example, when it comes to packaging, the 10 countries named above as well as Italy, Malta, and Romania ensure the complete sterility of the products used.

....

Germany, Norway, Spain, and Sweden request that the period after opening should be indicated on the container. In France, Spain, the Czech Republic, Norway, and Slovenia, manufacturers and/or distributors must create a product file which is sent to the relevant authorities before the product is placed on the market. Spain is the only country with a list of pigments solely approved for the Spanish market. In Italy, Belgium, Czech Republic, Liechtenstein, Luxembourg, Malta, Romania, Slovenia, Slovakia, Switzerland, the Netherlands, launching a tattoo or permanent makeup practice requires a special license or specific certificate of studies. In France, however, it requires a specific training period. In 2015, the European Commission issued further restrictions preventing the commercialization of certain substances present in tattoo and permanent makeup pigments.

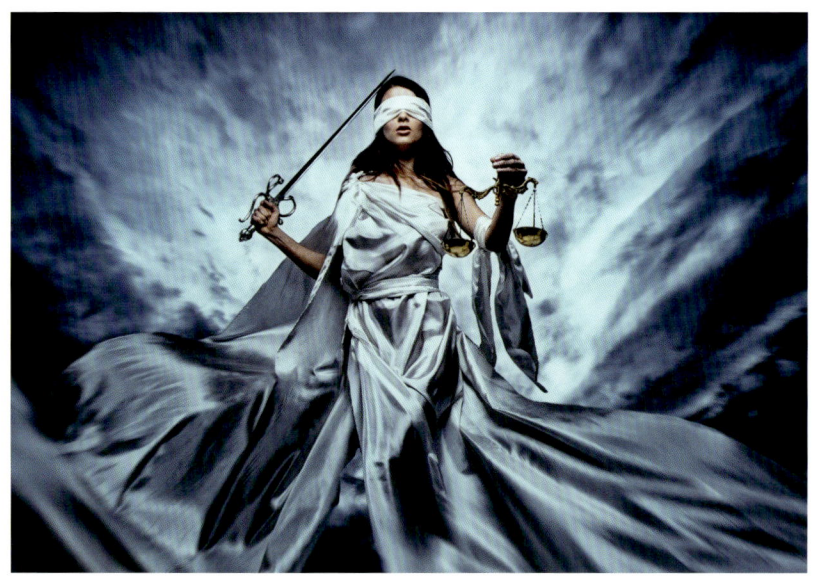

"The Annex XV dossier should address all substances listed in the Council of Europe resolution ResAP(2008)1 and potentially any 00 1(a) and 1(b) or as skin sensitizer. Due to the complexity and high number of substances concerned, we would like to discuss with ECHA the best way to prepare the Annex XV dossier, potentially with the involvement of some member states (e.g. by grouping substances on the basis of their hazard classes (skin sensitizers, CMRs), and the possibility to use Article 68(2) for CMRs in order to reduce the workload."

The complexity of the subject required the support and collaboration of certain member states including Denmark, Germany, Italy, and Norway.

The conclusions and risk assessments concerning hundreds of substances used in tattoo and permanent makeup products, together with the socio-economic impacts of these restrictions, will determine European legislative actions that will supersede each national legislation.

Finally, in 2017 the European Directorate for the Quality of Medicines and Health care (EDQM) published certain updates regarding the potential risk of toxicity of tattoo and permanent makeup pigments, entitled: Safer tattooing: overview of current knowledge and challenges of toxicological assessment.

This publication is intended to provide a general, updated framework concerning the potential toxicological risks of the pigments used, together will an assessment of recent scientific information regarding tattoo processes and subsequent tissue response.

4.2. DECLARATION OF CONSENT

This is the document that includes the contractual obligations of the client and the professional and protects both through a detailed disclosure of the risks linked to the agreed-upon procedure.

CLIENT	PROFESSIONAL
• It is the client's responsibility to analyze every part of the document provided by the professional and to sign it only after ensuring that they have understood what they have read.	• It is the professional's responsibility to create a document that is as clear and meticulous as possible, and for the procedure to be performed to be explained in detail, including the preliminary phase, the procedure itself, and the post-procedural phase, so that the client is aware of the risks and benefits.
• A client that is a minor may only undergo procedure with the consent of both parents, ideally identified through a family certificate.	• The professional declines responsibility for any lack of information about the client and for the risk of infection following the procedure which may be caused by the client's negligence in arbitrarily deciding not to adhere to the hygienic advice provided by the professional.
• If the client refuses to undergo an allergy test, they should sign the declaration of consent in the designated section.	
• The declaration of consent serves to inform the client of the potential benefits of the chosen procedure, while also mentioning the risks linked to the procedure itself. The client is responsible for their own individual health conditions (e.g. cases of immunodepression, highly aggressive procedures, or debilitation, malnutrition, acute or chronic diseases or recent surgeries, pregnancy or breastfeeding, allergies general skin diseases, congenital or acquired coagulation problems, seizures, the possibility of donating blood or organs within 6/12 months following the procedure, alcohol or drug use, the use of vasodilators, anticoagulants, or anti-platelet drugs, the presence of pre-cancerous lesions).	• As part of the declaration of consent, the professional will advise the client to undergo an allergy test at an appropriate medical facility to avoid allergic reactions to the pigment that will be used.

IN SUMMARY

The declaration of consent attests to the presence of:
- a qualified, certified professional practitioner;
- a practice that is furnished with the most up-to-date technical equipment and all the certifications relating to the products used;
- a practice that guarantees health authorizations and whose hygienic activities conform to legal regulation.

AFTER CARE RECOMMENDATIONS FOR THE CLIENT

- 4/6 hours after the procedure, wash with warm water and neutral soap. Dry the area by patting delicately.
- Spread a thin layer of protective, soothing cream, until completely absorbed.
- To keep the skin moisturized, repeat this process 3-4 times a day for 10-15 days.
- During the scarring phase avoid wearing synthetic garments or covering the area with gauze.
- Abstain from sun exposure or the use of tanning beds without total protection; do not bathe in saltwater or chlorinated water. Avoid saunas, steam baths, physical activities, and cosmetic products for the next 20 days.
- In case of itching, apply more moisturizer and avoid rubbing the affected area.

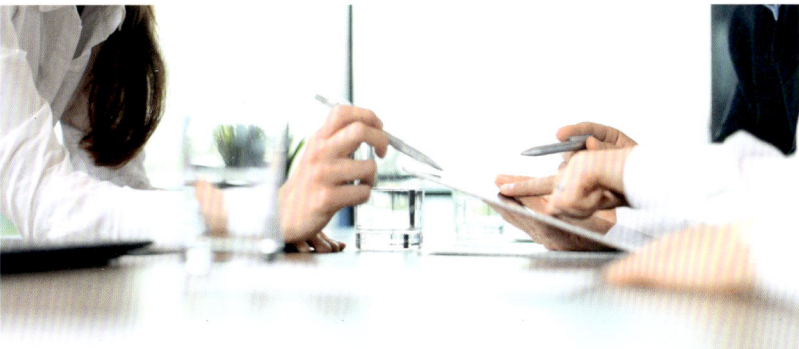

The declaration of consent in the following photos is valid in Germany. In other countries, adapt the declaration of consent to the applicable regulations. It is advisable to get legal consultation from your own insurance provider or attorney.

The declaration of consent must be accompanied by the customer record, a document which compiles all of the presences, technologies, equipment, and pigments used on each client and an agreement regarding data storage terms and protection.

DECLARATION OF CONSENT

DECLARATION OF CONSENT
FOR THE PERFORMANCE OF COSMETIC MICROPIGMENTATION

CLIENT

Last Name, First Name _____

Street, City, Post Code _____

Email _____

Telephone number _____

Dear Client,

You have chosen to undergo micropigmentation. Please read and follow these instructions. I use a standardized process to ensure the highest quality assurance and detailed and comprehensive consultation.

PREPARATIONS

Do not consume alcohol within a minimum of 12 hours before the pigmentation process. Please consult with your doctor before taking any pain medication. Please avoid extreme sun exposure for about one week before the treatment.

MICROPIGMENTATION WITH AMIEA COLORS

amiea colors are made of cosmetic- or pharmaceutical materials. They do not contain any human or animal ingredients, and do not come into contact with animal products during storage or transport. Furthermore, they are not tested on animals. amiea colors are dermatologically- and allergy tested. However, the risk of reaction to pigments previously used for pigmentation treatments cannot be excluded. This can lead to color change or an allergic reaction.

TIPS

The use of thin needle cartridges to introduce pigment may lead to irritation, light redness, and light swelling immediately after the micropigmentation process. Micropigmentation lasts for several years depending on skin type and color, but complete fading or a minimum duration cannot be guaranteed. It is possible for the color to become permanent and/or for removal to cause scars.

At the start of treatment, the client should check her pigmentation practitioner's certifications. The practitioner commits to following hygienic standards. Hygienic film should therefore be used to cover all work materials. The needle cartridges must be removed from their sterile packaging in view of the client. The expiration dates of the needle cartridges and colors must be heeded and documented. Colors from different manufacturers should never be mixed. Mixing colors must be done under hygienic conditions. The preliminary drawing must be done with the selected colors. The client has the right to check the process in the mirror at any time, and potentially to interrupt the process.

CONTRAINDICATIONS

Do not proceed with micropigmentation while the following contraindications are present: feverish infections, infectious diseases, antibiotics, pregnancy, lactation, menstruation, acute herpes, conjunctivitis, local infections, plastic surgery, chemotherapy or radiotherapy, unstable scars, skin diseases in the application zone, bacteria, viral, or fungal infections.

In the case of allergic reactions to the pigments, skin disorders (keloids, freckles, birthmarks, warts, melanomas, impetigo, hives), skin cancer, acute cardiovascular problems, taking of Macumar or other blood thinners, antidepressants, diabetes, HIV, and hepatitis, the client should not undergo micropigmentation.

NEW PIGMENTATION	REFRESHER APPLICATION
○ Upper eyeliner	○ Upper eyeliner
○ Lower eyeliner	○ Lower eyeliner
○ Thickening upper lash line	○ Thickening upper lash line
○ Thickening lower lash line	○ Thickening lower lash line
○ Eyebrow	○ Shape/color correction
	○ Tattoo

CONSENT

I confirm that I have read and understood the above information. All of my questions were answered comprehensively and in a manner which I could understand. I had enough time and opportunity to think over my decision. A local anesthetic which I have supplied may be applied.

I confirm that I have been fully informed of any potential contraindications, the treatment process, the potential risks of pigmentation, the necessary follow-up treatment, the pros and cons, as well as the options for removing micropigmentation and its associated risks. I explicitly agreed to the shape and color of the micropigmentation on the basis of a preliminary drawing.

I am of legal age and legally competent. The treatment proceeds at my own risk. The information is subject to data protection regulations and will be handled with strict confidentiality. I consent to the internal use and storage of my data. We assume no liability for the completeness of this declaration of consent.

Place, date, signature _____

Pigmentation practitioner
name & signature _____

COSTS

The treatment costs: _____

This amount includes a follow-up treatment within _____ weeks. If the client does not make an appointment for follow-up treatment, the appointment is void and the client bears the costs of the follow-up treatment. Refresher applications and changes within the next 24 months will be charged at 50% of the original price. Color and shape corrections costs depend on complexity.

FOLLOW-UP APPOINTMENT

The follow-up appointment is scheduled for _____ If you do not keep this follow-up appointment, we assume no liability and the guarantee becomes null and void.

Place of jurisdiction _____

Place, date, signature _____

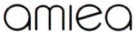

5

FROM MAKEUP
TO PERMANENT MAKEUP

5.1. THE HISTORY OF MAKEUP

How far back can we trace the history of makeup? Who first started using it? How are colors chosen? Did men wear makeup too? Who do you think sets trends? Who suggests a style for a given year? The creators of beauty are influenced by historical events, of course, not individuals. History, archeology, and the social sciences have uncovered the origins of makeup through the study of the traditions and daily habits of every population on earth which did not renounce the worship and cultivation of beauty. At the same time, developments in science (in terms of technology and materials) and, above all, in medicine, provide the basis for certain studies and for a deeper view of the history of makeup as an anthropologically and sociologically important component of human behavior, especially for women.

ANCIENT EGYPT AND MESOPOTAMIA

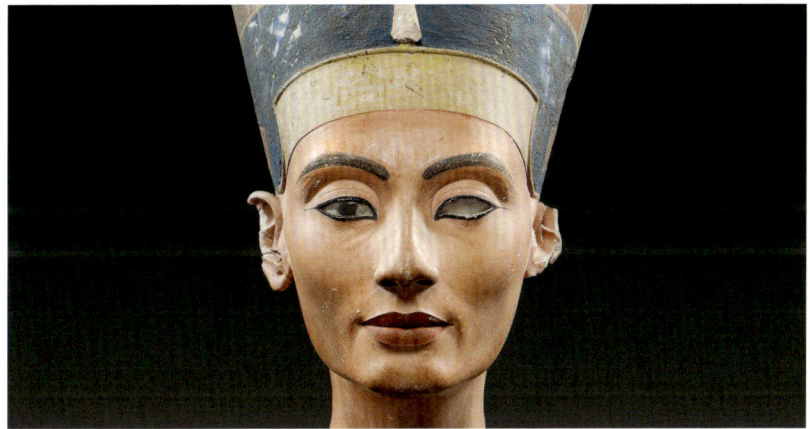

As early as 4,000 B.C, in ancient Egypt, compact green, red, white, and blue pigments, sticks of black kohl, and even creams and pomades were considered "divine substances". The Sumerian statuettes found in Ur show that the use of black eyeliner, similar to the "smoky eye" of today, was widespread throughout the entire Mesopotamian and Mediterranean region.

The Egyptians were the first to create a type of cosmetic using kohl, a dark powder created by grinding burned almonds, lead and copper, minerals, ashes, and ocher, and applying the resulting substances to the eyes using a little stick. This gave the eyes an almond-shape look that was considered very attractive.

It is said that queen Nefertiti used kohl not only to achieve an enchanting and seductive look, but also for its protective and therapeutic value: according to Egyptian doctors, the makeup also protected wearers from eye infections.

GREEK AND ROMAN TIMES

The most important thing for Greek women was to show their virtue and purity through the paleness of their faces, which they achieved using something extremely poisonous: basic lead carbonate (white lead). In the third century B.C., it was fashionable among Roman women to wear hairpieces made of long hair and layered curls, dyed with ocher powder for a reddish-blonde look. These hairstyles framed eyelashes and eyebrows made up with a substance made from burned ants, similar to kohl, and lips painted with red lead.

They whitened their faces and arms with white lead or chalk, and rimmed their eyes with dark soot. Donkey's milk was used to whiten and soften skin – Popea, the wife of Emperor Nero, famously bathed in it – then the woman's cosmetae (slaves skilled in aesthetics) would cover their mistress with cerussite, a cream made from lead oxide, to keep the skin fresh. Meanwhile, Greek women used a sacred plant named Anchusatinctoria (henna) or phukos (a type of seaweed) for their red color.

THE MIDDLE AGES AND THE RENAISSANCE

It may seem surprising, but even during the dark, hyper-religious era of the Middle Ages, both men and women continued to wear makeup, although they relegated the practice exclusively to special occasions. It's no coincidence that the first Treatise on Historical Cosmetics ("De Ornatu Mulierum", or "On Women's Cosmetics") was written around the 11th century, by Trotula de Ruggiero, of Salerno. Against the will of the Church, which preached extreme humility and condemned any aesthetic embellishment associated with prostitution, people continued to whiten their complexions during Feudal times using dangerous concoctions made of lead, vinegar, honey, and arsenic. Only with the Renaissance, and the exaltation of canonical beauty by Botticelli, Michelangelo, and Rafael, did aesthetics regain their value. The use of lapis lazuli to draw blue veins, red blush applied to the cheeks and red lead for lips, and soot to contour eyes and eyebrows were all intended to highlight the extreme whiteness of the face, hands, and teeth. Fashion called for a voluptuous, sensuous, and prosperous femininity, which was perfumed with oils and essences from the Orient and the West Indies, recently discovered by Christopher Columbus in 1492. Water, however, was feared because of the dangers of cholera epidemics.

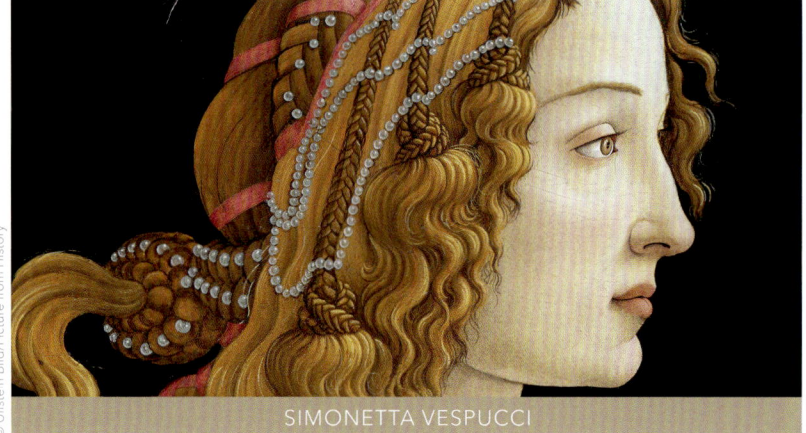
SIMONETTA VESPUCCI

18TH AND 19TH CENTURIES

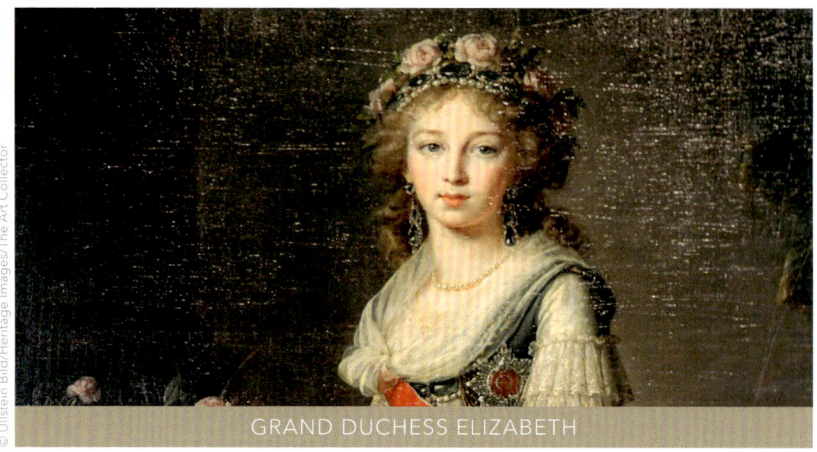
GRAND DUCHESS ELIZABETH

Although in the 18th century, the ladies of French nobility were dedicated to the pursuit of an "absolutely white" complexion, by the Victorian period in England, the use of face makeup began to be associated with the dishonorable practices of prostitutes and actresses, based on the idea that a ruddy face, or worse, a tan, were markers of the lowest social classes, meaning the "workers". The dangerous mix of lead oxide and arsenic covering the faces of young women gave them an ethereal, luminous complexion, but soon caused their skin to shrivel up, weaken, and become wrinkled, especially if they did not protect themselves from the sun with veils and parasols. Soon, this was replaced by the widespread use of face powder or finely ground rice, applied to the face and neckline. These new powders were mixed with natural ingredients like oats, honey, egg yolks, and rose petals, and finished off with the ever-more sophisticated aromas of perfumes from French masters. In 1830, Queen Victoria's coronation in England inaugurated a period of austerity and extreme morality, in which the aesthetic use of makeup was sacrificed in favor of rigorous styles featuring muted, sober colors on the face and a preference for black clothing. Only in the second half of the 19th century, thanks to developments in science and medicine, did the chemical industry begin mass-producing eyeshadows made from lead and stibnite powders, and lipsticks made from mercury sulphides. All of these ingredients were banned soon after, when they were revealed to be highly toxic; white lead was banned in 1913, for example.

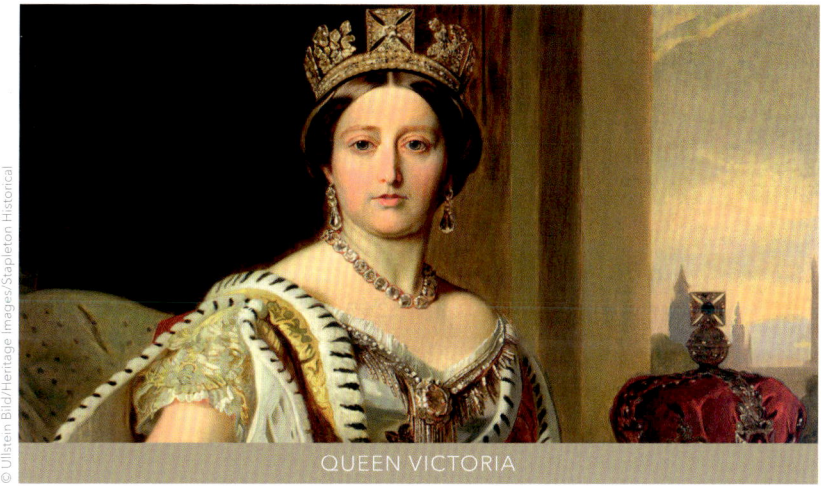

QUEEN VICTORIA

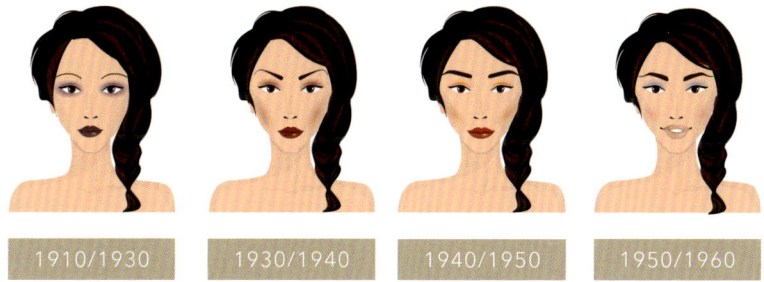

1910/1930 1930/1940 1940/1950 1950/1960

THE TWENTIETH CENTURY AND THE MAKEUP INDUSTRY

The twentieth century established makeup as a feminine ritual for everyday beauty. In 1930, women from every social class emulated Greta Garbo and Marlene Dietrich, both considered unparalleled

icons of contemporary female beauty. Helena Rubinstein (1903), Coty (1904), Harriet Hubbard (1907), Max Factor (1909), L'Oréal by Eugène Shueller (1909), and Elizabeth Arden (1910) were pioneers of international makeup. Everything changed in 1910: with the increased distribution of cosmetic products, especially by three companies in the USA - Elizabeth Arden, Helena Rubinstein, and Max Factor - and the appearance of emerging groups like Revlon and Estée Lauder, the sector was revitalized, emphasizing color over pallor.

Enchanting, seductive eyes were emphasized by thin, sloping brows, lips became heart-shaped,and the natural contours of the face were re-shaped, and covered in foundation which accentuated shapes and hid blemishes (Max Factor's 1914 pancake foundation, available in 12 shades, remained popular for decades). But it was in the 1920s that Coco Chanel revolutionized the idea of color, setting the trend of tanned skin, even if artificial, and overthrowing the ideal of the luminously "white" and ethereal lady. In the early 1930s, the Seventh Art, meaning cinema, heralded the definitive success of creative makeup, which gave rise to professional makeup artists who exported the myth of the Hollywood divas, which every woman emulated and which every man dreamed of.

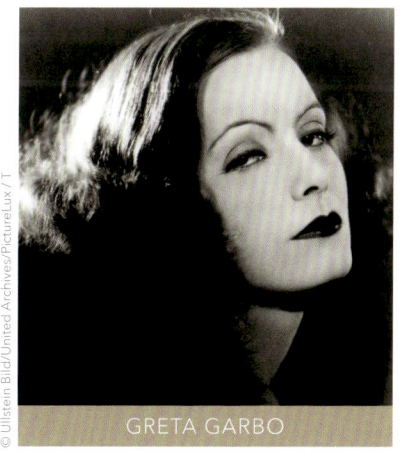

GRETA GARBO

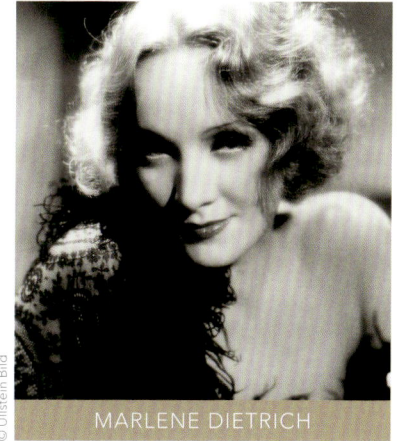

MARLENE DIETRICH

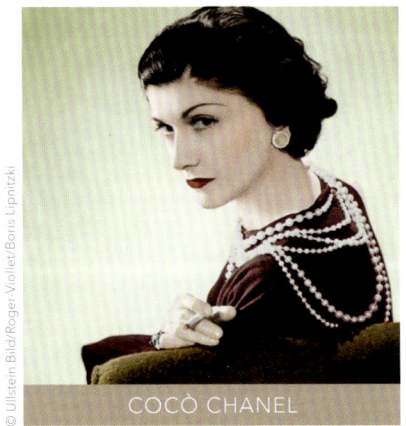

COCÒ CHANEL

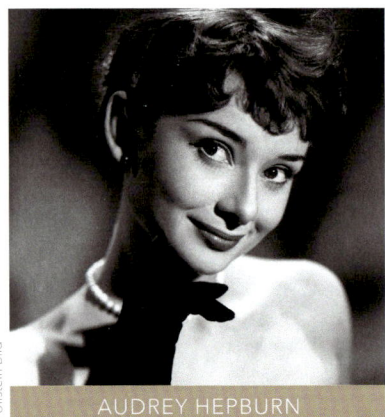

AUDREY HEPBURN

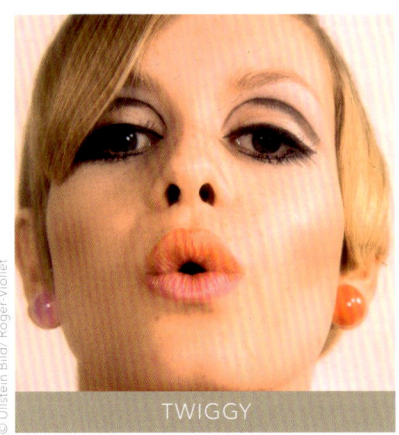

TWIGGY

from sales of the first makeup removers, cleansing milks, the first lotions for face and body, and early sun lotions for beach vacations, which were made from glycerin, lanolin, sunflower oil, and beeswax. Natural vegetable products were soon replaced by cheaper substances from the petrochemical industry (mineral oil, Vaseline, paraffin).

THE 50s AND THE ECONOMIC BOOM OF THE 60s

After the two world wars, there was a period of reconstruction and a longing for renewal that erupted in a true explosion of color. The flawless complexion responded to the demand for women in the 1940s and 1950s to be perfect wives and mothers (and in Italy, they had just won the right to vote). In fact, the beauty sector boomed during this period, including the door-to-door sales popularized by Avon. These were also the years in which movies celebrated the fresh-faced beauty of Audrey Hepburn, whose carefully blended shades of makeup framed a signature cat-eye look that led to the huge popularity of winged liner. A few years later, Twiggy, the model, turned the daring and revolutionary trend of miniskirt into the iconic look of the 1960s.

WOMEN'S EMANCIPATION IN THE 70s

The Seventies can be described in two words: exasperation and excess. Hair teased with brushes and hairspray, very colorful eyes, false lashes, iridescent lips, and pastel tones were mandatory for any woman who wanted to affirm her civil rights.

These rights were increasingly important in politics, and companies responded with sale strategies that targeted women, profiting

THE EXAGGERATED CONSUMERISM OF THE 80s AND 90s

But beauty isn't about economy, and makeup sales spiked in the Eighties, as trends called for more and more emphasis on dark eyes and magnetic gazes, accentuated with layers of eyeliner and eyeshadow in dazzling shades of blue, green, and purple. Women reached for bold lip colors, like lacquer red or Valentino red. The disco years called for mica, a metallic mineral powder, which was applied to the eyelids and the body for a shimmering look.

By the Nineties, increasingly specific products appeared, like creams and ointments to combat cellulite, which soon reached an apex and took over the market.

THE 2000s

In the 2000s, the arrival of the internet meant that trends shifted abruptly and followed one after another. In fact, it's impossible to define a single global trend during this period; instead, the focus was on a mix of styles and cultures, with icons and models who embodied very broad ranges of beauty. This decade saw everything from a very pronounced "American" style of makeup to a more subtle "Italian" style, and on to the endless combinations of eyeliner and red lipstick that define the "French" look.

This was also when the first "influencers" appeared: the makeup artists or models whose social media channels enriched and populated YouTube and Instagram, offering a variety of looks to viewers young and old. Products also reflected this new style: Korea invented BB creams, which were soon available in stores around the world, along with multicolored foundation sponges, highlighters, and primer. These are products that nobody had even heard of just a few years before, and which weren't easy to find. Permanent makeup also took off in this period, offering new equipment, pigments, and above all, techniques that differed greatly from what had until then been known as cosmetic tattooing, and often left people with strangely colored eyebrows.

THE 2010s AND COSMETIC SURGERY

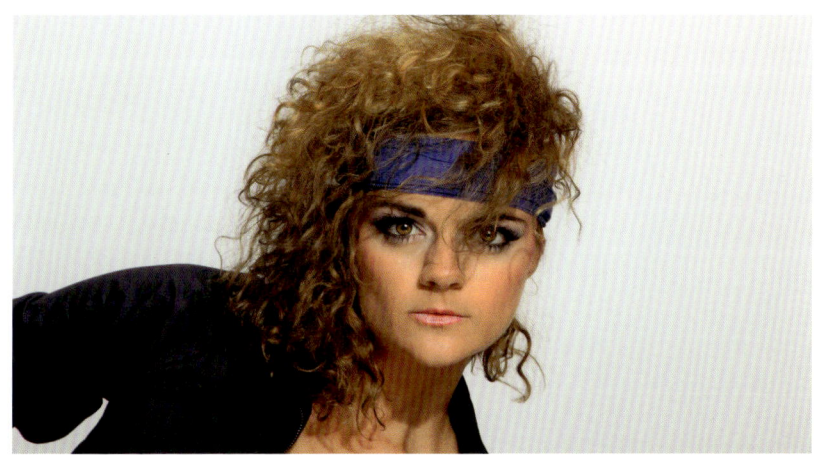

Specific products are giving way to permanent or semi-permanent solutions, in the form of cosmetic surgery: plumped lips, breast implants, face lifts, and rejuvenated features. This is the era of cosmetic surgery use and abuse, which actually began in the United States in 1963, with the first silicone implants. It wasn't until the 90s, however, that people turned to botox injections and filler to reduce wrinkles. The concept of "permanent makeup" continues to gain traction as the latest solution to a problem. This opens new and interesting possibilities in the history of everyday makeup for women, who find themselves busier and busier.

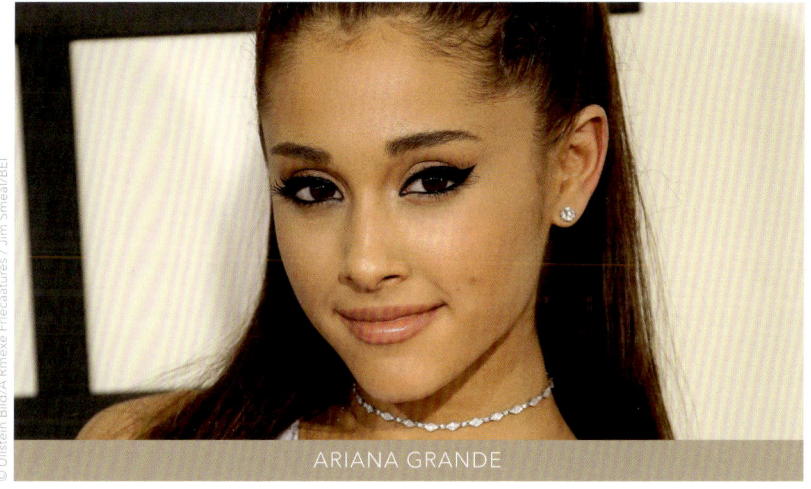

ARIANA GRANDE

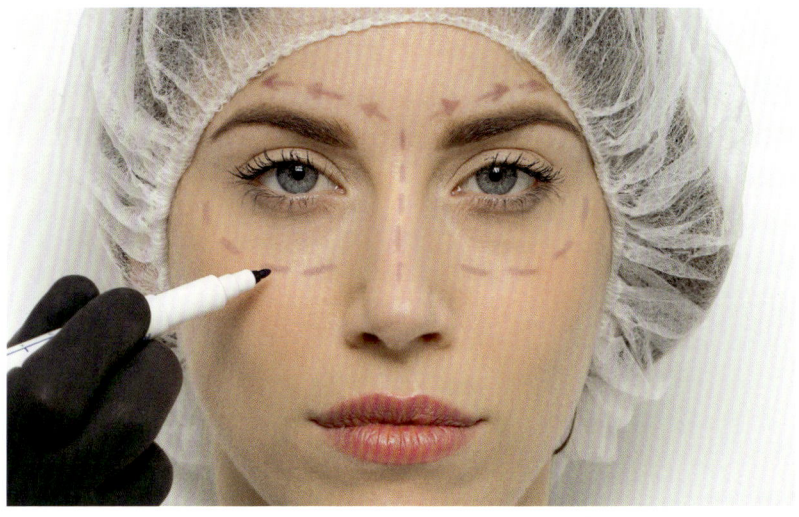

5.2. THE HISTORY OF PERMANENT MAKEUP

Let's take a deeper look into this topic, and identify the point at which makeup becomes "definitive" or "permanent", in order to understand future possibilities.

In 1987, after years of medical experience, the German doctor Ulrich K. Kesserling applied permanent camouflaging to reduce the appearance of the scars resulting from surgery to reconstruct the shape of the areola and nipple following a mastectomy: thus, medical or breast tattooing was born.

In layman's terms, the practices used in decorative or ornamental tattoos were transferred for medical use, through the final application of permanent makeup (PMU) to complete a surgery.

Thus, cosmetic, embellishment techniques were put to the service of science thanks to qualified and skilled tattoo artists, who could apply color below the surface of the skin to correct blemishes in the face or body and to improve appearance and resolve psychological concerns relating to personal appearance (aesthetic discomfort).

Over time, the various specializations took shape: semi-permanent makeup and visagism-based tattoos (eyes and eyebrows), scalp pigmentation (to resolve hair and scalp problems, removing discomfort and collateral effects of pharmaceutical procedures, keratin fibers, hairpieces, etc.), and aesthetic micropigmentation (for scars or vitiligo or other skin spots). By the end of the 1990s, tattooed makeup had undergone a decisive change, moving away from the idea of the tattoo gun and instead asserting itself as a practice characterized by delicate, precise, and deep application. As technological tools continue to advance and consumers favor more and more a natural look, the 2000s onwards sees the rise of the permanent makeup professional, who is very specialized and whose practice differs greatly from tattoo artists who perform creative, colorful lines using artistic and creative drawings. Instead, the permanent makeup professional takes a scientific approach, adopting even paramedical criteria with techniques and methodologies developed from cosmetic surgery, and using pigments which can be applied deeply, but always "externally". On the face, for example, the professional carefully draws and modifies the features of the eyes, lips, and eyebrows, for a natural effect. The professional may also shade in the scalp to recreate a shaved look, or apply pigment to the areola to hide any unpleasant blemishes. Now, just a decade later, the fields of application seem wide open: dermopigmentation has recently been paired with surgery, in synergy or applied in parallel, to reconstruct or re-create, according to a more modern perspective and philosophy on life, the "color of well-being" or the "magic of beauty", meaning what nature has created, thus re-establishing aesthetic balance and providing an immediate, positive psychological effect for the clients.

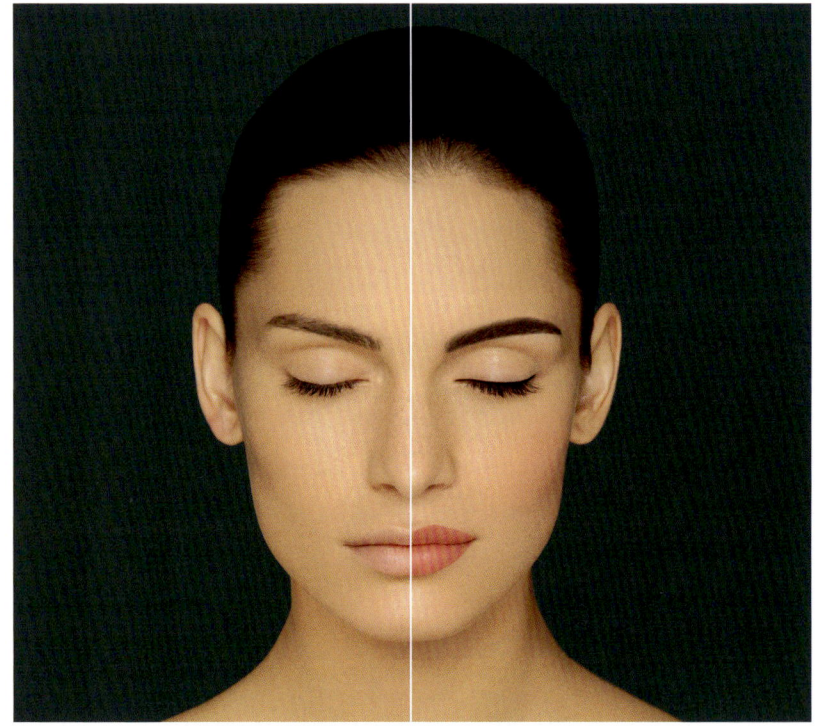

6

BASIC UNDERSTANDING OF VISAGISM

Over the years, each dermopigmentation professional develops their own operating protocol, a sort of "user's guide" to refer to, which is based on their experiences and what they have learned during training.

A qualified technician works according to three fundamental guidelines:
- optical illusion
- custom
- basis for comparison

6.1. OPTICAL ILLUSION

An optical illusion tricks the eye into seeing something that's not there: so that what is not real seems real, or more simply, so that things seem different from what they are.

Dermopigmentation proceeds from the same principle: if a person has no eyebrows, it is the job of the professional to create the optical illusion in which eyebrows appear where there are none.

Dermopigmentation can have radical effects on the non-verbal expressions of the gaze or the lips, tricking the eye that beholds them. "The trick is there, you just can't see it," is a catchphrase among skilled magicians: the professional must turn magic into reality, without performing work that is invasive.

A simple game can explain the concept of optical illusion even more aptly: at first glance, figure B seems longer than figure A. A closer look, however, reveals that they are actually exactly the same: but while the first evokes a sense of closure, the second on benefits from a sense of openness, which appears to modify its dimensions.

If the intention is to re-size the gaze, the tail of the eyebrow should appear more closed; if the goal is to visually enlarge the forehead,

make it more open. Moving the vertex of the eyebrow outwards therefore makes the forehead seem larger; while moving it slightly inwards has the opposite effect and makes the forehead seem more narrow.

Makeup is about optical illusion; through the use of color and shading, we can create shapes, magnify details, make lips more seductive, and enhance the gaze.

This is how an image can distort the observer's perspective and disorient them: the same image allows the viewer to see a friendly little pig, but turning it upside down reveals an owl with outstretched wings.

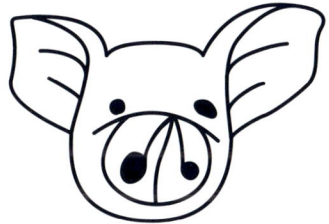 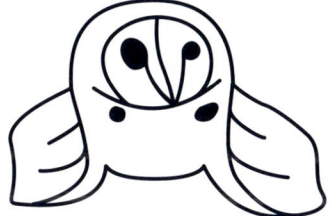

6.2. CUSTOM

From a legal standpoint, a custom refers to a repeated behavior within a collective. Using this basic definition, we can state that a custom is an established way of operating and proceeding. A custom means reinforcing a habit, insisting on a practice, preserving a tradition.

Permanent makeup, especially permanent makeup for the eyebrows, cannot avoid taking into consideration the habits, fashions, and traditions of the country where it is performed. Seeing a man walking around wearing pants is absolutely no cause for confusion in most Western countries. But if the same man wore a kilt in an Italian city, he certainly would not go unobserved. If we were to decontextualize this man and set him in Scotland instead, where the kilt is part of local, traditional clothing, his walk would no longer cause any curious glances.

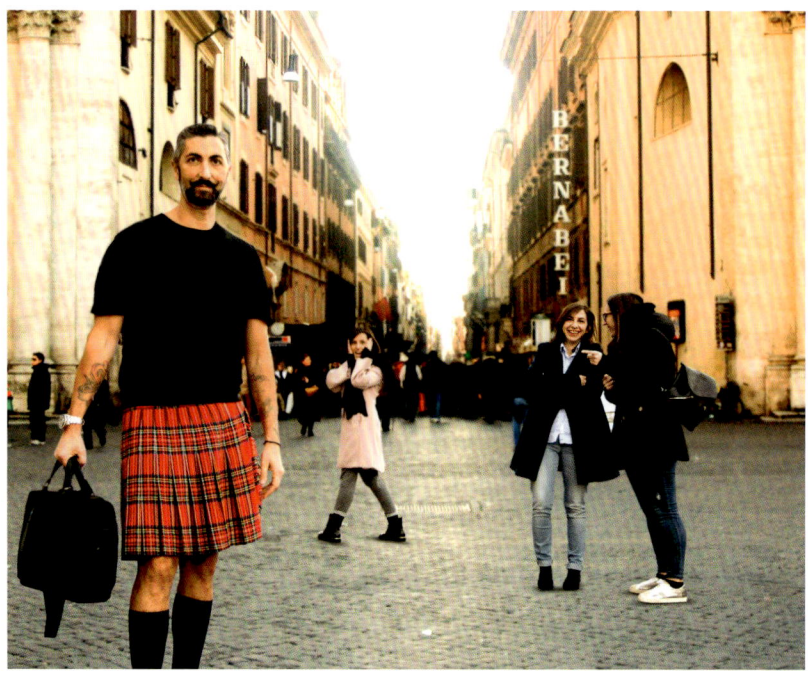

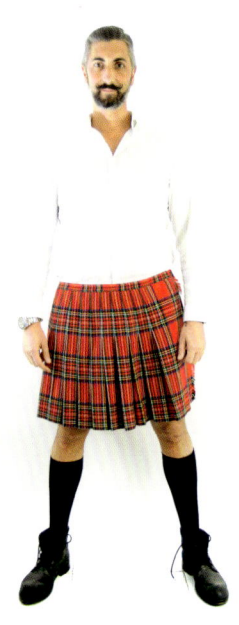

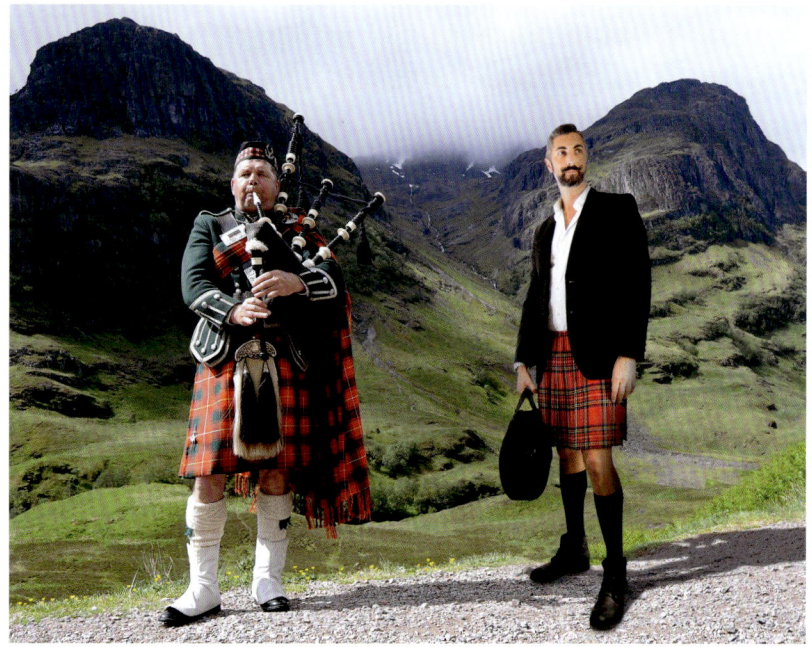

The same considerations apply to permanent makeup. In Italy, eyebrows often share the structural characteristics of the one shown in Fig. A.

Drawing a completely horizontal eyebrow (Fig. B). or which differs greatly from visagistic norms in Western countries would quickly reveal the illusion, and produce a certain confusion in whoever saw it. Custom can undo an optical illusion, and proceeding out of context can invalidate its effects.

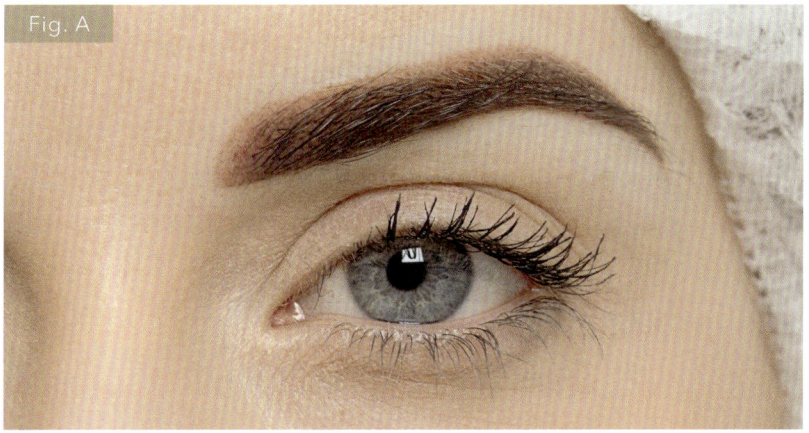

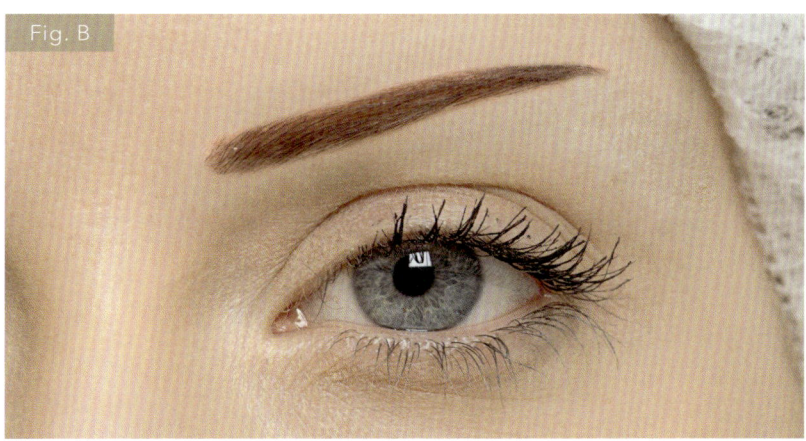

"The skin is a vehicle for emotions.
The epidermis reveals the essence of emotions to the world.
Years of research and experimentation have taught me to
understand and love skin, and to respect its character.
My knowledge lies in the use of pigment,
my faithful companion, which allows me to
restore the skin's natural beauty, enhance
its details, and hide imperfections.
So that emotions can once again flow freely."

TONI BELFATTO

6.3. STANDARDS OF COMPARISON

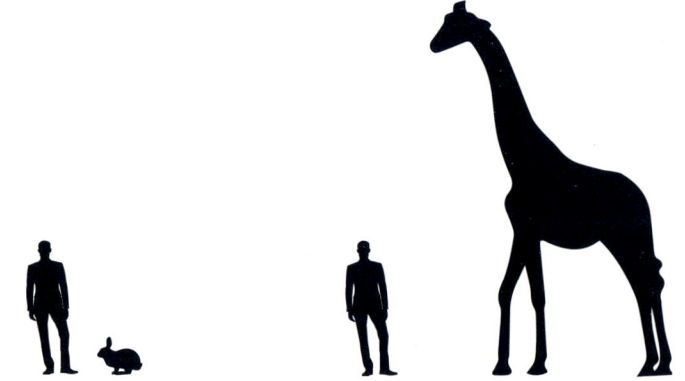

Expressing a preference, in any context, presupposes that there is a range of alternatives from which to choose. You can't state that you prefer meat to fish without having tasted both, or that you find one winter to be particularly harsh if you can't compare it to the previous one.

A comparison can only happen if there are standards to be placed side by side.

If we entered a white cube without walls or furniture, we could not be considered tall or short, thin or fat by an external observer, since there would be no standard of comparison to place us in reference to. If another person were to enter the white cube, the differences between us would then become salient.

A man certainly seems large next to a rabbit, but would immediately seem tiny if the rabbit were replaced by a giraffe.

This is the most important principle in permanent makeup. Making any visagism-based assessment of a client means understanding their appearance; only after understanding it and making the necessary comparisons, can we proceed.

If a person wants to make their eyes seems larger, the eyebrow above it needs to be made smaller, so that the eye, when compared to the eyebrow, appears bigger.

6.4. EYEBROWS

6.4.1 STATISTICS

This graphic shows the number of people around the world who undergo permanent makeup to correct imperfections, enhance their gaze, define their lip shape, correct discolorations, or hide scars. The most requested procedure in permanent makeup concerns the eyebrows, with nearly 70% of users.

The arch of the eyebrow is the part of the face that has the most impact on non-verbal expression: any work on the eyebrows therefore implies a desire to improve how we communicate with others. 20% of clients choose permanent makeup for the lips, and the remaining 10% have it applied to their eyes.

EYEBROWS 70%	LIPS 20%	EYES 10%

A deeper look at the reasons for which 70% of clients choose procedures on the eyebrows reveal: 50% of these clients choose permanent makeup for the eyebrows to increase the density of their brows and change their shape. Another 30% aim to correct prior work and the remaining 20% seek to correct alopecia, scars, or to counteract the thinning process.

INCREASE IN DENSITY AND CHANGE IN SHAPE 50%	CORRECTING PRIOR WORK 30%	ALOPECIA, SCARS, VARIOUS THINNING 20%

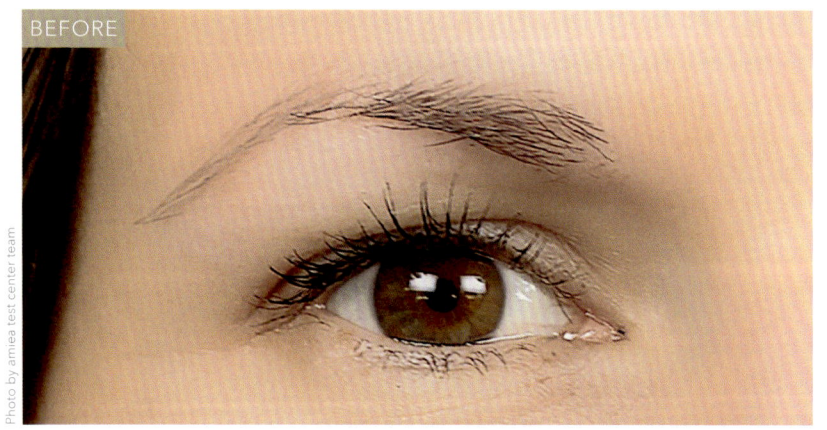

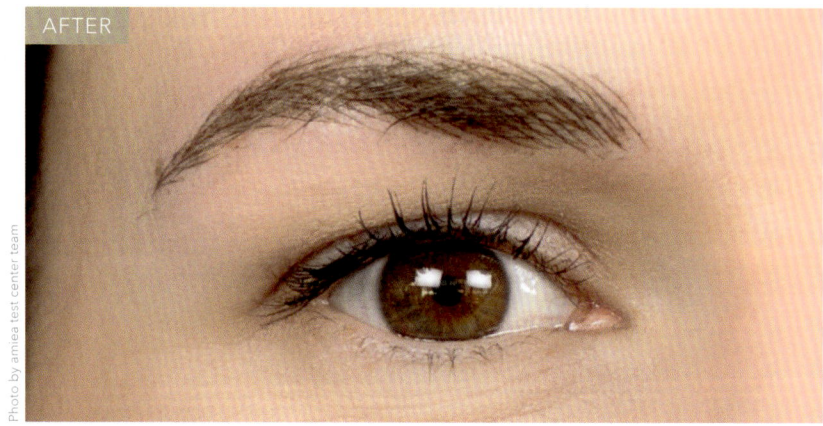

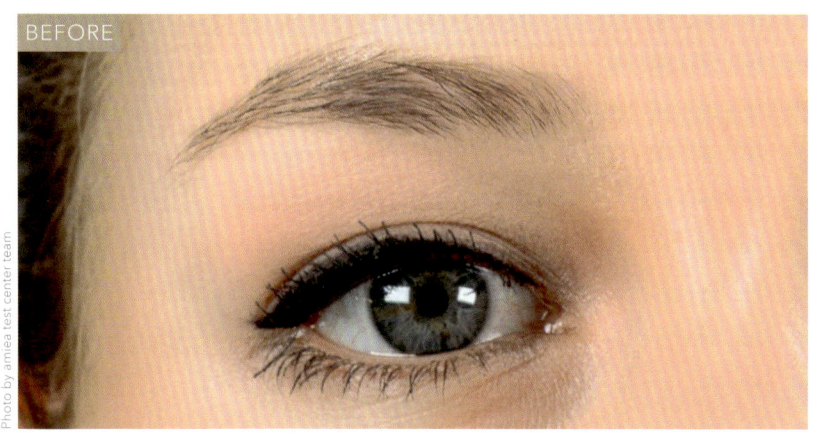

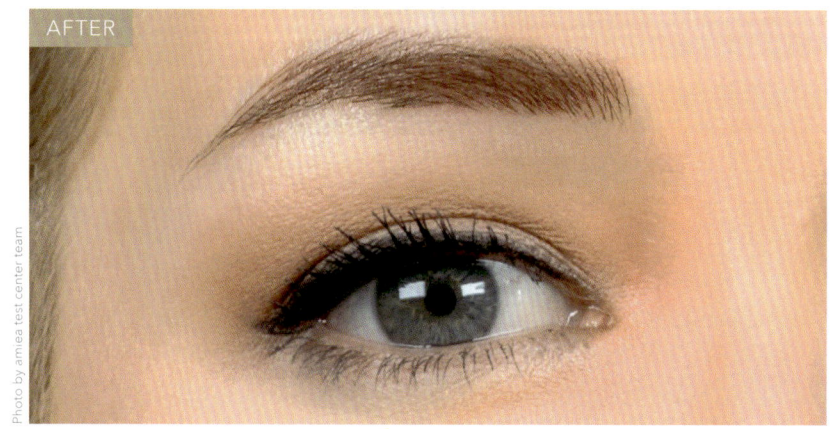

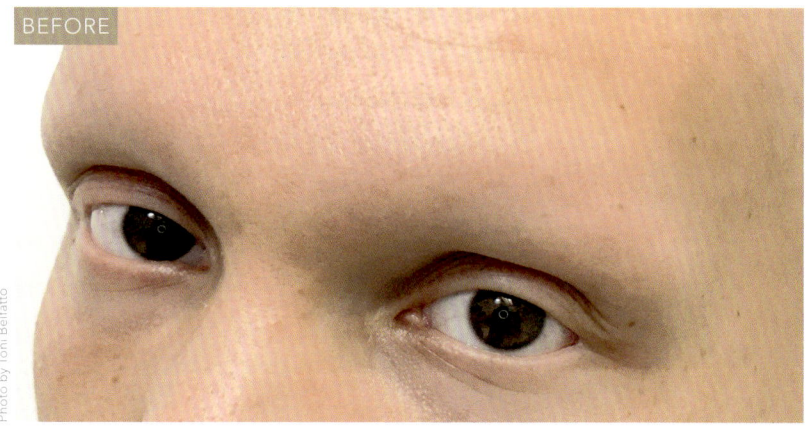

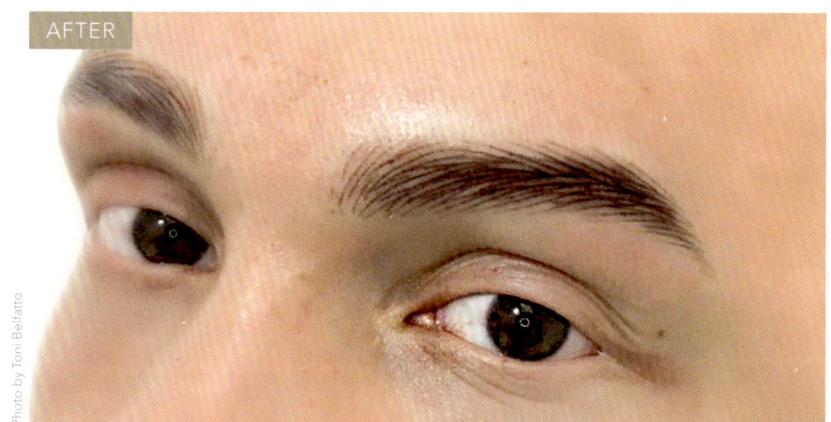

6.4.2. EYEBROWS: ANATOMY AND TERMINOLOGY

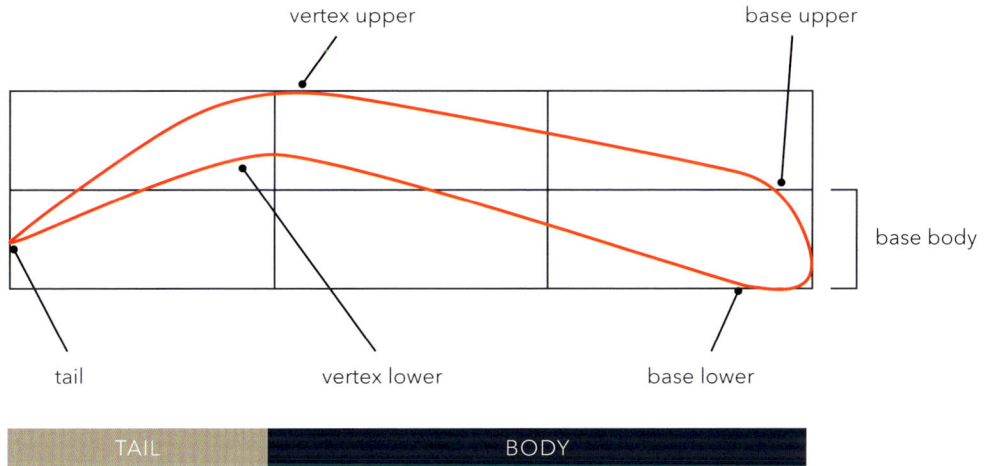

The arch of the brow is made up of two areas: the body and the tail. The body constitutes two thirds of the entire eyebrow; the remaining third belongs to the tail. The first part of the eyebrow is called the base of the body, and it can be divided into the lower base and the upper base. The body is thicker at the base, then gradually narrows out towards the tail.

Between the body and the tail, there is the vertex (both lower and upper), the highest part of the entire eyebrow when looking at it horizontally. The vertex can be shaped differently, depending on whether the goal is to soften the gaze or make it more aggressive, make it more common or more distinctive. The vertex will therefore be softer if the intent is to soften the gaze, more angled if the intention is to communicate a sense of rigor, or more straight if no particular expression is to be conveyed. Meanwhile, the tail should never be lower than the body: this is to avoid the risk of an empty, inexpressive look.

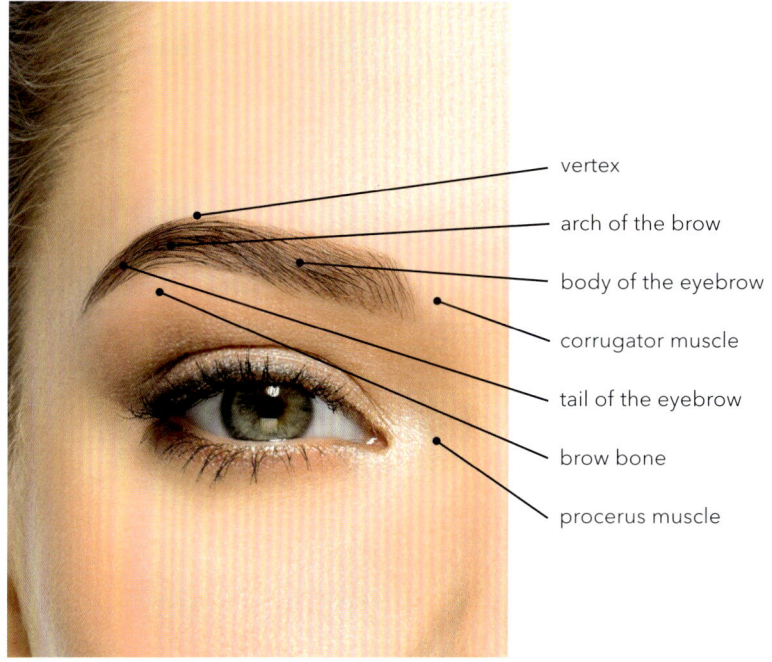

The brow bone, which is below the vertex and the tail, can be enhanced with highlighter to make the brow even more attractive. Shading should be concentrated towards the lower part of the body and the tail, while the upper part should be lighter, since light normally illuminates the upper area, making a darker shade there stand out too harshly. The shading should be lighter in certain areas to correspond with the illuminated part of the natural eyebrow, in which hairs are thinner and lighter in the upper contour.

"The skin is the part of you that interacts with the world first, comes into contact with others first; it is the "clothing" of your spirit and your body's natural defense."

TONI BELFATTO

6.4.3. IDEAL POSITION OF THE EYEBROW

THE X-POINT RULE

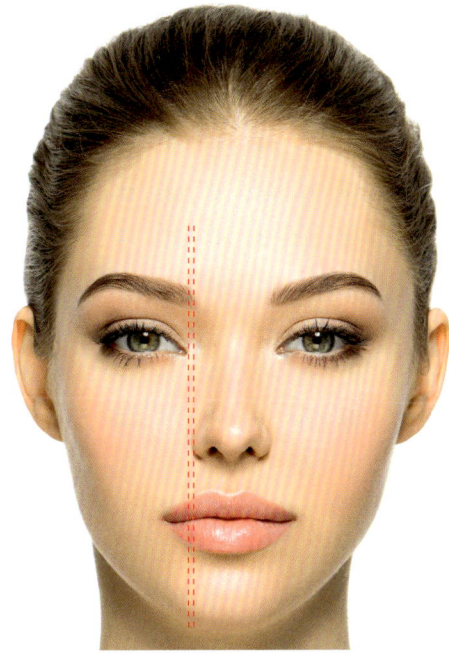

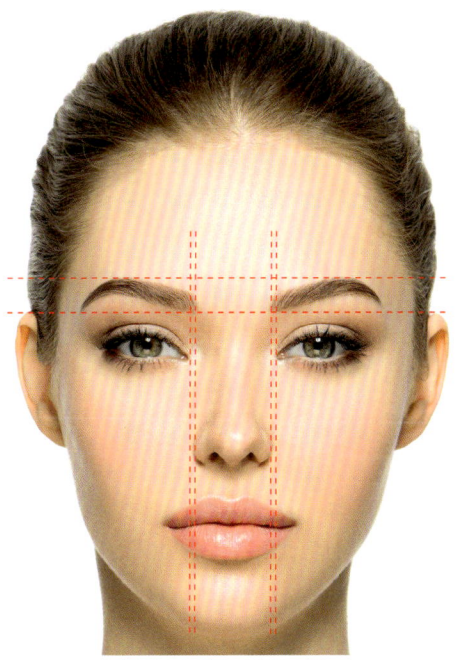

The X-point is a reference point which corresponds to an imaginary line that starts from a fixed element (the nose or the eye). Two of these reference points, placed in parallel to each other, create a space called a range, within which the base of the eyebrow is inserted. The base can be positioned closer to the nose or the eye, or in the center. The starting point of the eyebrow can be positioned based on the client's preference, as long as the aesthetics of the face is always preserved since any choice will lead to inevitable changes in the face's non-verbal expression: an X-point that is closer to the nose will create a harder, more decisive look, while an X-point place closer to the eye instead creates a softer, more open look.

In figure 2, the lower horizontal line defines the height of the eyebrow's starting point. It can be found by tracing it along an imaginary line that runs parallel to the ceiling and the floor. Another line placed parallel this one, which is positioned higher, will serve to define the vertex. which is the highest point of both the eyebrows.

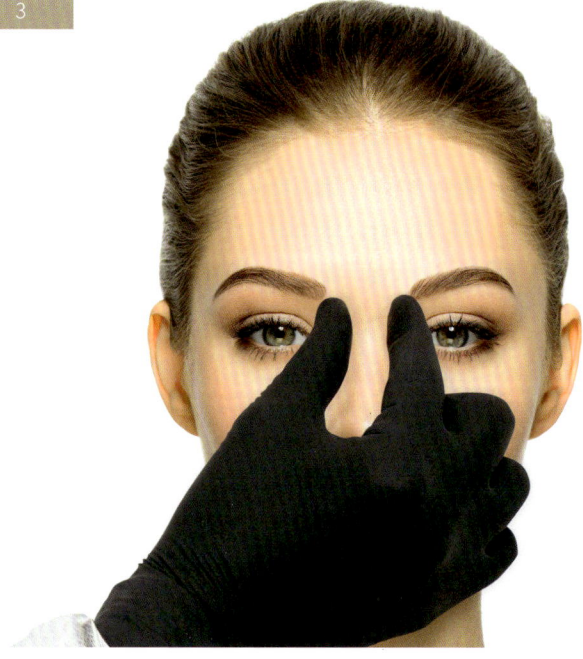

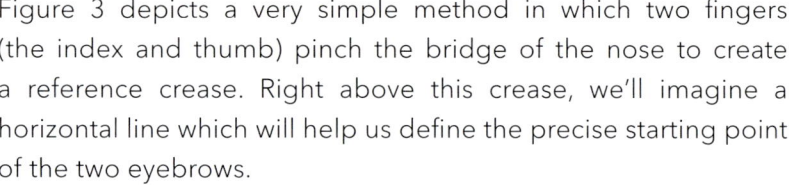

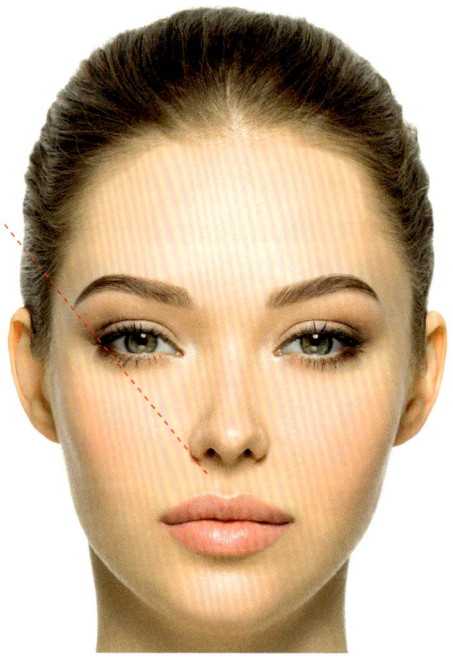

Figure 3 depicts a very simple method in which two fingers (the index and thumb) pinch the bridge of the nose to create a reference crease. Right above this crease, we'll imagine a horizontal line which will help us define the precise starting point of the two eyebrows.

Now we can identify the first reference lines which will show us the position of the vertex and the length of the tail, respectively. The first line starts from the wing of the nose and touches the outer corner of the eye, defining the furthest point where the eyebrow's tail can end.

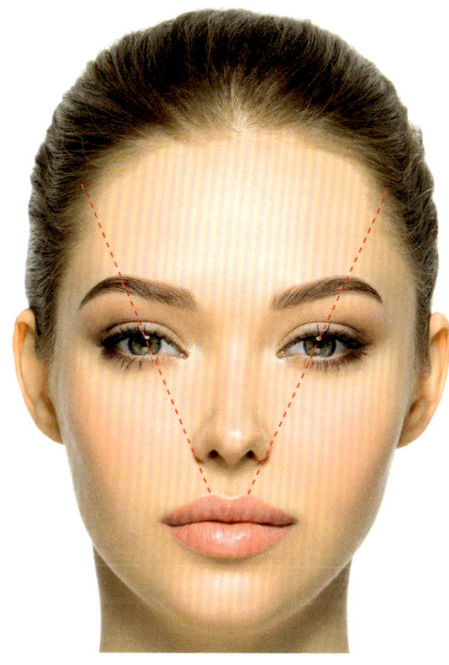

The line that starts from the side of the nose and runs through the pupil defines the position of the highest point of the eyebrow, the vertex. To correctly define the vertex, the client should be staring straight ahead.

6.4.4. GEOMETRY OF THE EYEBROW

When drawing both male and female eyebrows, it is important to minutely understand and study the base of the eyebrow body. Some basic geometry comes in hand here: mathematical geometry can help us avoid differing points of view, since as everyone knows, mathematics has no room for opinion!

According to Leonardo da Vinci, an inverted isosceles trapezoid should fit between the two eyebrows in order to give them a sense of openness. In a man, the trapeze may look more like a rectangle, but it must maintain a certain aperture in order not to look extremely closed off.

Given that the base is the element with the most impact on the eyes' non-verbal expression, determining the beginning of the base requires extreme care. Two extremely straight eyebrows give the impression that the person is angry or severe. Drawing a pointy trapezoid with the eyebrows angled inwards would inevitably reinforce the harsh expression. On the other hand, a totally rounded base for the eyebrows would give the expression a sense of vacancy.

Da Vinci's study helps give the gaze a natural expression that is aesthetically pleasing. Of course, the professional should align their understanding of visagism with the client's preferences, but they should never go against good sense or compromise their personal work philosophy.

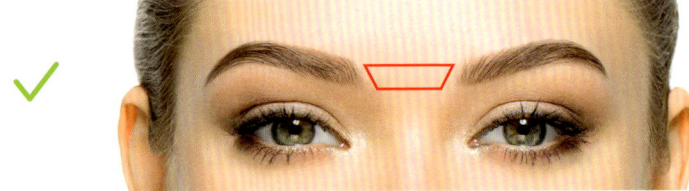
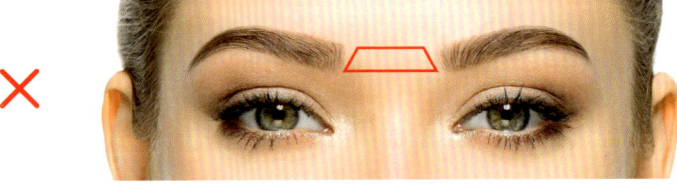
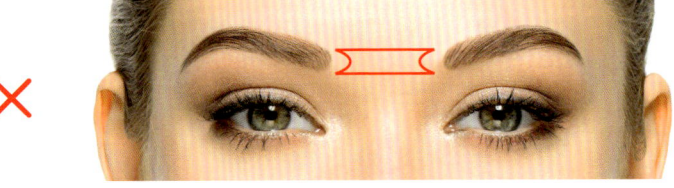
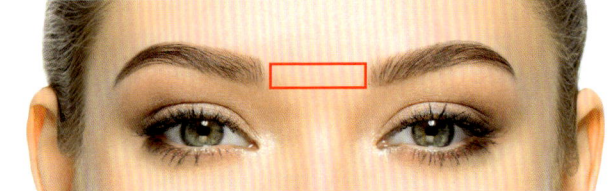

6.4.5. GUIDELINES: THE 5 REFERENCE POINTS

Before beginning any sketch, you should have a clear vision of what you want to achieve for the client, and never leave anything up to improvisation.

There are five specific reference points that will help you achieve the desired results as accurately and quickly as possible. The first two points serve to lay out the base of the body and its thickness, while the other two indicate the height of the brow and the width of the vertex, and the last point determines the length and thickness of the tail. Once these five points are determined and drawn in, all you need to do is connect them in order to see the chosen shape, and if necessary, make corrections and adjustments.

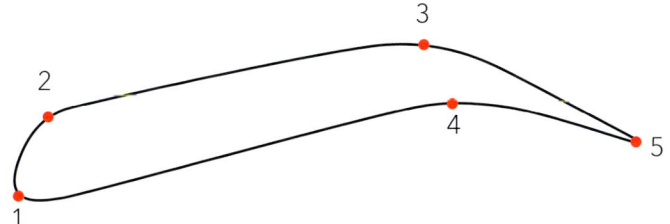

The base of the eyebrow begins with an initial, vertical guide. The wing of the nose does not always coincide with the inner corner of the eye: in this case, it's best to draw two guides: one vertical guide from the wing of the nose, and another vertical guide from the interior angle of the eye. This results in a technical range where you will position the base of the eyebrow depending on what kind of gaze is to be achieved. For a harder look, the eyebrow should begin at point A; for a softer look, the eyebrow should begin at point B. After having drawn in the first brow arch, according to a careful morphological study of the structure of the face, the professional's proposal can be tailored to fit the client's tastes: only once the client is completely satisfied should the professional begin sketching in the second eyebrow. We will use vertical, horizontal, and oblique guidelines to operate safely and meticulously.

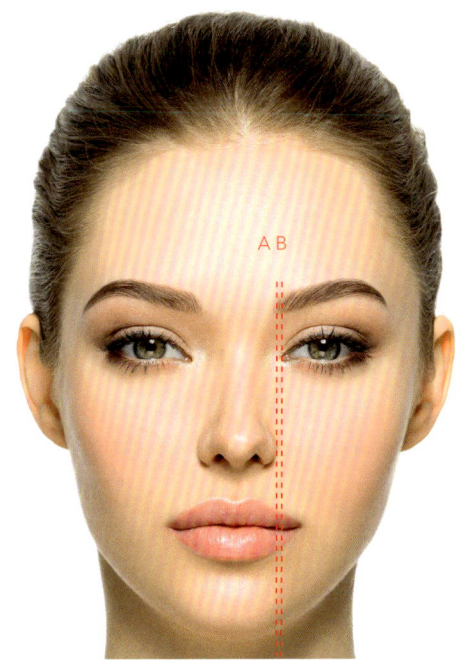

1 VERTICAL GUIDELINE

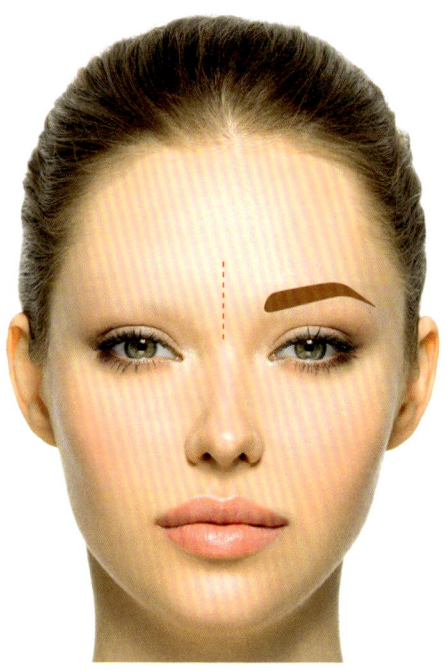

Using a sterile, single-use sketching tool and the pigment chosen for the procedure, trace a vertical line at the center of the face, using the forehead, eyes, and nose as reference points. This guideline will be useful for verifying that the distance between the two eyebrows is correct and centered according to the part of the face in question.

2 FIRST HORIZONTAL GUIDELINE

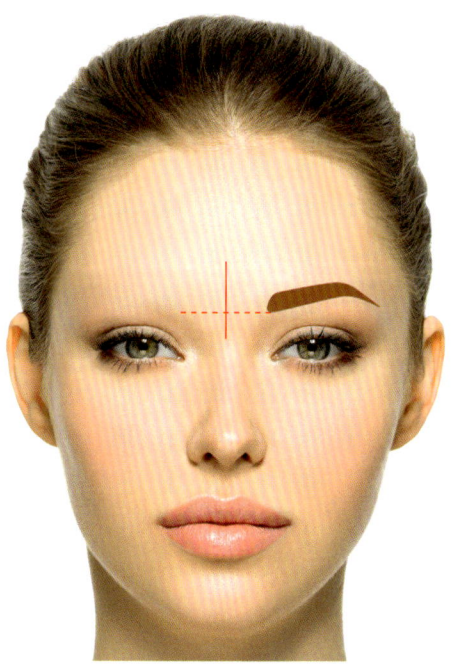

Next, we establish the first horizontal guideline, which is a line that runs parallel to the ground; it starts from the previously drawn eyebrow and leads to the point chosen for the beginning of the second eyebrow. The first horizontal guideline serves to ensure that the eyebrows are placed at the correct height compared to the eyes.

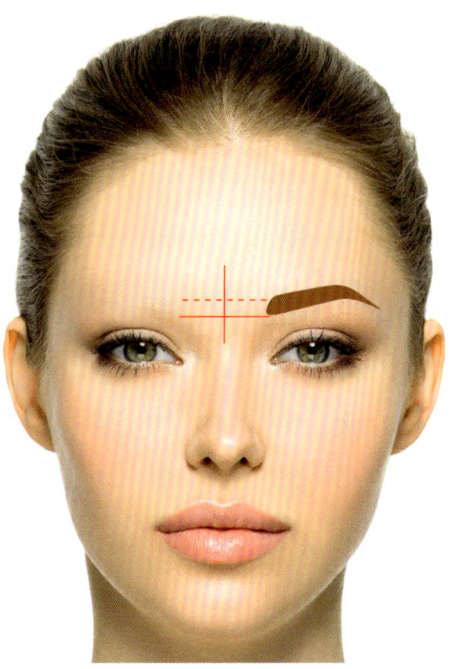

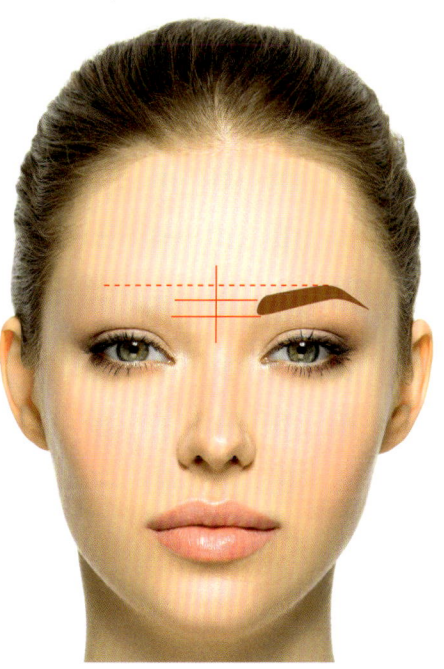

The second, upper horizontal reference point indicates the maximum height of the base of the body of the eyebrow and therefore the width of the base of the eyebrow.

The third horizontal guideline concerns the vertex: a line that runs parallel to the floor and connects the brow arches and determines the highest point of the entire eyebrow. The vertex is one of the most important parts in characterizing a face's non-verbal expression, which is why the original intentions should be considered very carefully.

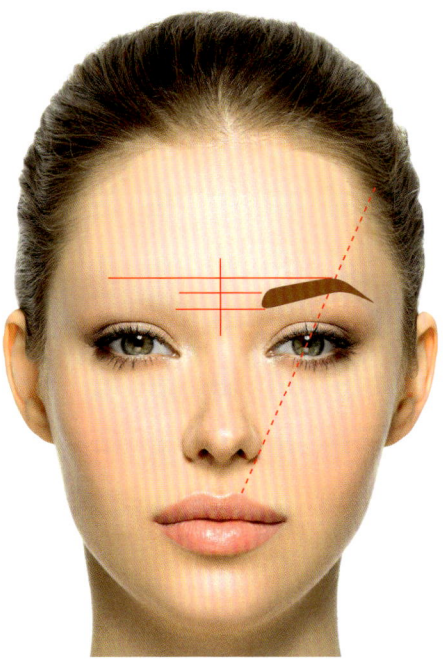

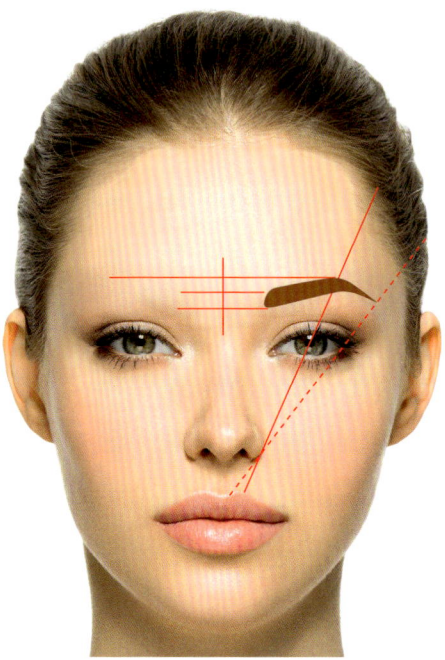

Now it is time to determine the innermost or outermost position of the vertex, not just its height. The best way to prevent the client from continuously moving their eyes is to firmly place a finger in front of their face, at a distance of about 40 cm, and ask them to stare at it to align the center of the pupil. Only then should you begin tracing an imaginary oblique line that starts from the wing of the nose, passes through the center of the pupil, and therefore indicates the correct placement of the vertex. Repeat the same process for the other eye.

The second oblique guideline determines the length of the tail of the eyebrow. Starting from the wing of the nose once again, trace a second imaginary line, which this time passes through the outer corner of the eye, indicating the maximum length of the tail.

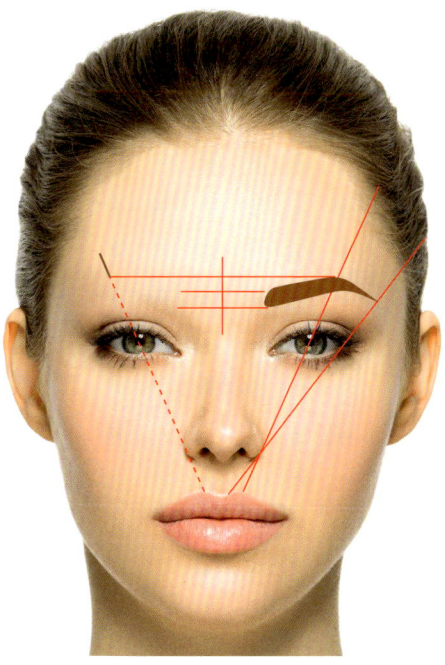

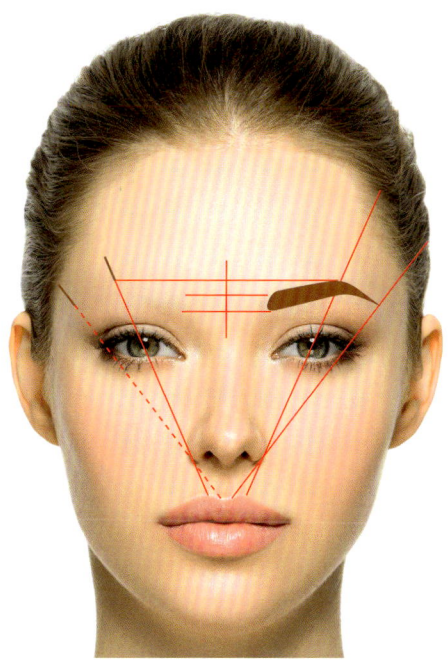

Proceed to mirror this guideline by sketching the first oblique guide on the client's right eye area. The criteria for sketching the guides on the first eye will be expertly repeated for the second eye. The wing of the nose and the center of the pupil will indicate the correct position of the vertex.

The wing of the nose and the outer corner of the eye will allow us to determine the length of the tail. These criteria only serve as a general rule, however, as they may not be appropriate for clients with very large noses, or noses that are too small. The professional must account for many, extremely different variables; the important thing is attaining the certainty and flexibility that make an excellent sketch possible.

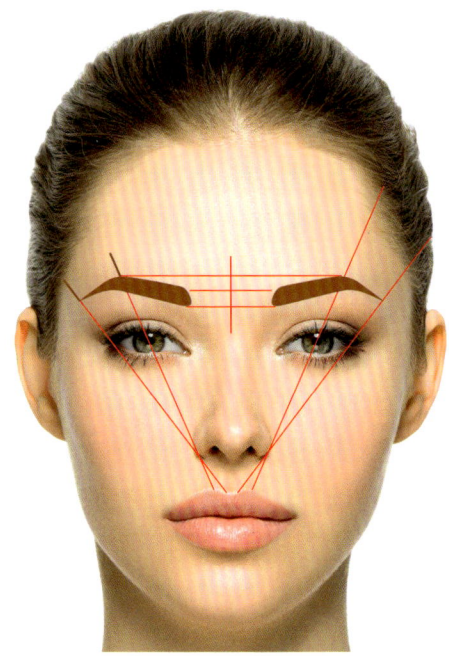

Once this is done, we'll have a grid within which we can quickly position the second eyebrow.

Using these reference points creates a symmetrical and accurate sketch, which should be checked using two fundamental tools in the sketching phase that allow for both a direct an indirect view of the results.

A frontal observation of the client affords an initial, direct view; using a mirror and a camera afterwards grants an indirect view, which will guarantee the quality of the final results.

"As it is impossible to build an architectural masterpiece without a good foundation, it is impossible to learn how to make beautiful permanent makeup without a serious basic training."

OLGA KRAVCHENKO

6.4.7. THE MIRROR

Makeup artists use mirrors for two main reasons:
- there are fewer obstructive elements (the field of vision is restricted to the focus point, and any differences can be spotted immediately);
- there is a double distance (from the subject to the mirror as well as the distance reflected within the mirror, granting a macroscopic view).

When painters use a long paintbrush they do so for the same reason: for a macroscopic view of what they are painting. Then they use a smaller paintbrush and move closer to the canvas when they need to concentrate on details; and they take a step back again to return to that macroscopic view. One particular mirror is created ad-hoc during the sketching phase.

This mirror is smaller in size, and a vertical and horizontal line are drawn on it, as well as many vertical and horizontal lines in slightly lighter colors.
This grid serves to check the distance from the main vertical line. The main horizontal line serves to make sure that the layout is completely parallel to the floor. This kind of mirror is without a doubt an important tool to limit the risks of an incorrect sketch, although of course each case is to be considered individually.

The grid provides precise references, but use your judgment when using it: for example, if one of the client's eyes is bigger than the other, it follows that this eyebrow should also be bigger than the other.

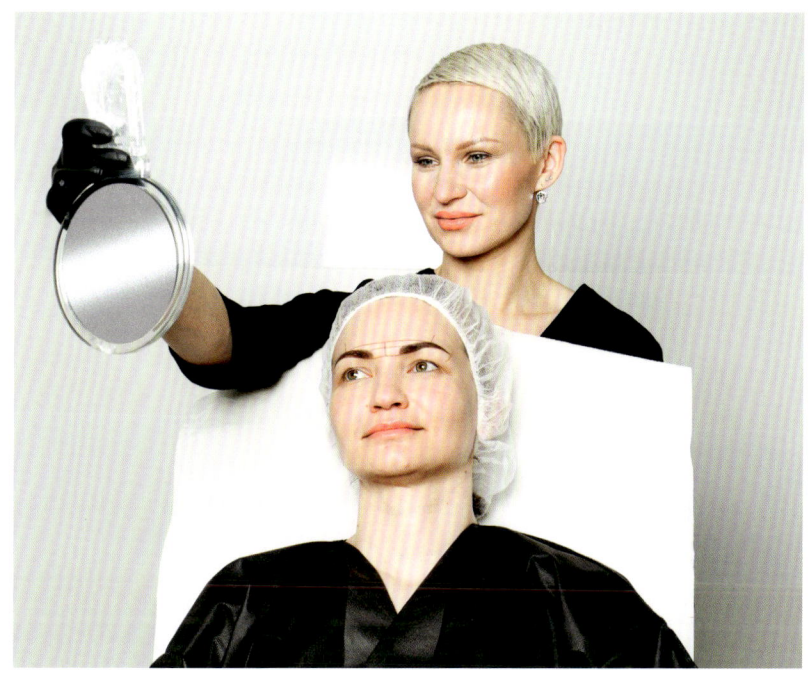

6.4.8. PHOTOGRAPHY TEST

Another element provides the absolute certainty of being able to proceed with confidence: the photography test. In this case we will also use a camera with a grid: the photo should be taken with the subject standing in front of a light background to avoid any distracting elements, and the lens should be focused at the subject's eye level.

Combining all of the application methods above allows the position of both eyebrows to be seen correctly.

This ensures that the sketch will be correct, and therefore that the desired results will be achieved.

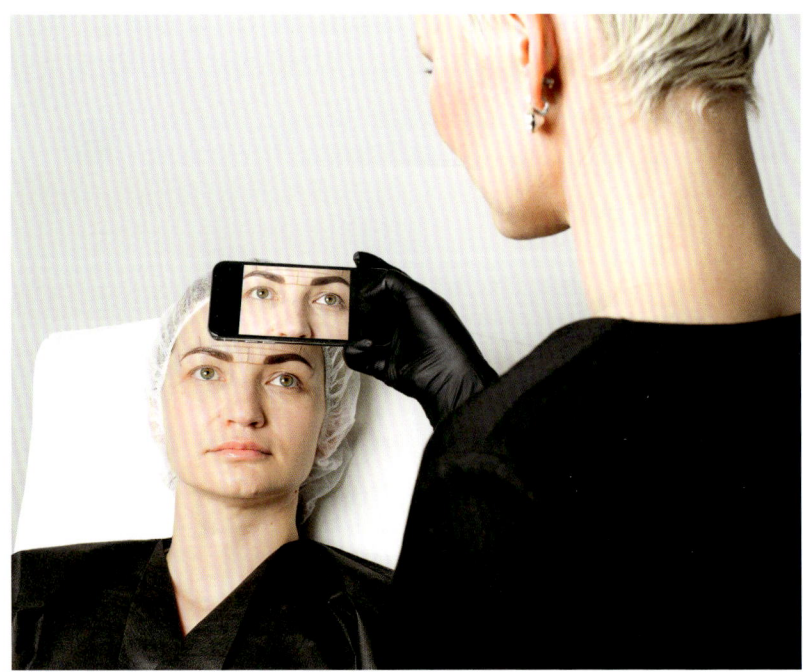

"The face is a beautiful picture created by nature, we don't have to redraw it completely, but just add a little emphasis."

ELENA NIKORA

6.5. LIPS

6.5.1 STATISTICS

DEFINING THE OUTLINE 40%	RECONSTRUCTION 40%	SCARS, VARIOUS DISCOLORATIONS 20%

Full, soft, and velvety lips: these are some of the adjectives used to emphasize the mouth's seductive power. It is considered the most sensual part of the face. Permanent lip makeup is said to be the most difficult procedure, both from a technical standpoint as well as in terms of color; in fact, the mouth requires particular attention, both in terms of caring for it and in especially makeup, where the risk of creating a vulgar, unnatural lip line is always present. An inappropriate color, excessively enlarging the contours of the lips, or a lip line that is too obvious would make even Michelangelo's Madonnas look vulgar.

Lips can suffer devastating damage from herpes, which can permanently compromise the mucous membranes in the same way as scarring can. Lips can also lose their definition if their color is too light, or if they are irregularly shaped. Additionally, some clients may simply want fuller, more sensual lips.

The application techniques used to shape the mouth can vary based on each client's personal and subjective desires. When the shape of the lips is perfect, but the client wants to make the contours more pronounced, they may request a pencil-effect lip liner.

Filling in the mucous membranes with pigment corrects discoloration, or places more emphasis on the lips using color.

Correcting significant asymmetries or increasing the mouth's volume without changing its shape is called reconstruction.

The hyper-realistic technique is definitely the most convincing, because it allows the client to highlight the beauty of her own lips using just lip gloss.

The statistics for lips speak for themselves: 40% of people choose to make their lips more defined, while another 40% seek to correct problems with the color or shape of their lips, or correct prior work, and the remaining 20% seek the procedure because of scars or discoloration.

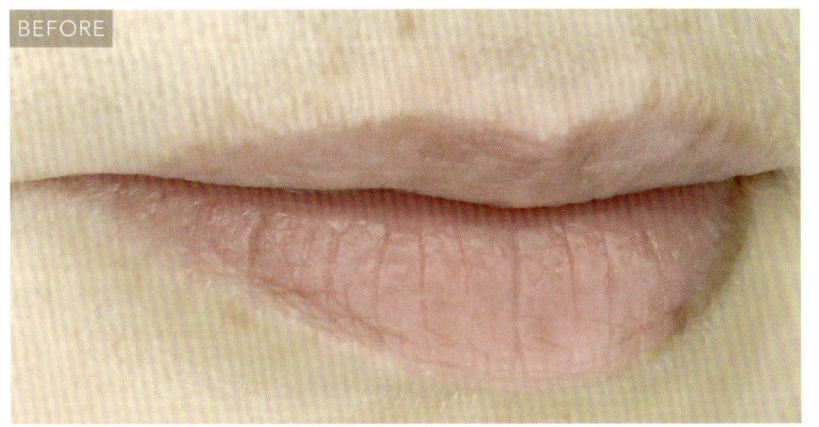

BEFORE

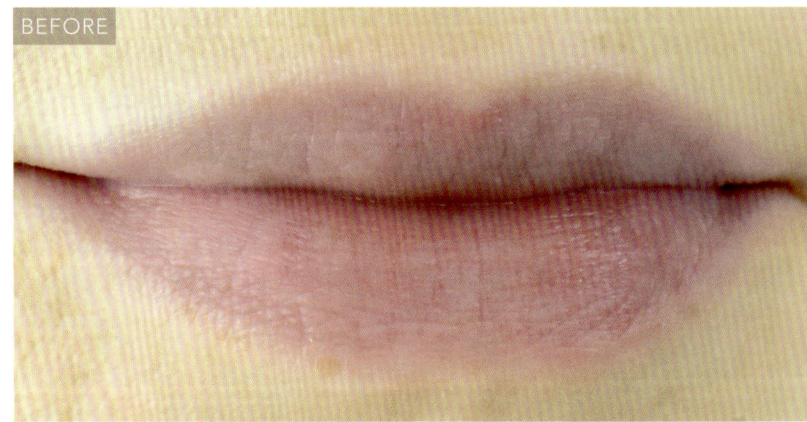

BEFORE

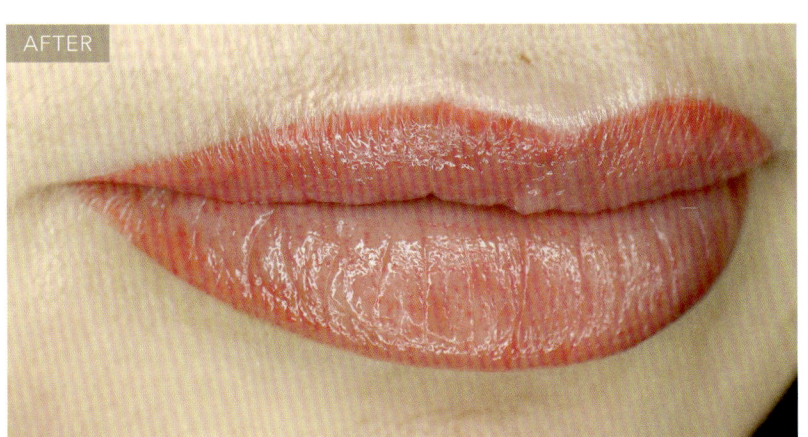

AFTER

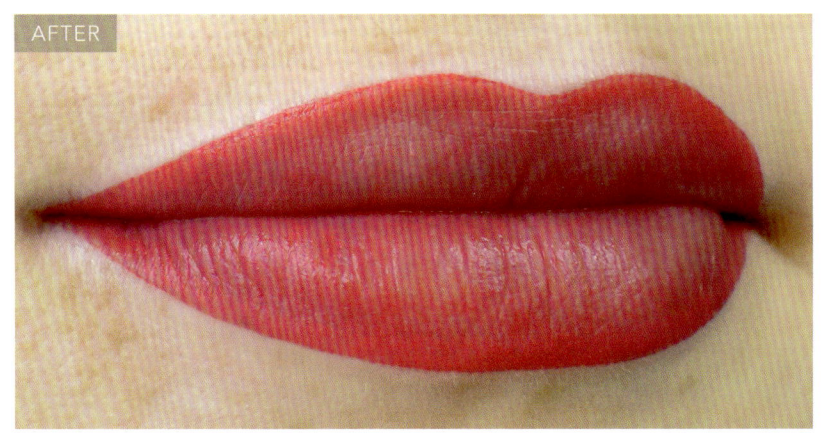

AFTER

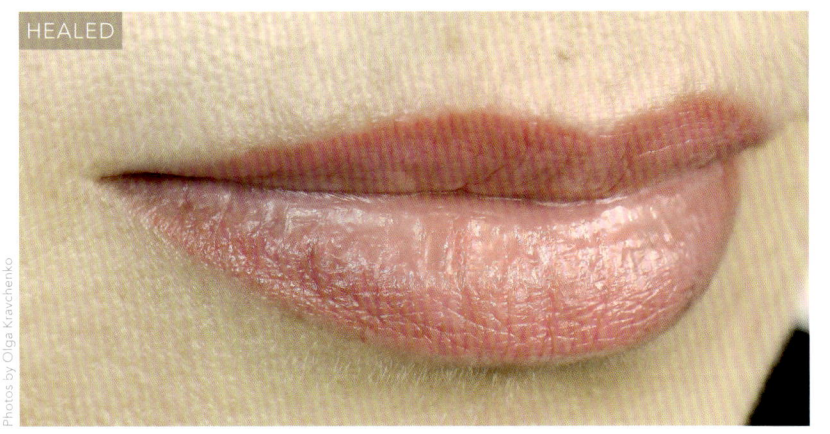

HEALED

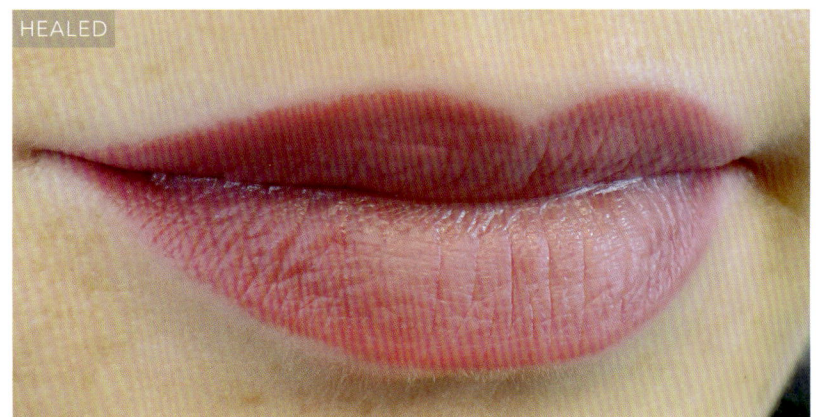

HEALED

Photos by Olga Kravchenko

6.5.2. LIPS: ANATOMY AND TERMINOLOGY

ANATOMY OF THE LIPS

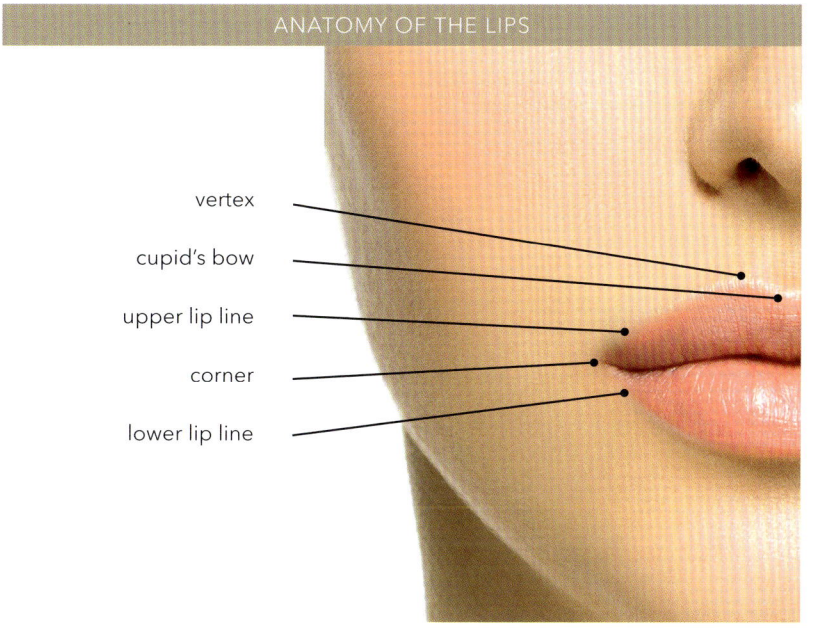

vertex
cupid's bow
upper lip line
corner
lower lip line

LIP TERMINOLOGY

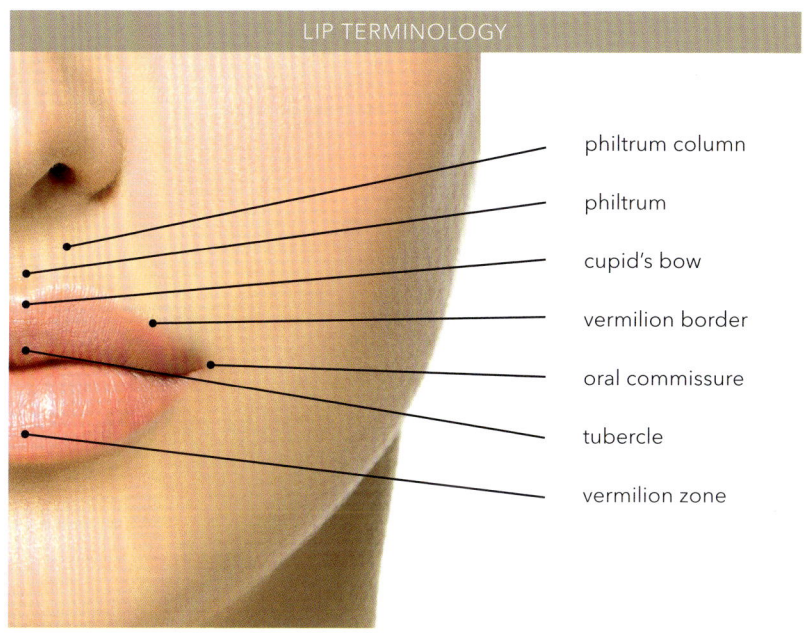

philtrum column
philtrum
cupid's bow
vermilion border
oral commissure
tubercle
vermilion zone

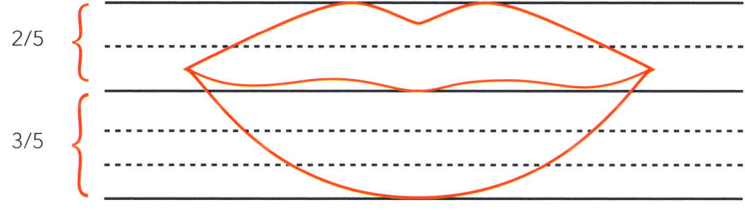

2/5

3/5

Normally, the upper lip is smaller than the lower lip. The mouth could be represented as the following fractions: 2/5 upper lip and 3/5 lower lip.

6.5.3. THE GUIDELINES

1 PHILTRAL COLUMNS

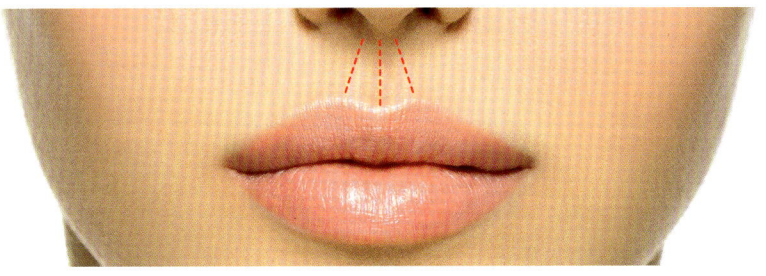

Proceed with the sketch. Start by following the philtral columns, which, if positioned correctly, should coincide with the highest vertex of the Cupid's bow: draw two little marks to see if the distances from the center are the same.

2 CUPID'S BOW

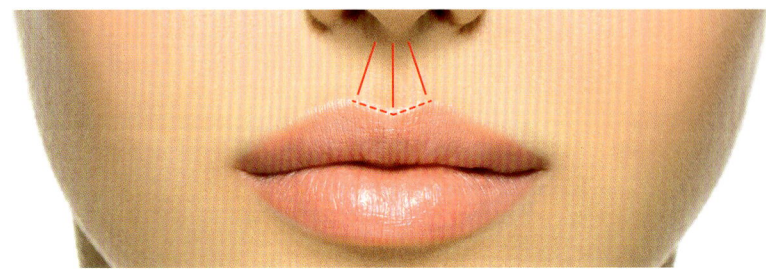

Draw a saturated line connecting the central part of the Cupid's bow with the right and left vertices: the result should look like an open "V".

3 LOWER REFERENCE POINTS

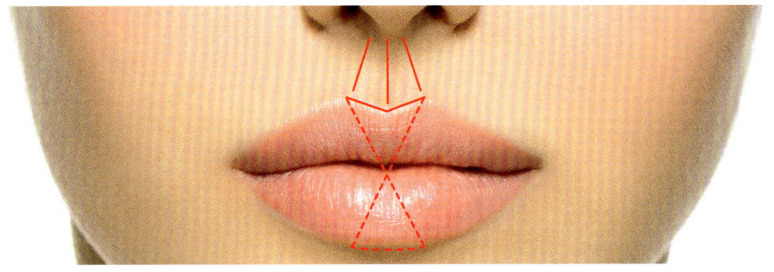

This image shows where to imagine an "X", which if extended downwards, will help us identify the two lower reference points, which we'll connect to create the lower curve.

4 UPPER ANGLES

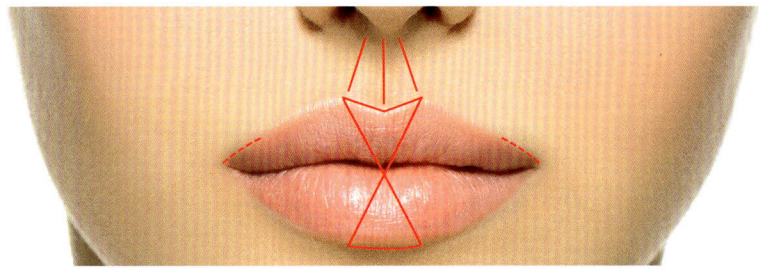

Next, trace two lines in the upper lip, one in the external right corner and on in the external left corner, before repeating this step on the lower lip.

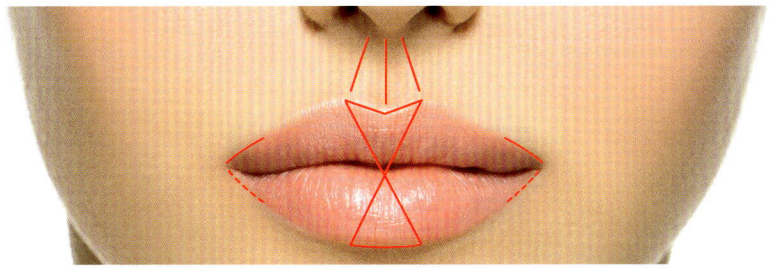

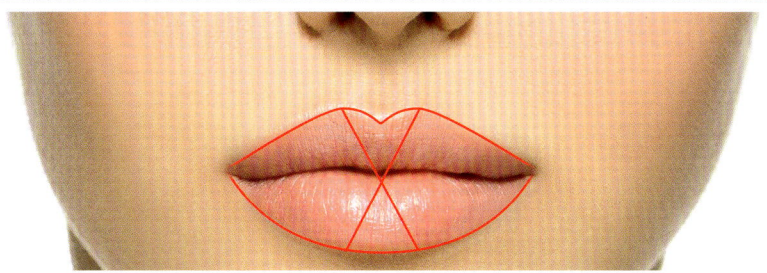

Connect the dots, just like in the puzzle game, to reveal the desired lip shape.

The first sketch may not be perfect. That is why it is important to work in front of a mirror, and analyze the results with the client. Only when you are sure of having obtained the best shape should you proceed to mark out the outline.

IMPORTANT NOTICE:

In case we want to correct asymmetry or to give the lip more volume, it is allowed to draw the contour slightly outside of the client's mucous membrane, but never exceeding 1-1.5mm.

NOTE: After finishing the sketch, it is important to check the lips to avoid making any simple mistakes. Make sure not to overly enlarge the top part, since the color will be perceived differently because of the light, even if it is the same pigment. It will be lighter on the outside of the lip, and darker on the inside of the lip's mucous membranes (Fig. A).

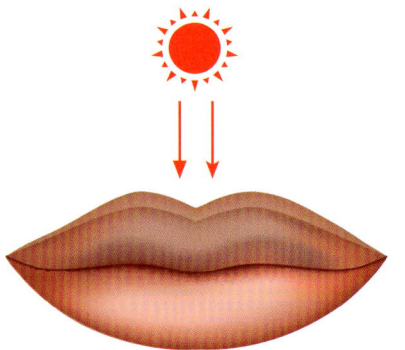

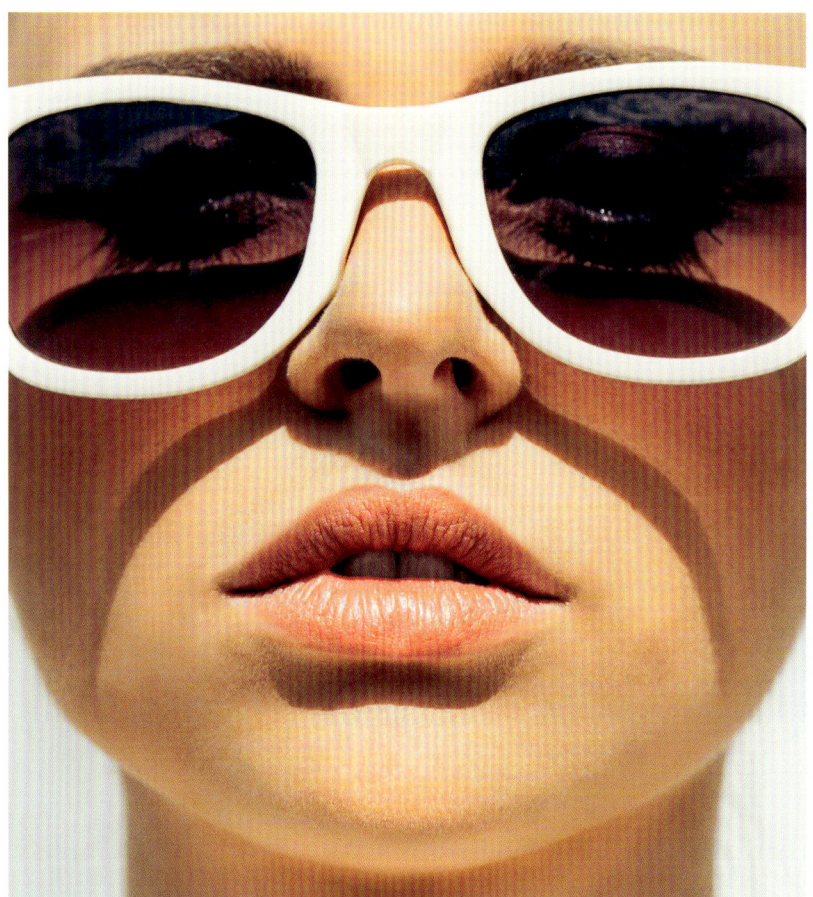

6.6. EYES

6.6.1. STATISTICS

It is immediately clear that 50% of clients choose to have permanent eye makeup applied in order to change the appearance of their gaze, make their eye shape more defined, or deepen or brighten their look.

30% of clients seek to replace their daily makeup application, while the remaining 20% suffer from cases of alopecia or wish to correct asymmetries or low-quality prior procedures.

CHANGING THE APPEARANCE OF THEIR LOOK 50%	REPLACING BASIC MAKEUP 30%	ALOPECIA OR CORRECTIONS 20%

6.6.2. EYES: ANATOMY AND TERMINOLOGY

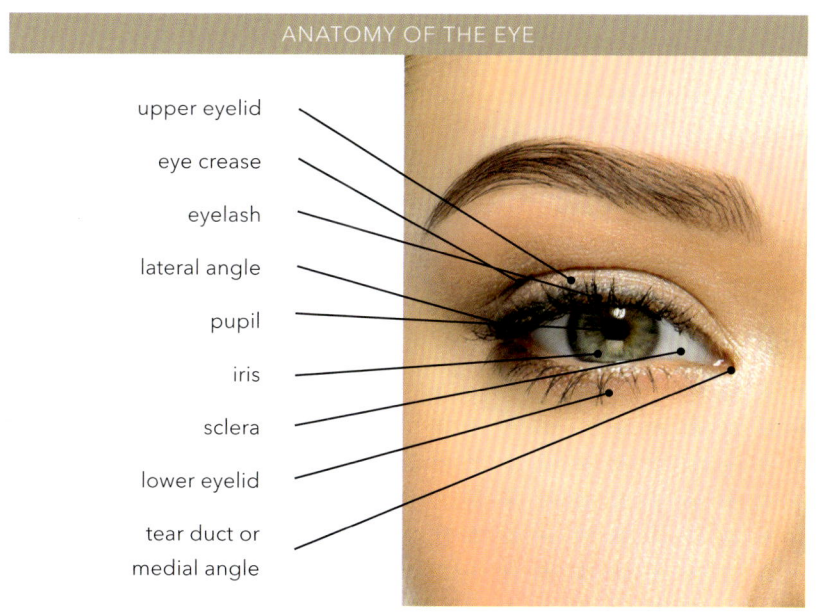

ANATOMY OF THE EYE

upper eyelid
eye crease
eyelash
lateral angle
pupil
iris
sclera
lower eyelid
tear duct or medial angle

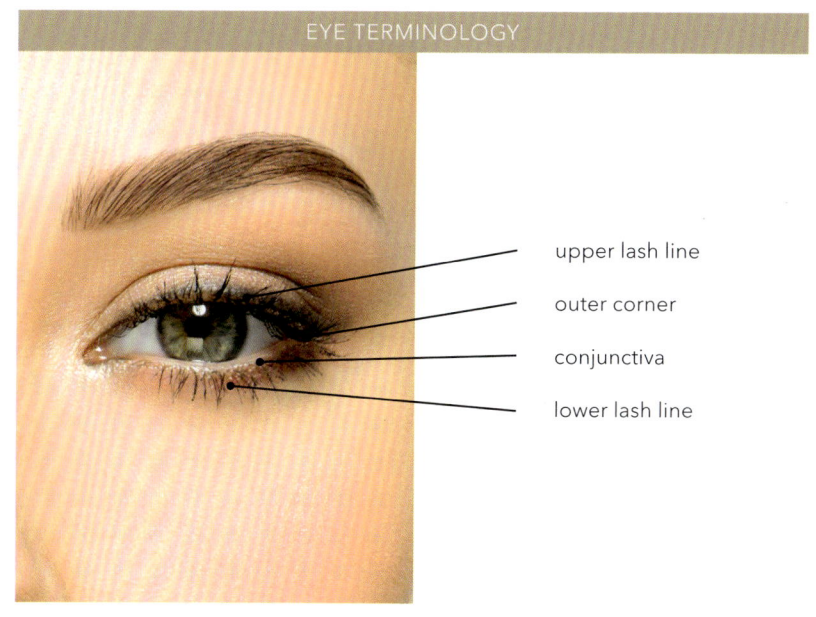

EYE TERMINOLOGY

upper lash line
outer corner
conjunctiva
lower lash line

6.6.3. THE GUIDELINES

For simplicity's sake, we'll narrow down the different eye shapes into three categories:

Imagine a horizontal line that runs from the inside corner of the eye to the outside corner: this is called the X Point.

If the inside corner lines up with the outside corner, this is a neutral eye (Fig. A), which has neither an ascending nor a descending shape. If the outside corner: is higher than the inside corner, this is a positive eye (Fig. B). In a negative eye, the inside corner is higher than the outside corner (Fig. C).

Understanding eye shapes is useful for being able to immediately understand what can be corrected, and for choosing the procedure that is most suited to enhancing each client's look.

A neutral eye can freely be transformed by being made positive, elongated, or widened, without flouting the principles of visagism. In this case, eyeliner begins not from the outside corner of the eye, but a few millimeters before it, exactly along the line of the X-point (Fig. D) in order to create the illusion of a positive eye.

For an eye that is already positive, there is no need for eyeliner to extend the lower rim of the eye upwards. Instead, eyeliner that extends horizontally, rather than vertically, is preferable, which aims to widen the eye instead of lengthening it (Fig. E).

For a negative eye, eyeliner is best extended upwards, giving the eye a positive look which eliminates the droopy appearance of the negative eye. In this case, eyeliner begins a few millimeters before the outside corner of the eye to make the eye seem a slightly less neutral (Fig. F).

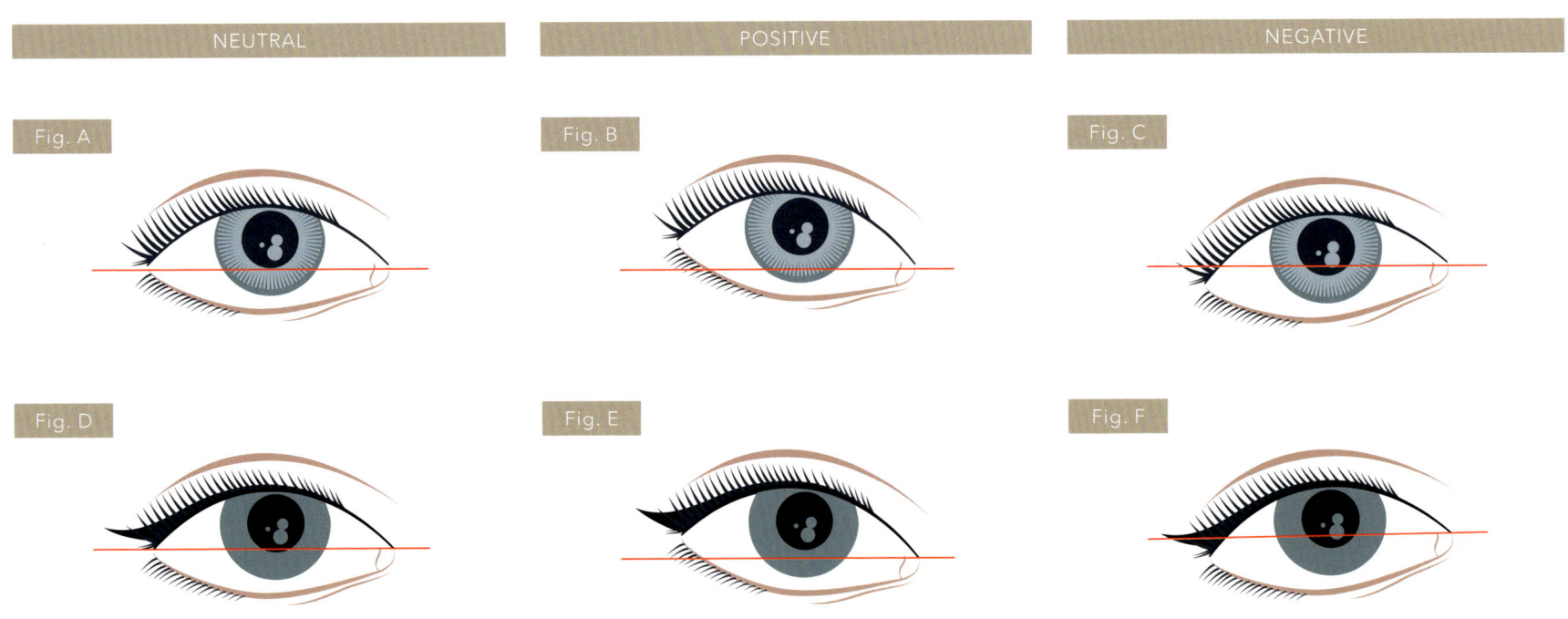

NEUTRAL · POSITIVE · NEGATIVE

Fig. A · Fig. B · Fig. C

Fig. D · Fig. E · Fig. F

6.7. SKETCHING TOOLS

A good sketch ensures that the procedure is performed accurately, without forgetting crucial elements, and most importantly, without improvising.

Each dermopigmentation professional should acquire the right tools for correctly executing this delicate stage of the process.

Here are the basic, indispensable tools for the job:
- tweezers to remove hair: epilate the area outside the sketch, in order to remove most of the hairs that get in the way. More hair is then removed when the choice is made, so that the brow area is left perfectly clean. Don't forget to sterilize the tweezers according to the rules for maintaining hygienic tools outlined in chapter 3.
- Marking tools: choose a sterile marker, a special makeup pencil or an amiea mixing pen with single-use sterile tips for drawing the sketch. In some countries only sterile, single-use markers are allowed for this purpose;
- cleanser/disinfectant: usually, green soap or tattoo soap is used here, normally diluted with 80% water;
- cotton balls or pads: soaked with green soap, these help clean up minor color smudges;
- small cups to hold the color: used as sterile capsules in which to mix the color;
- the chosen color;

- a medium-sized mirror and a large mirror, for both a microscopic and macroscopic perspective;
- a mixer: to perfectly blend the different pigments used in the procedures;
- protective sheaths: to protect the handpiece and console from cross-contamination.

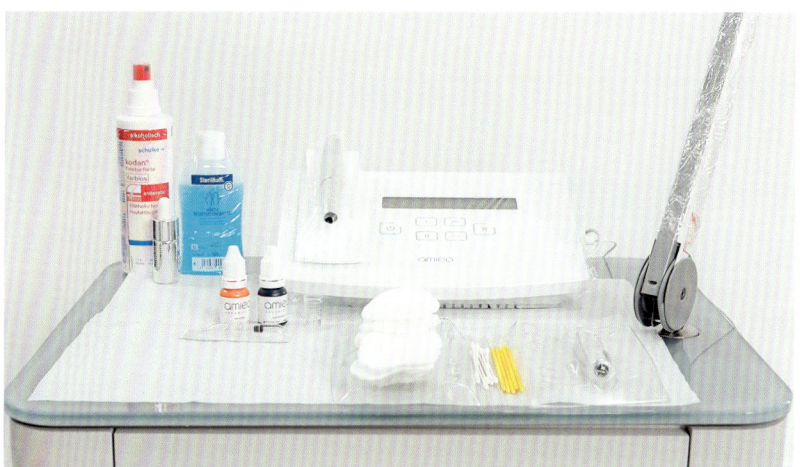

7

BASICS OF MICROPIGMENTATION

The handpiece is the main character in the art of micro-pigmentation. But it can't play its part without a skilled hand guiding it and allowing it to achieve different kind of lines, saturation and different effects, even when using the same needle and the same color.

Below are the key criteria at the heart of micropigmentation:
- pressure
- speed
- needle frequency
- number of needles
- color dilution
- angle
- direction
- alignment
- diameter
- needle setting
- timing

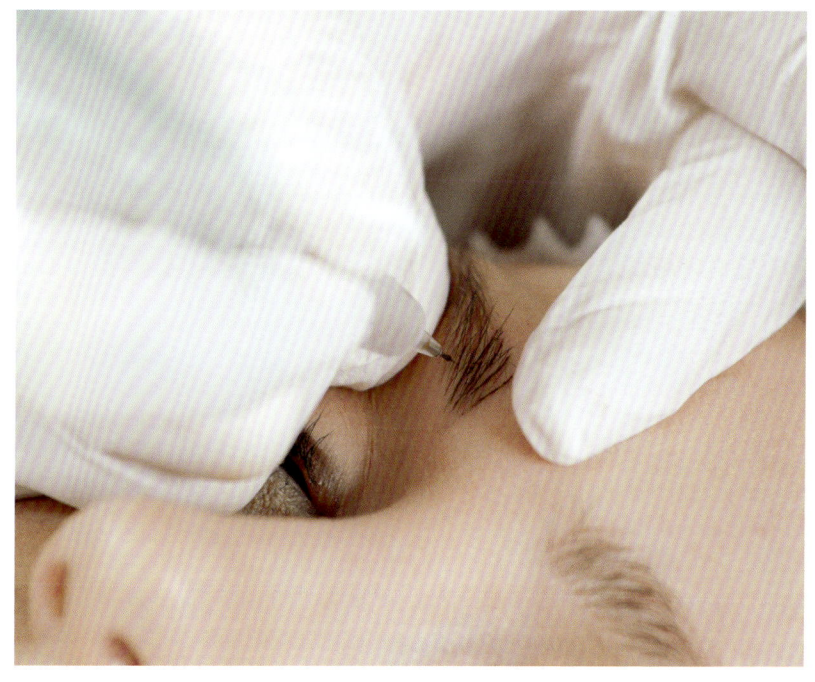

7.1. PRESSURE

The hand can create different kinds of pressure, depending on whether the professional wants to push a needle into the epidermis, dermis, or hypodermis.
In case we are working in the epidermis using light pressure, color will fade out completely after the first 30/40 days exfoliation.

Too much pressure, which pushes the color into the hypodermis, inevitably causes bleeding during the color application, inappropriately diluting the pigment and making the color fade over the following days.
Because of the greater presence of fat cells, there is also the risk that the color could migrate and create hypertrophic scars.

The correct pressure allows the needle to deposit the color in the dermis.

Does more pressure equal more or less ability to write on a paper?

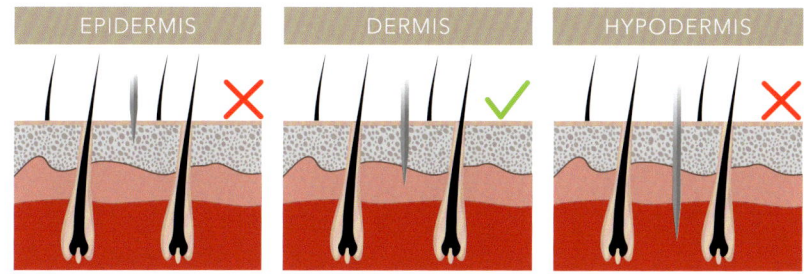

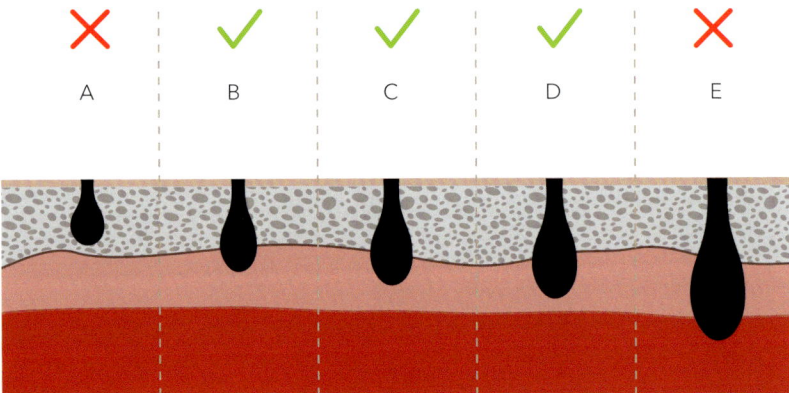

Let's say we draw 5 dots with 5 different levels of pressure: each dot represents a little column of color. In the first and fifth dots, the wrong pressure was applied, as explained above: the needle stopped in the epidermis in the first column (A) and penetrated the hypodermis in the fifth column (E). The other three levels of pressure (B, C, D) can all be considered equally correct, since they all placed the color in the dermis. The final result can vary, however, based on the pressure used. It is precisely because the three dots were created with different levels of pressure, based on their depth in the dermis, that we see variations in the intensity of the color. When the first layer of the epidermis undergoes cell regeneration, from outside we'll see that the first dot (B) has 0.5mm of color, the second dot (C) has 1mm of color, and the third dot (D) has 1.5mm length. To achieve a more visible, meaning more defined, effect, the needle must penetrate the deepest layer of the dermis; for a more delicate effect, it should stop in the more superficial layers.

7.2. HAND MOTION

The motion of the hand is another variable in permanent makeup. Think about a speed of around 10km/h, with a maximum speed of 30km/h: the faster your hand moves, the less ability you have to make a mark because of the continuous vertical oscillation (bps) of the needle. The speed of your hand therefore has a fundamental impact on the final results. If you move at 10km/h, you'll be able to create a saturated line because the needle will be able to create more dots in a particular area; as the speed of the professional's hand increases, reaching 30km/h for example, the effect will be more transparent because the needle won't have had enough time to deposit color.

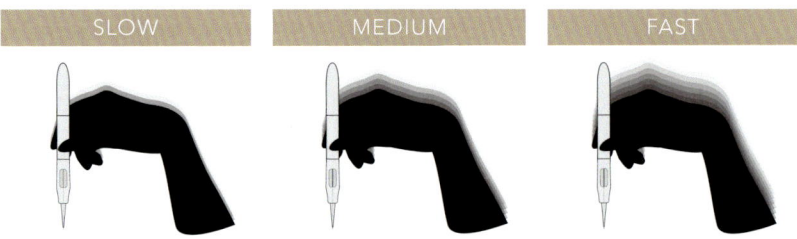

Let's try a different example. Imagine a motorcycle whose motor is leaking oil: if it is slowly traveling down the street, it will leave a continuous trail of oil; if instead, its speed increases, the trail will be irregular and dotted.

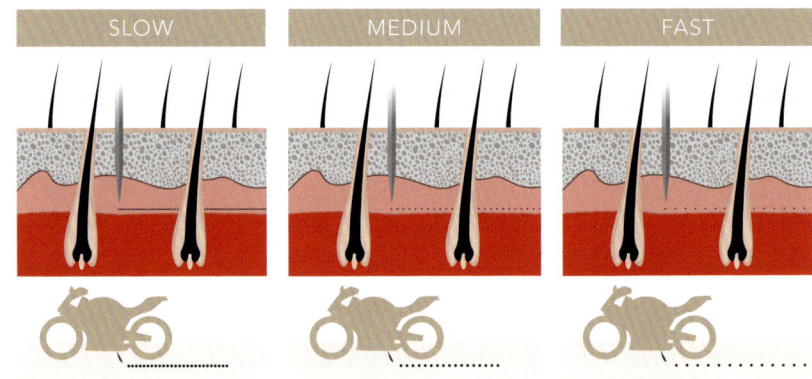

7.3. NEEDLE FREQUENCY (BPS)

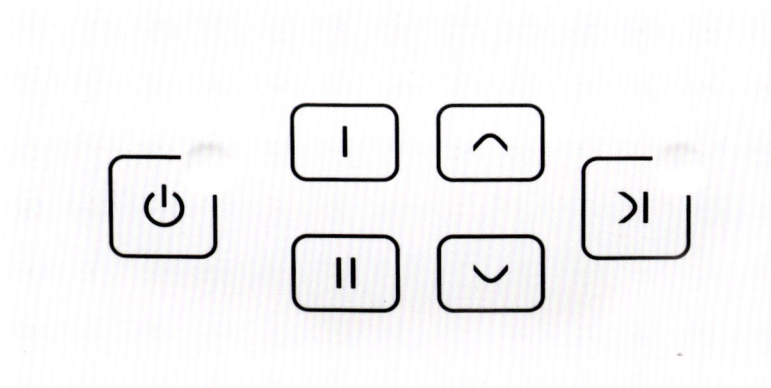

The handpiece can function at 50-150 beats per second (bps), simply by increasing or decreasing the frequency using the control unit, where it is marked with a + or -. This feature is comparable to a car's accelerator, in that it enables the needle to operate faster or slower. By increasing the needle frequency and maintaining constant hand pressure and speed, the ability to make a mark increases. Imagine that the hand moves at 10km/h, and the handpiece performs 100 beats per second. Maintaining the speed of 10/km but increasing the beats per second would leave the dermis more saturated with color. A full, saturated line is created by a higher needle frequency. To achieve a lighter, more faint line, the needle frequency should instead be lowered.

7.4. NUMBER OF NEEDLES

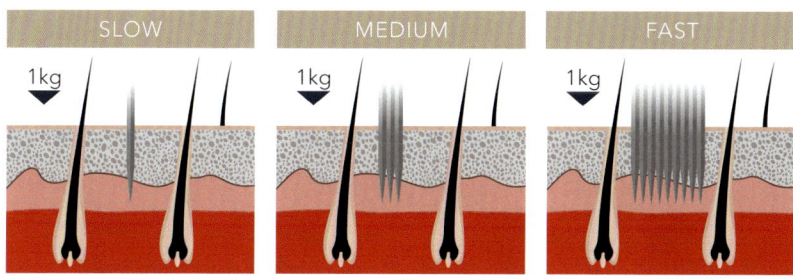

As shown in the diagram, different kinds of needles can be used:
• with 1 tip
• with 3 tips
• with 7 tips

Keeping pressure, speed, and frequency constant, increasing the number of needle tips decreases the ability to make marks; because increasing the surface area of the needles' penetration decreases the depth they can reach.
A larger needle therefore requires more pressure to achieve the same result as when using a smaller needle at a lower pressure.

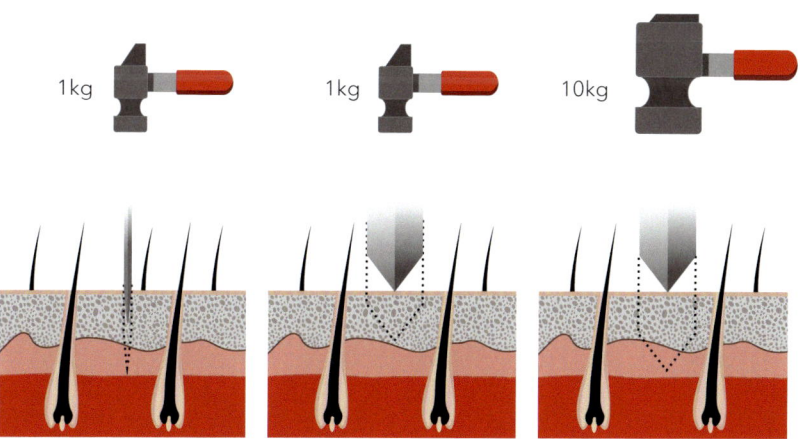

If you were walking over snow with stiletto heels, each individual step would be extremely difficult, since the tendency would be that of sinking into the snow. But if you put on snowshoes, walking would become much easier, and your pace would increase, because you would remain comfortably on the surface of the snow.

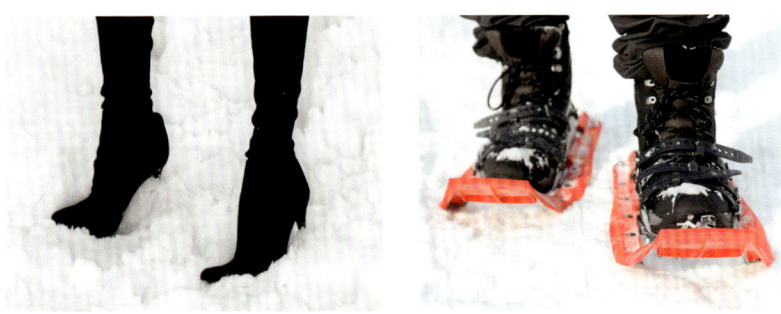

7.5. COLOR DILUTION

It doesn't matter if the line is made with a pure or diluted color; what matters is that the ability to create a mark is inversely proportionate to the dilution of the color; the more the color is diluted, the less you can make a mark.

Consider the "stray" hairs for example: to make them appear lighter and therefore more faint, the color should be more diluted than with thick hairs.

dilution

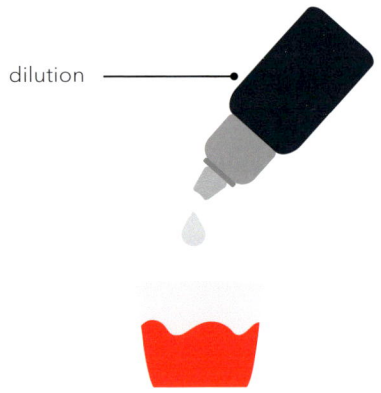

7.6. ANGLE

The angle at which the needle enters the skin is also important. This figure shows three different angles: but which is the correct angle for each type of procedure? And why?

The histological aspect of the skin determines the answer to these questions. In an oil reservoir, the pumps of the oil wells run perpendicular to the ground to extract the petroleum. This is because of the physics of the Earth's pressure on the layer below the crust, which draws everything towards the surface. The complete inverse occurs at the surface: the law of gravity, as we know, pushes everything downwards. If we tried to make a hole with a drill angled at 90°, the Earth's pressure would cause the oil to spurt out up to 30 meters high. If instead, the hole is created at a 45° angle, the pressure would still push upwards, but the petroleum would exit more slowly, and with a weaker force. The same process occurs in the skin because of pressure inside the body.

Making a hole with a needle angled at 90°, causes more bleeding; to avoid this, use an angle of 45°/ 60°. Scalp pigmentation is the exception. In this case, the needle may actually need to penetrate at 90°, depending on the procedure, the work surface, and the application techniques being used.

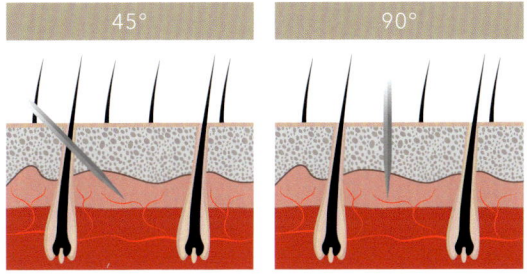

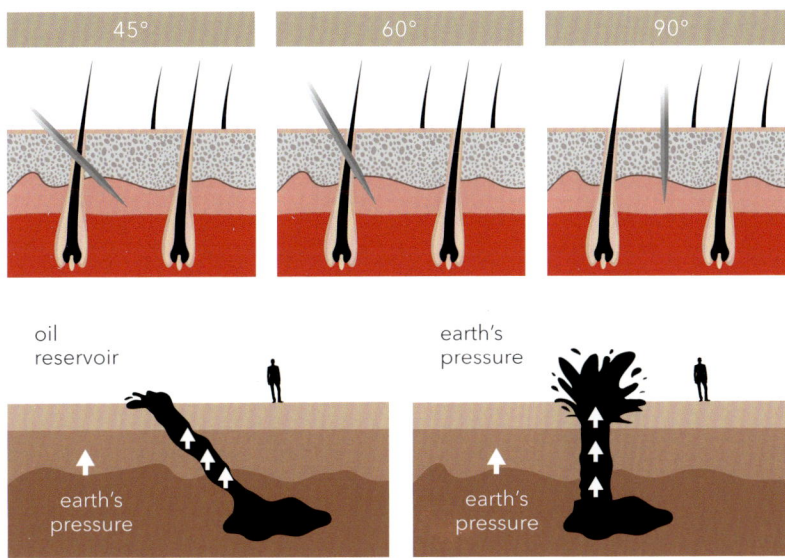

7.7. DIRECTION OR ORIENTATION

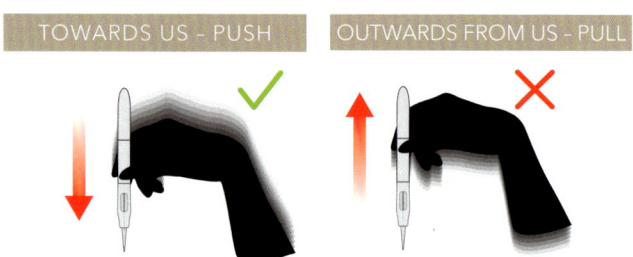

Once you've chosen the best angle, determine in which direction to move the needle. The professional can push the needle towards themselves, or away from themselves, and from left to right or vice versa. The direction is crucial, but to understand which direction is correct, understand that a needle has a body and a taper. The taper is the point, which is the narrowest part, where the needle is tempered. Imagine having to hang a large and heavy frame on a wall: you wouldn't use a small nail if you didn't want to risk having it fall.

You're more likely to use the kind of dowel specifically created to bear the weight of a large frame. To avoid ruining the plaster, it's best to make sure to create the hole with the right drill bit. It would be best to first make a small, 2-gauge hole, then enlarge it with a 5-gauge bit, and only then proceed to use an 8-gauge bit to finish the job without damaging the wall.

The same principle holds for the skin. Always insert the thinnest part of the needle, never the thickest. If you are working with a 45°/60° angle and you choose to work towards yourself, you would first start with the tip and only then expand the mark by using part of the body of the needle. If you are working at 60° and therefore are working outwards, the skin won't be pierced by the tip but by the body: this would create a cut, which would then form a scab.

The professional should always work towards themselves, and always try to have the needle tip enter first, then the body.

7.8. ALIGNMENT

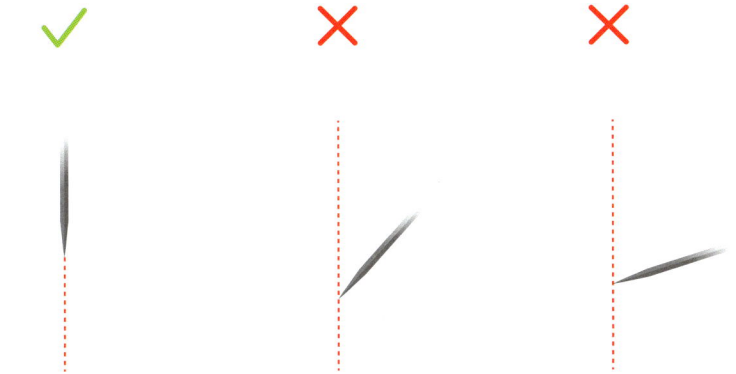

The needle should always be aligned with the line it needs to trace, maintaining a 45° angle and working towards the professional. This means the needle is aligned towards the hair to be drawn, towards the lip contour being created, towards the eyeliner, or towards any other line in a tattoo.

Failing to correctly follow this guideline means risking marks that are too thick because too much pigment accumulates in them. The goal is always to make lines of pigment that have the same thickness as the needle.

7.9. NEEDLE DIAMETER

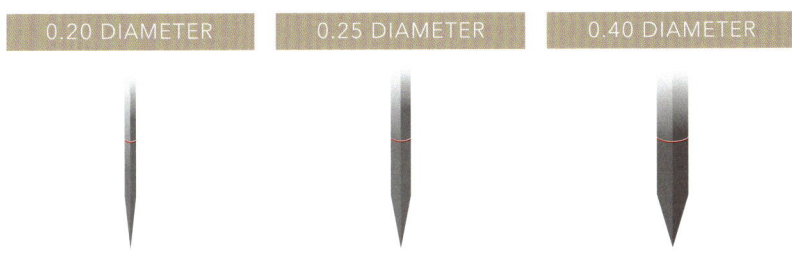

0.20 DIAMETER   0.25 DIAMETER   0.40 DIAMETER

Remember that needles can have different diameters, but to obtain the most natural results possible it's best to use needles with small diameters, even if they are harder to use at first. Over time, the pigment placed in the skin inevitably migrates and a very thin hair will become ever so slightly thicker. Traditional needles have diameters ranging from 0.30 to 0.40 mm, while needles made for permanent eyebrow makeup can be found with a diameter of 0.20 mm.

A very fine needle gives definition to hair strokes, which allows lines to remain crisp even several months later.

7.10. SETTING THE NEEDLE

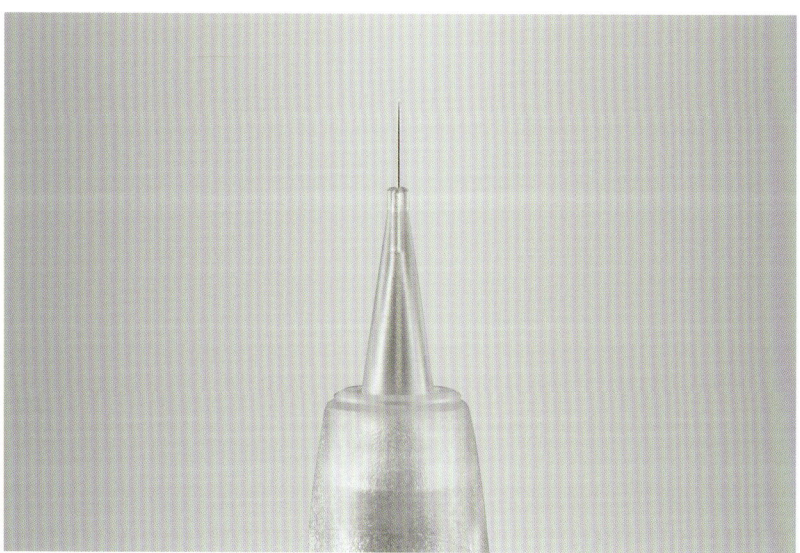

The needle should be about 1.5mm long. Only 1/3 of the needle will enter the skin, meaning around 0.5 mm, while the other 2/3 (1mm) remain outside. Regardless, setting the needle and continuously monitoring it during the procedure only partly ensures that it only penetrates the dermis.

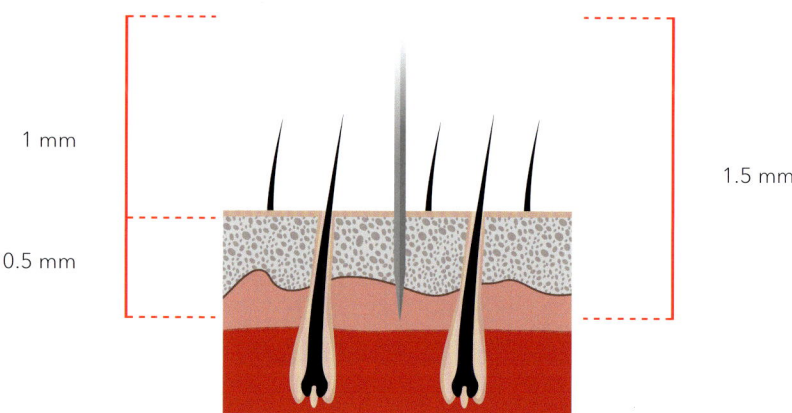

1 mm

0.5 mm

1.5 mm

8

RULES FOR CREATING
PRECISE LINES

8.1. BODY POSTURE

A perfect line comes from the right posture of the body, hand, and fingers. The body's weight should be as balanced as possible when aiming to create a precise line.

If the professional were to be neatly divided in two, both parts of the body should fall to the left and right at the exact same time.

If you work with your ankles or legs crossed, you can't expect stability. Legs should be planted, and facing the same way, in order to correctly distribute the weight of the body (Fig. A).

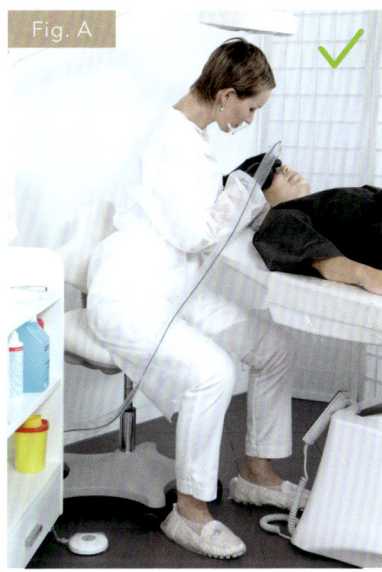

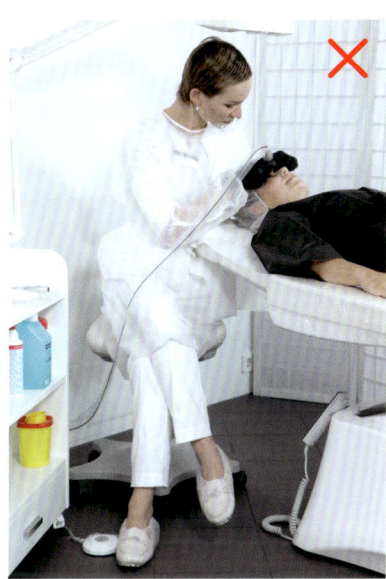

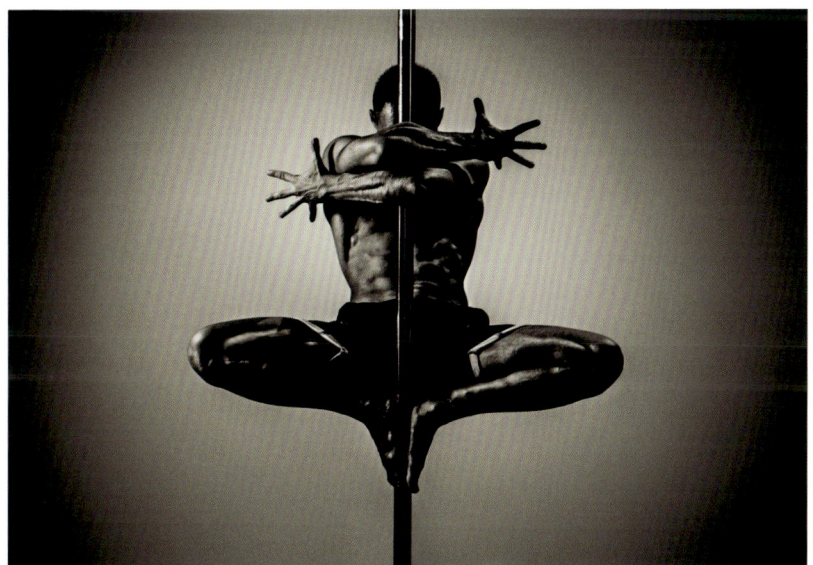

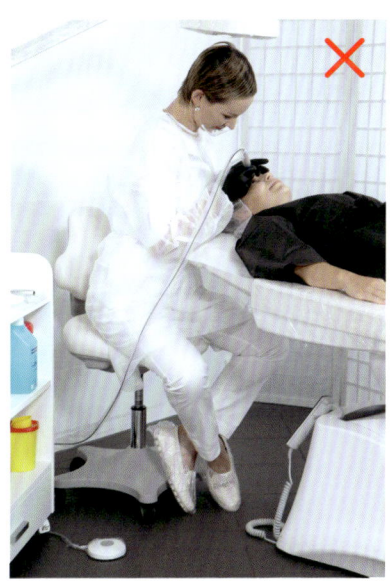

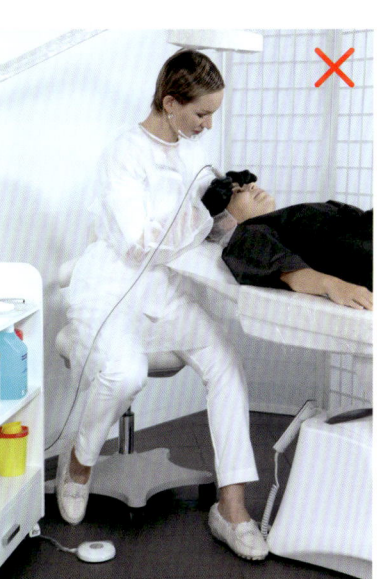

8.2. HOLDING THE HANDPIECE

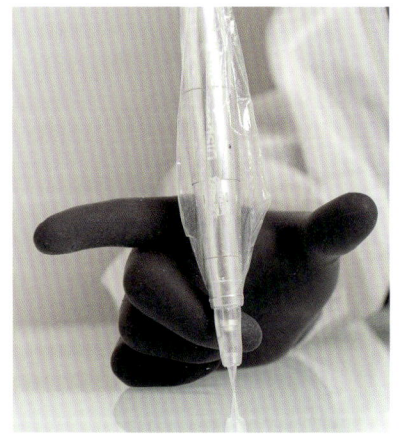
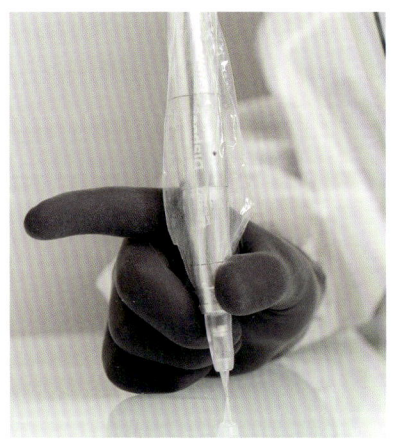
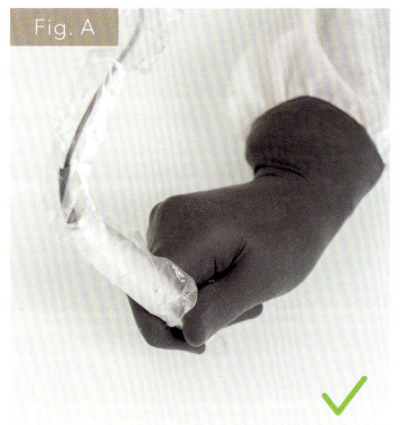
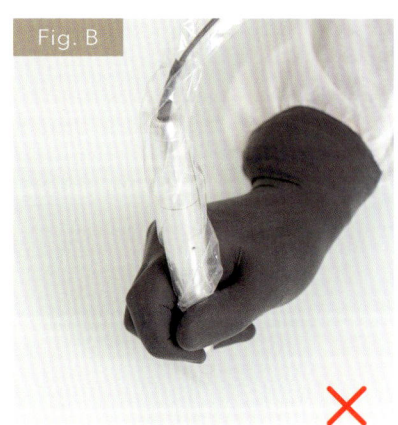
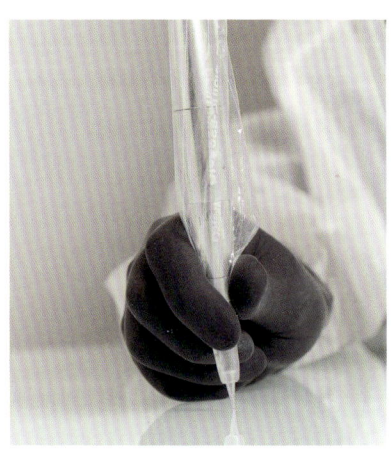
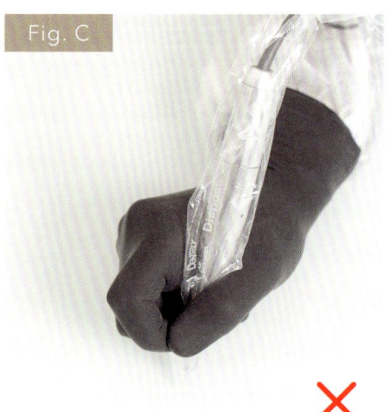

To use the handpiece correctly, use a secure and stable grip. Use three fingers to hold it: the middle finger supports the handpiece, and is the finger that will usually bear the typical dermopigmentation professional callus. The thumb serves to keep it stable and still, while the index finger guides it.

You'll notice that where the handpiece rests is very important: in order to achieve the correct angle, it's best to hold it on your second knuckle (Fig. A). Often, out of habit or for convenience, we let the handpiece slide into the crease between our thumb and index finger or at the first knuckle. This position won't allow us to sustain the correct grip and angle, and will lead to sloppy lines (Fig. B-C).

8.3. HAND POSITION

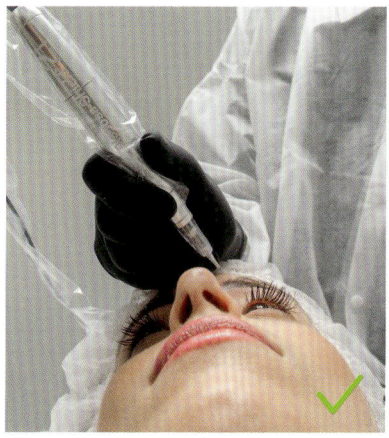
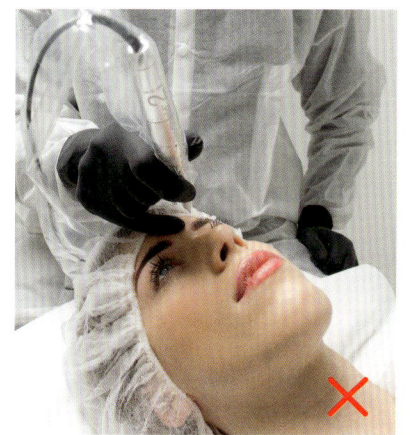
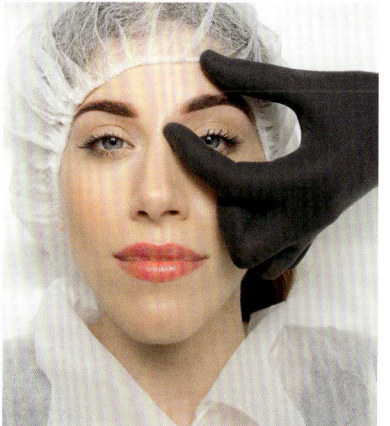
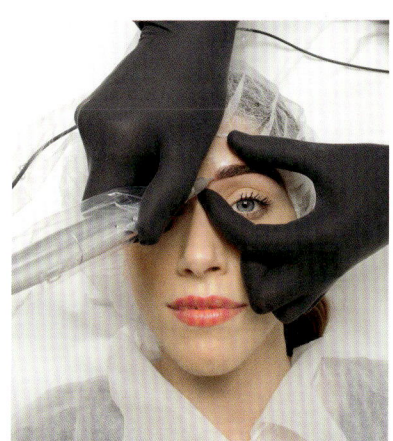

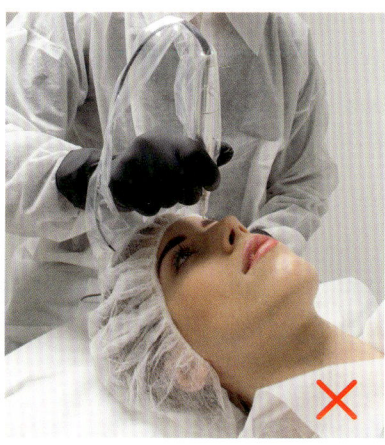
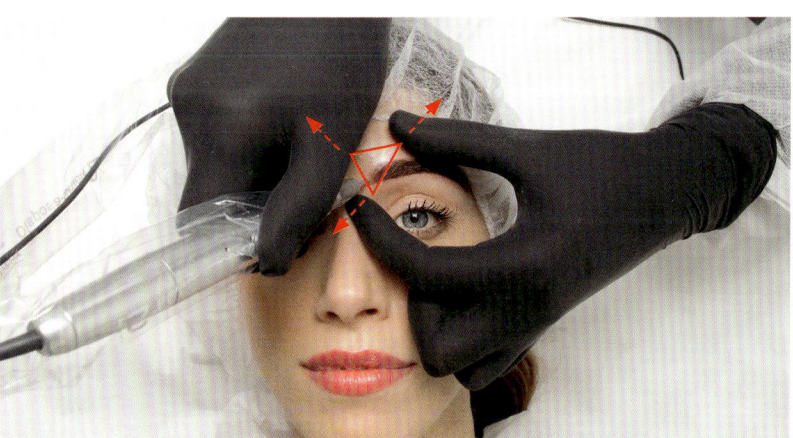

Don't underestimate the position of the hands. The hand which the professional uses to hold the handpiece must stay firm, whether resting on the client's forehead, cheek, head, or lips. The entire side of the palm should be in contact with the body part in question in order to achieve the right tension for the needle to be able to reach the skin with the best possible precision.

The other hand is mostly used for holding the skin taut in the area being pigmented, and to feel the vibrations created by the needle's entry into the skin to understand if it is reaching the epidermis, the dermis, or the hypodermis. This creates a triangle of tension between the hand holding the handpiece and pressing on the skin, and the other hand which holds the skin taut. The professional works within this triangle.

8.4. THE PROFESSIONAL'S POSTURE AND POSITIONING

During permanent makeup procedures, the professional will assume different positions in relation to the client, in order to maintain the parameters they've studied and practiced constant, and to work as nimbly and comfortably as possible.

EYEBROWS

When working on the client's left eyebrow, the professional will be seated behind the client, resting their right hand firmly on the client's forehead and rotating from time to time to the client's left to ensure that the needle remains aligned with the hairs, according to the different direction and orientation in which each hair grows (Fig. A).

When working on the right eyebrow, the professional will instead still be seated behind the client, but will rest their hand on the client's cheek, and rotate the client's head depending on the direction and orientation of hair growth (Fig. B).

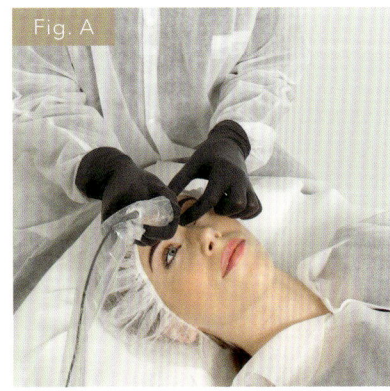
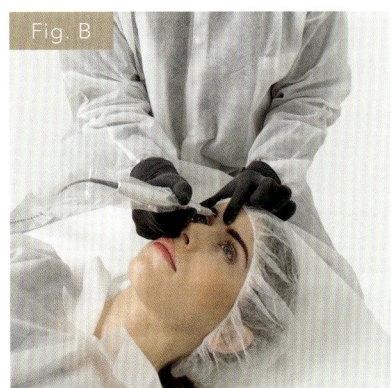

We recommend changing your grip on the handpiece, holding it from a higher position in order to more easily reach the inside of the lip without changing the angle. Working on the client's right side means their face will be turned to the left, the professional's hand will once again rest on their jaw, and grip the handpiece from lower down as before.

Meanwhile, the left hand plays a key role in maintaining tension in the lips, which will undergo different degrees of stretching depending on the technique being used (Fig. C).

LIPS

When working on the lips, the professional will be seated to the right of the client, and maintain this position throughout the entire procedure. Start from the left side of the mouth, rotating the client's face towards the right in order to rest your right hand on their jaw. As you move towards the center, the client's face will be turned upwards, and your hand will rest on their chin.
Note: if the chin protrudes compared the jaw, the hand holding the handpiece will be higher and therefore further away from the contour of the mouth, therefore running the risk of not depositing pigment as evenly as along the sides.

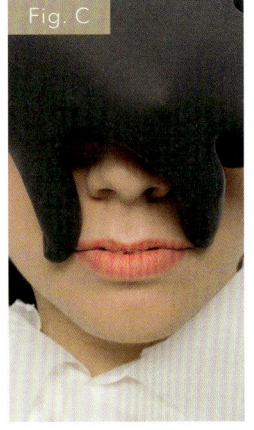
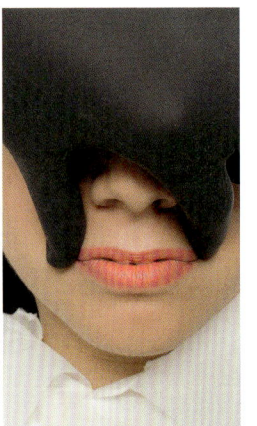
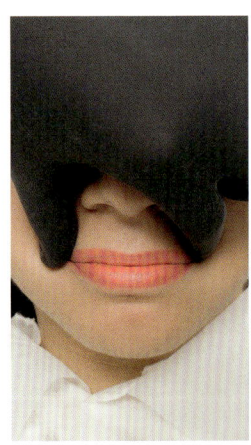

EYES

As with the lips, when working on the eyes the professional will also be seated to the right hand side of the client, and will remain there for the procedure on both eyes (Fig. D).

Their grip on the handpiece will change however: its tip will face the professional when working on the client's left eye, but it will be pointed outwards when working on the right eye (Fig. E).

The position of the left hand plays a key role during procedures on the eyes. since it will serve to hold the eye area taut to allow the needle to penetrate perfectly. This prevents any vibrations due to involuntary movements from the client.

The thumb will pull the skin on the upper lash line towards the professional, while the index stretches the skin in the opposite direction. The space between them is where the handpiece will perform the pigmentation (Fig. F). For the lower lash line, proceed with the tension created above, as shown in the photos, then use the right hand to hold the lower part taut, trying to open the eye to work on the lash line more comfortably (Fig. G).

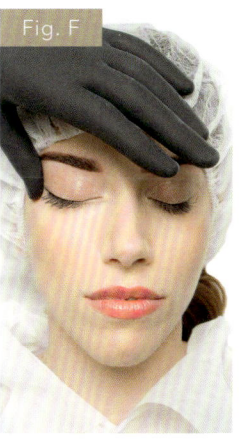

Fig. F

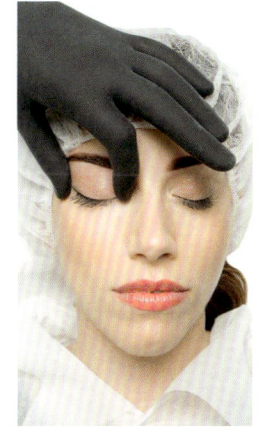

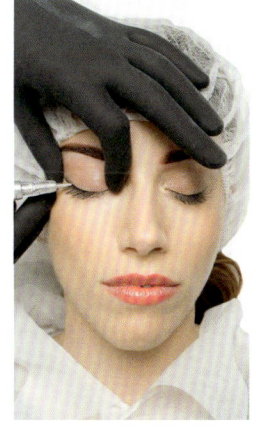

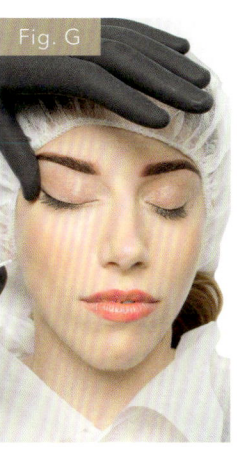

Fig. G

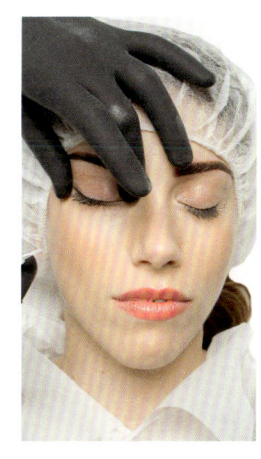

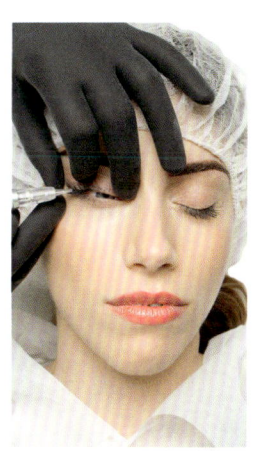

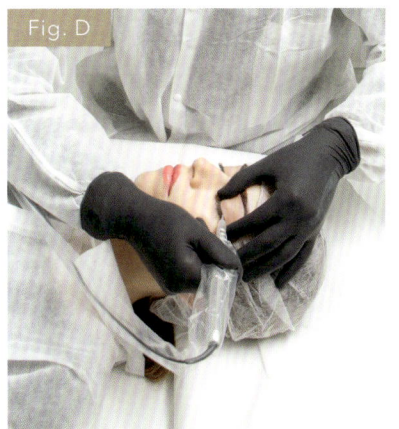

Fig. D

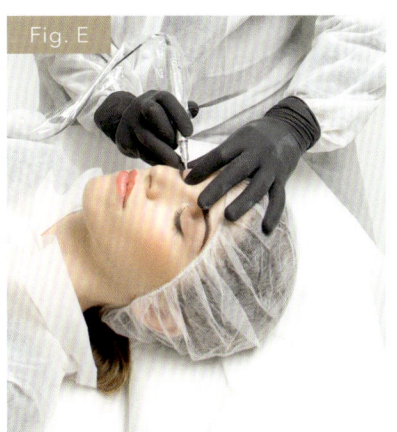

Fig. E

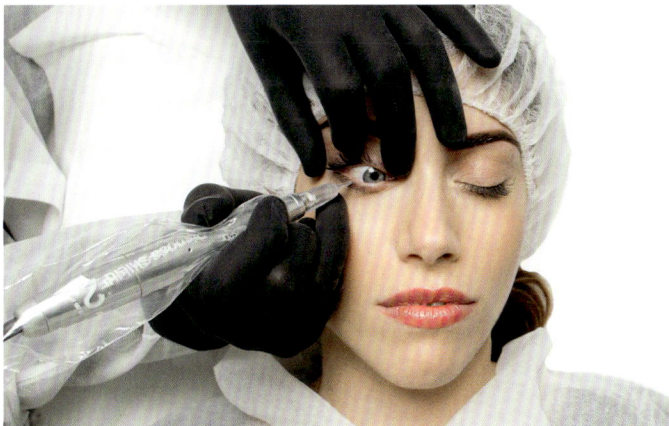

8.5. DRAWING VERTICAL LINES

Drawing vertical lines has to do with the alignment of the hair. The human brain reads an image (or in the case of dermopigmentation, a line), and commands the hand to create what it sees.

After drawing one vertical hair then another and another, the hand gets used to the same, repeated movement. Your hand needs to be able to perform the same movement repeatedly in order to create perfect lines, instead of shaky ones.

In an eyebrow, each line won't always be vertical: you may need to turn the client or your own body in order for the needle to vertically align with the hair it needs to create.

The hand will always perform the same, continuous movement; it is the surface on which it creates the lines that may change.

8.6. JUNCTURE POINTS

In many cases, the lines you'll draw will be relatively long (lines on the lips may reach 3-4cm): it is important for these lines not to appear fragmented and reveal the point at which movement paused. The most common error is to start a line, leave it, then pick it up again: doing this creates what are technically known as juncture points. Juncture points can be seen through an accumulation of color caused by the needle entering and exiting at the same point. To avoid creating juncture points, once a line is begun it should be continued as far as the professional can go, while reducing hand pressure: the needle will therefore leave the skin in a tapered off manner. Then, when picking the line back up, start 2-3 mm before the end of the line, and proceed in the opposite manner: using a light pressure at the beginning, then normal pressure until the most transparent point. The accumulation of the two faded lines will create the same color as the parts of the line created using constant pressure.

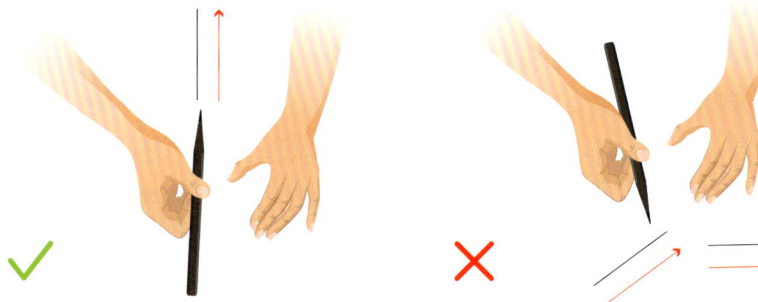

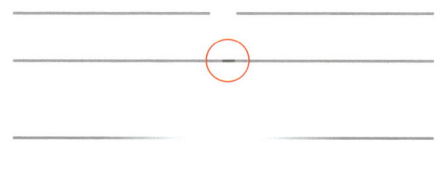

8.7. DRAWING A HAIR

The dermopigmentation professional's methods of observation are crucial in performing a procedure.
A macroscopic view of an eyebrow allows us to observe obvious elements like its shape and color. But the microscopic view is what allows professionals to register essential details.

Creating an eyebrow that is truly a "work of art" means perfecting the shape, the choice of pigment, and defining each individual hair as much as possible. A hair isn't just a line; it's a perfectly executed line.

A hair has a graphic shape (Fig. A):
• the first part, with a lighter color and tapered thickness;
• the center part, or shaft, with a deeper color and more thickness;
• the final part, which is more similar to the first in color and appearance.

Dividing it up likes this prevents us from perceiving it as a rigid entity that is uniformly thick throughout (Fig. B).

Don't even think about drawing a hair with a more pronounced area near the root, since the root is in the skin and therefore isn't visible (Fig. C).

Another common, major error is creating shaky lines by not achieving consistent depth (Fig. D).

To create a perfect hair, you must perfectly understand the histological aspect of the skin: only then can you predict what will happen inside the skin when the needle penetrates it and deposits pigment.

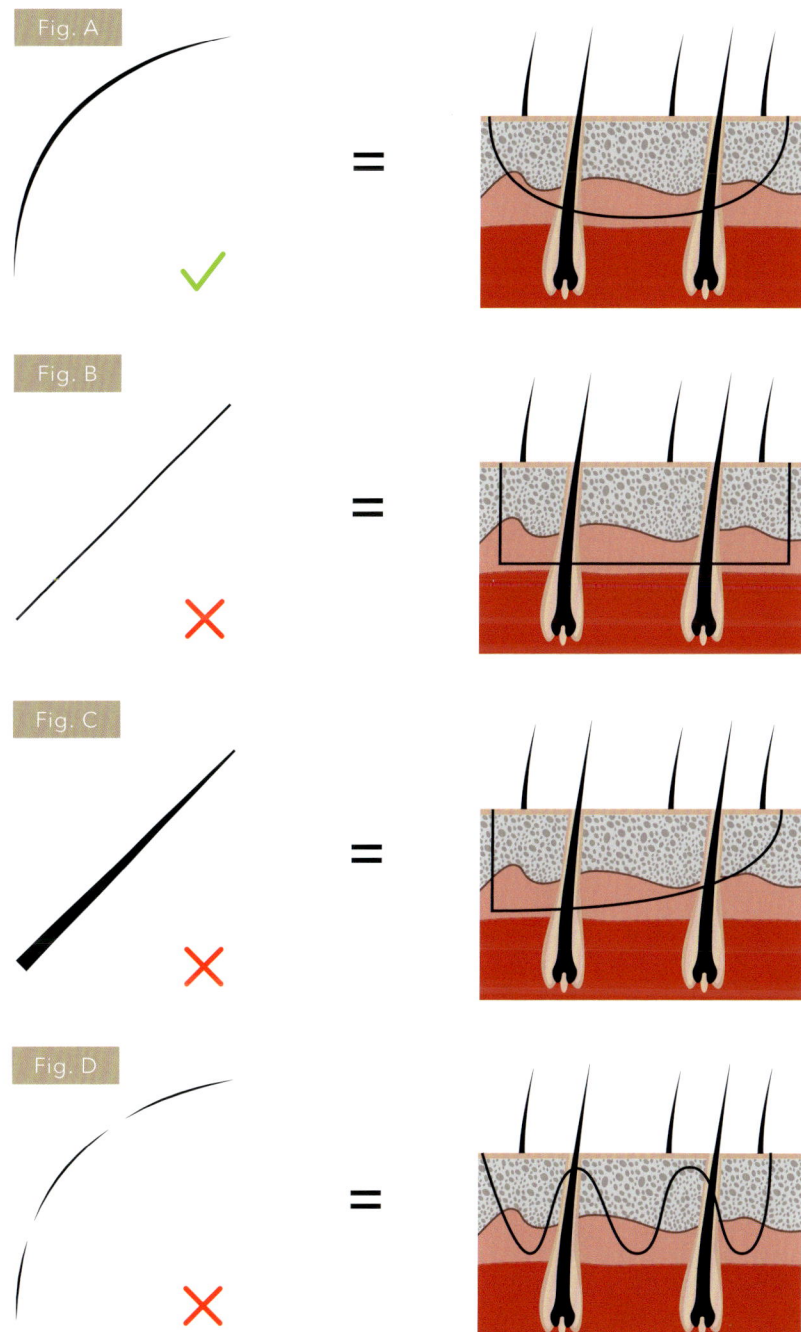

Look at Fig. E for how to perfectly create a hair: zones 1 and 3 are created using a unidirectional movement and tapering off pressure, zone 2 is created with a bidirectional movement with constant pressure in the dermis. Only by following this procedure can a hair be drawn realistically and blend in with the others.

Using very thin needles is crucial: it is usually best to use needles with a tip that is less than 0.20 mm in diameter. The needles used for hyperrealistic techniques have tips measuring 0.17 mm in diameter, to avoid structural changes in the color over time and allow the hair to maintain a constant appearance.

Don't be tempted to draw in hairs with 3-point needles because they seem easier to draw with. Within a few months, the hairs' appearance will change considerably because of the inevitable migration of the color, creating an unsightly increase in thickness as well as blurring in a way that compromises the initial look.

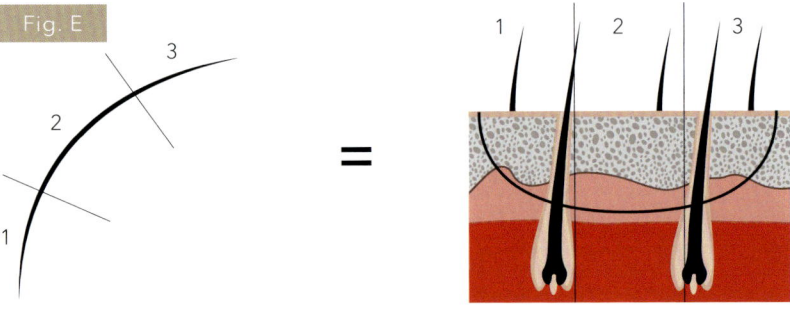

8.8. THE AIRPLANE TECHNIQUE

The motion of the hand is key in creating a hair. If we traced this movement, it would create shape very similar to that of an airplane's take-off and landing. The way the needle LANDS and TAKES-OFF shows us how to create the oblique parts while maintaining a constant depth in the dermis and completing the airplane's TAXIING down the runway.

Together, these movements and the take-off and landing patterns they create, produce an exciting, hyperrealistic eyebrow.

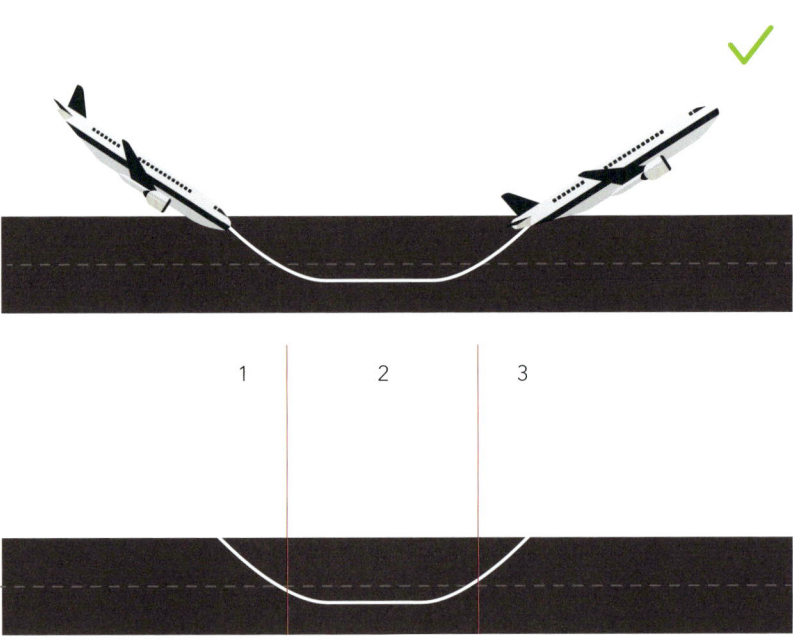

Moving the hand in a different way than described above could lead to an undesirable accumulation of pigment in the hair's start and end points, creating an unnatural effect.

To better understand which movements to avoid, we can picture the difference in take-off and landing between a helicopter and a plane: the helicopter moves straight up and down in a vertical manner. In permanent makeup, using the airplane movement for the needle deposits pigment evenly in the dermis, creating a hair that is uniformly thick in its entire length.

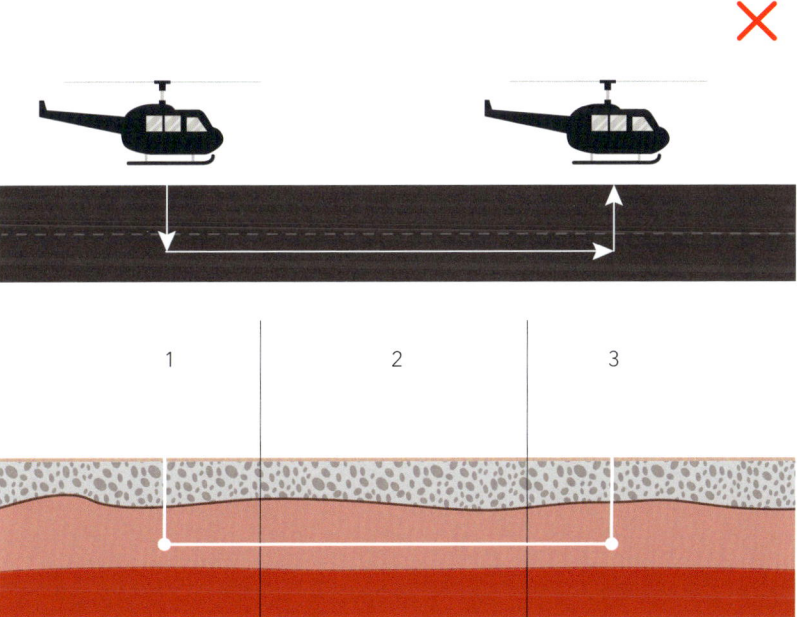

9

NEEDLE CLASSIFICATION

ROUND					FLAT					

LINER		SHADER		FLAT		MAGNUM		SLOPE	
NANO N[1]	o	3-POWER	⠿	4-FLAT	••••	5-MAGNUM	⠿	3-SLOPE	⫴
NANO N[2]	o	5-SHADER	⠿			9-MAGNUM	⠿	5-SLOPE	⫲⫲
NANO N[T]	⊙	5 -POWER	⠿					5-V.SLOPE	⫲⫲
1-MICRO	•	7-ROUND	⠿					10-DITTO	⫲⫲
1-LINER	•	7-POWER	⠿						
3-MICRO	⠿								
3-LINER	⠿								
3-OUTLINE	⠿								
5- ROUND	⠿								

Needles can be divided into two main families based on how they are welded.
- ROUND
- FLAT

ROUND needles are welded together in a circular manner, while FLAT needles are welded in a line. The welding can be done using silver or tin, depending on the quality of the needle. The shafts are made from surgical steel, as are the needles: at the end of the shaft is where the needles are welded.

The ROUND family can be further divided into two groups:
- ROUND liner
- ROUND shader

Liners are used to create lines and shaders are used for shading. The difference again comes from the welding. To create a liner needle, the needles are welded together more tightly so that the tips are so close together that upon entering the skin, they create a saturated line. In shader needles, the spacing is wider, so the needles can retain more color and release a more blurred,

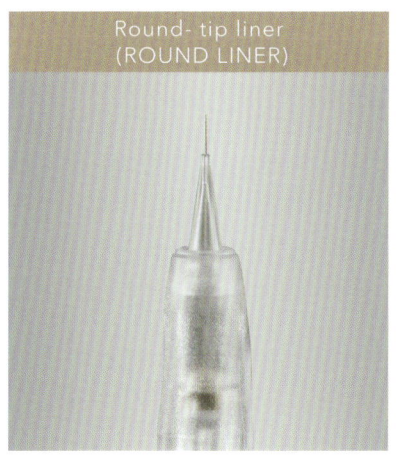

Round- tip liner
(ROUND LINER)

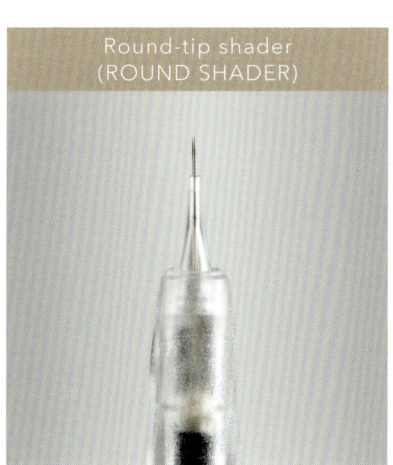

Round-tip shader
(ROUND SHADER)

less sharp line upon penetration. In addition to the needle name, a number (3, 5, or 7) indicates the number of needles welded together. So a liner needle for creating thin lines may have 3 tips, while a medium liner has 5, and a thick liner has 7 tips. Each needle has a body and a taper (or tip): the body is used for measuring the diameter of the needle while the taper forms the needle's final point. The diameter, multiplied by the number of needles, indicates the thickness of the line the needle will create. 3-Liner will create intense shading, while 5-Shader creates medium shading and 7-Round creates light shading. ROUND needles always have an odd number of needles in order to create a circle (1, 3, 5, 7).

The FLAT family can be further divided into groups:
- classic flat tip
- magnum
- soft
- slope

- Flats are generally used to create shading with different gradient effects. In the world of micropigmentation for the face, they take on various roles. They are used to create gloss effects on the lips, points of light, or three-dimensional effects in the eyebrows. Unlike magnums, they leave a more transparent mark; this is key in their use, since inserting them horizontally could create very defined lines as often occurs in the microblading specialization.
- Magnums on the other hand, are flat, superimposed needles. They always consist of an odd number of needles placed one above the other: the lower part contains more needles than the top.
- The slope is used to create more compact shading. This configuration creates three points with different levels of intensity since it consists of needles of different lengths, welded together obliquely in descending lengths.

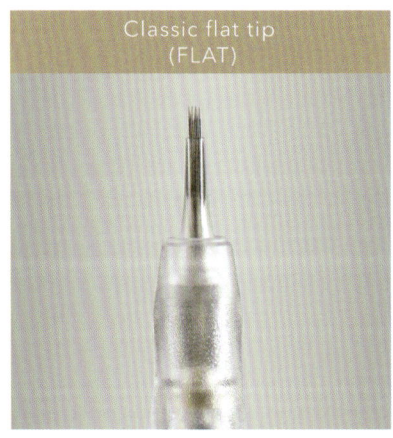
Classic flat tip (FLAT)

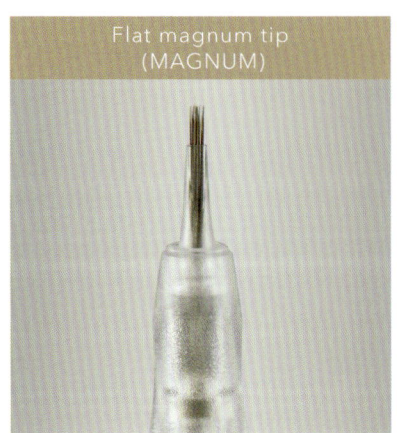
Flat magnum tip (MAGNUM)

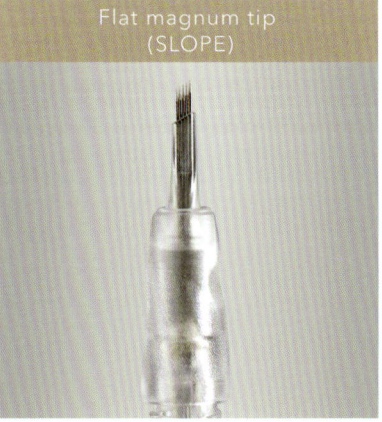
Flat magnum tip (SLOPE)

These needles are used to create gradient shading, in which more saturated parts are created by the longer needles and less saturated parts are created by the shorter ones. They are sometimes also used directly to create lines and hairstrokes, as with microblading. These needles have more saturation capacity than flats, since the double row of needles hold more pigment and don't leave transparent areas between each needle.

They are mainly used in procedures that require significant areas to be colored in, as with paramedical tattoos, for vitiligo, areola reconstruction, or creating a lipstick effect on the lips.

KEY

SPECIALIZATIONS

The following icons indicate the 4 areas of specialization within dermopigmentation, along with the descriptions of the needles and field of application.

- = PERMANENT MAKEUP
- = PARAMEDICAL TATTOOING
- = SCALP PIGMENTATION
- = BODY TATTOO

DIFFICULTY LEVEL

The icons describe the procedures that are best-suited for BEGINNERS (LOW) to ADVANCED PROFESSIONALS (MEDIUM) AND EXPERT PROFESSIONALS (HIGH).

- = LOW, recommended for beginners
- = MEDIUM, recommended for advanced professionals
- = HIGH, recommended for expert professionals

NEEDLES

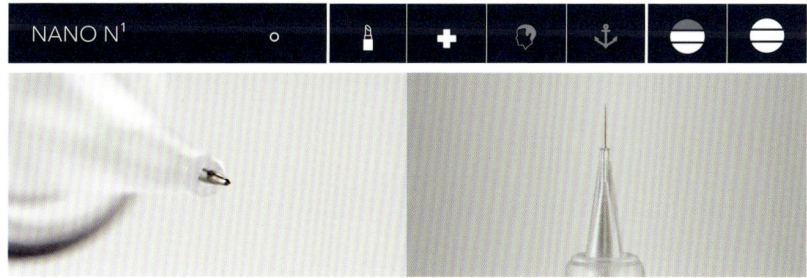

Procedure scope: precise, defined hairstrokes, precise contour of the lips, full lips, capillaries in areola procedure

Skin type: sensitive, dry skin types

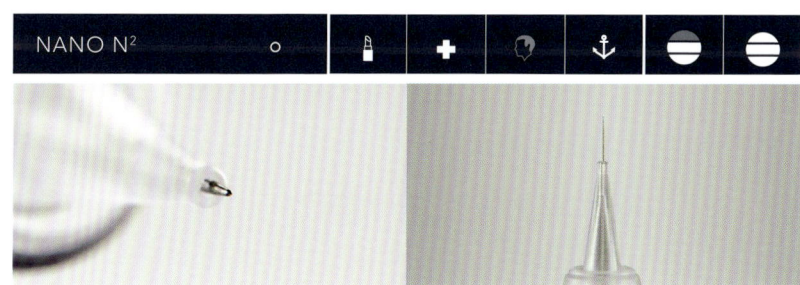

Procedure scope: fine hairstrokes, precise contour of the lips, full lips, capillaries in areola procedure, shading techniques

Skin type: combination/normal/oily skin types

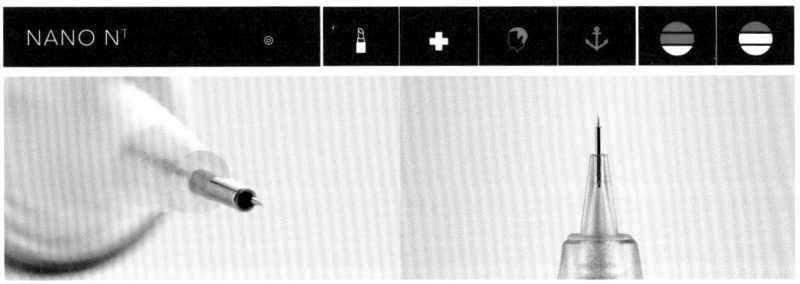

NANO Nᵀ

Procedure scope: precise, defined hairstrokes, precise contour of the lips, full lips, capillaries in areola procedure

Skin type: all skin types

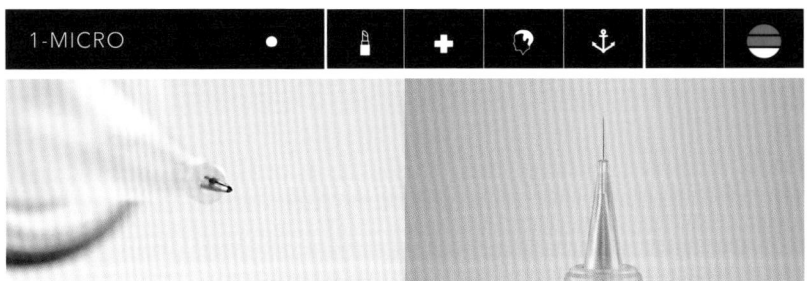

1-MICRO

Procedure scope: lip liner, eyeliner, shading techniques including full lips, lining techniques

Skin type: all skin types

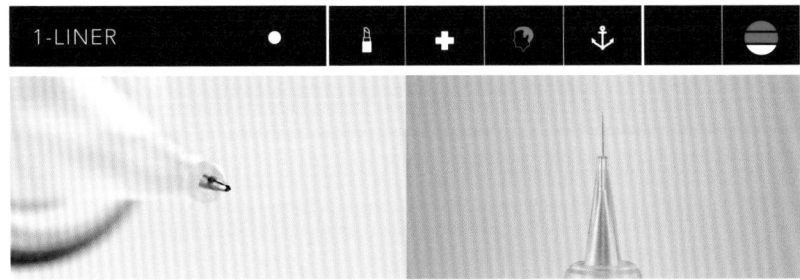

1-LINER

Procedure scope: eyeliner, eyebrow shading, lip smoothing contour and shading techniques

Skin type: all skin types

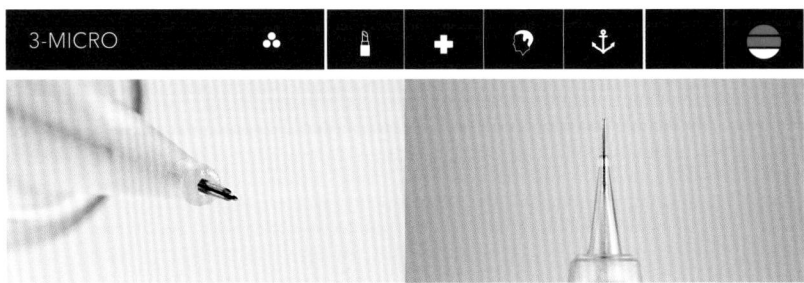

3-MICRO

Procedure scope: eyeliner, eyelash enhancement, eyeshading, eyebrow shading techniques, lip contour, full lips; areola, scars

Skin type: all skin types

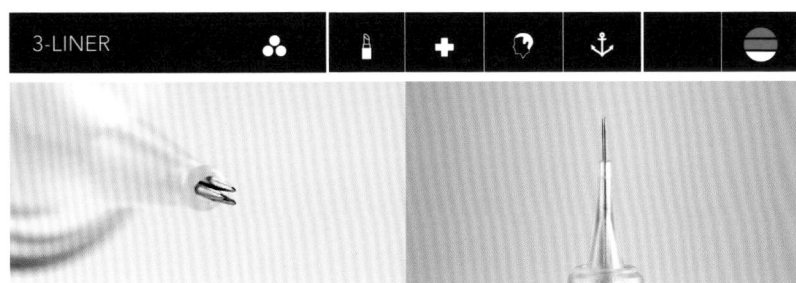

3-LINER

Procedure scope: thicker hair strokes, eyeliner, eyelash enhancement, lip contour, shading techniques, including full lips

Skin type: all skin types

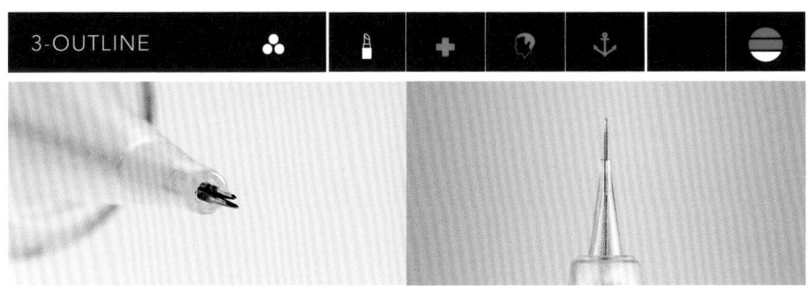

3-OUTLINE

Procedure scope: eyeliner, eyelash enhancement, eyebrow shading techniques, lip contour, full lips

Skin type: all skin types

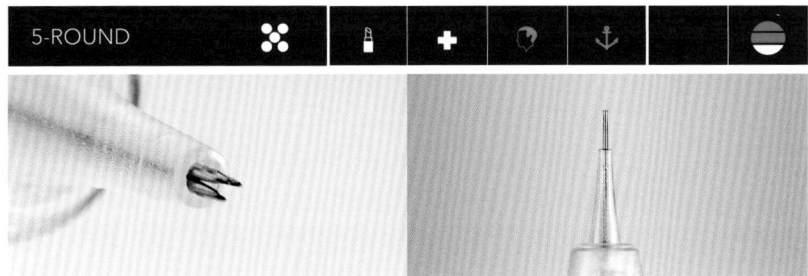

5-ROUND

Procedure scope: shading techniques in general, smooth not defined lines

Skin type: all skin types

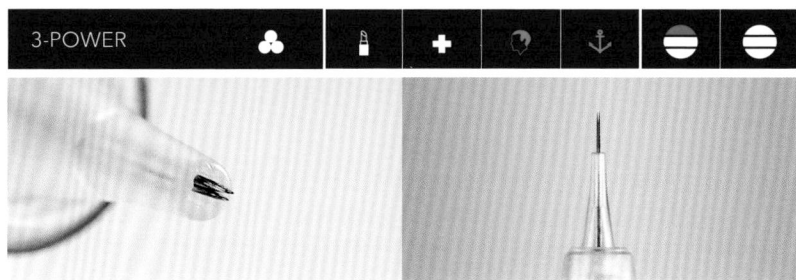

3-POWER

Procedure scope: eyeliner, eyelash enhancement, lip contour, full lips; areola, scars

Skin type: combination/normal/oily

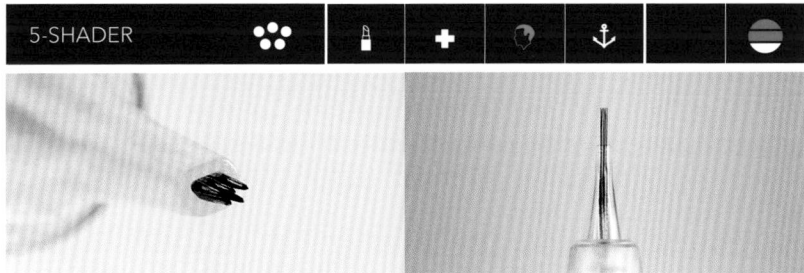

5-SHADER

Procedure scope: shading techniques in general in all areas

Skin type: all skin types

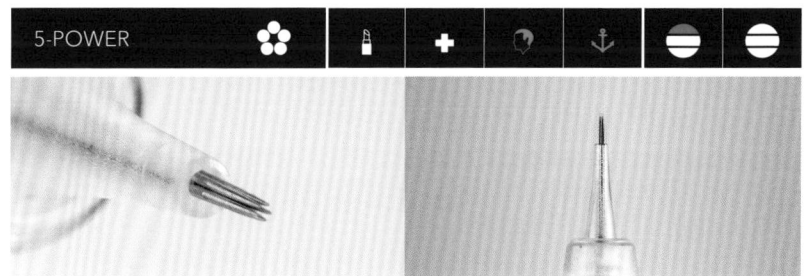

5-POWER

Procedure scope: shading techniques in general in all areas, especially body; lip contours

Skin type: all skin types

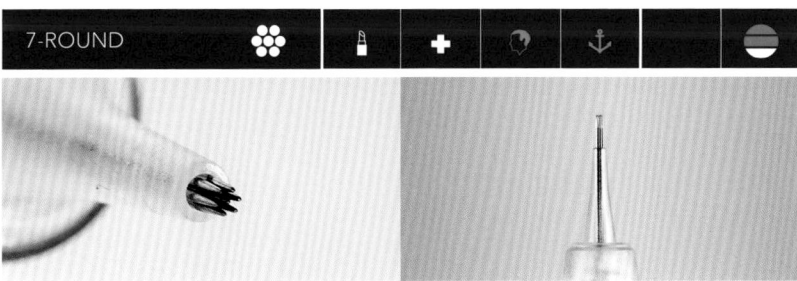

7-ROUND

Procedure scope: shading techniques in general in all areas, especially body

Skin type: all skin types

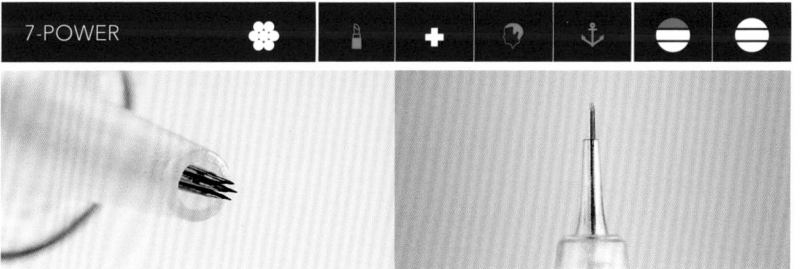

7-POWER

Procedure scope: shading techniques in general in all areas, especially body

Skin type: all skin types

4-FLAT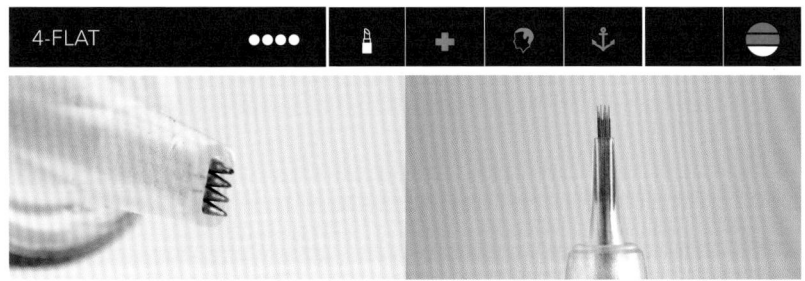

Procedure scope: eyebrow shading techniques, eyeliner, eyelash enhancement, eyeshadow, lip contour, full lips; areola

Skin type: all skin types

5-MAGNUM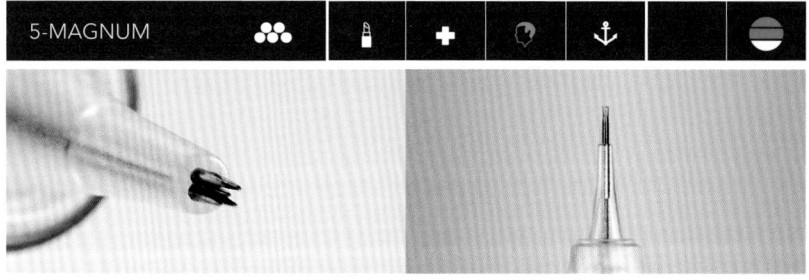

Procedure scope: shading techniques in general in all areas

Skin type: all skin types

9-MAGNUM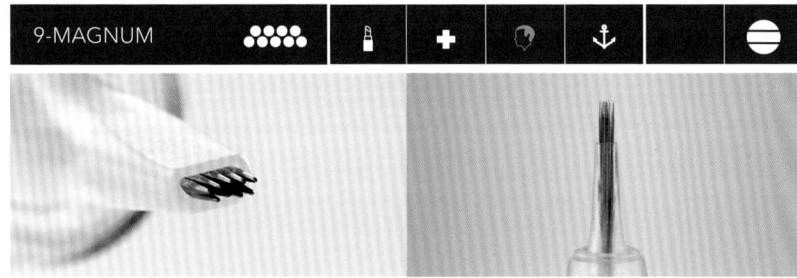

Procedure scope: shading techniques in general in all areas, especially for lips, areola, scars

Skin type: all skin types

3-SLOPE

Procedure scope: hairstrokes, eyebrow shading techniques, eyeliner, eyelash enhancement, eyeshadow, lip contour, full lips, areola

Skin type: all skin types

5-SLOPE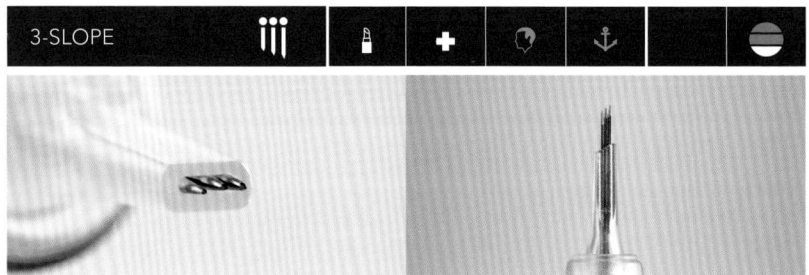

Procedure scope: shading techniques in general in all areas, contour lines

Skin type: all skin types

5-V.SLOPE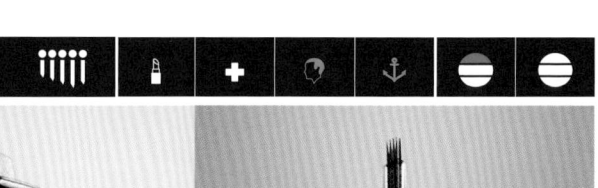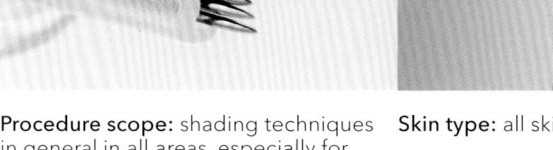

Procedure scope: shading techniques in general in all areas, especially for lips, areola, scars

Skin type: all skin types

144

10-DITTO

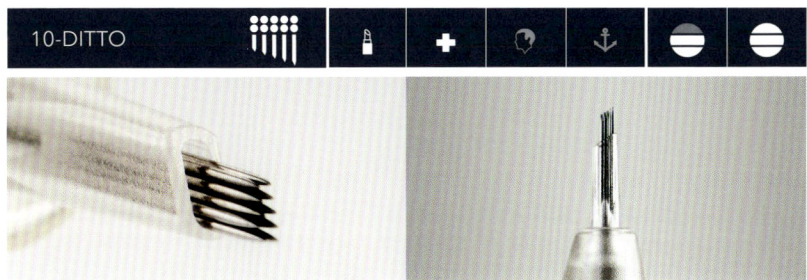

Procedure scope: shading techniques in general in all areas, especially for lips, areola, scars

Skin type: all skin types

10

COLORIMETRY VS THE SCIENCE OF PIGMENTS

"In color, I see the material's attempt at catching light." Plato

For painters, understanding the possibilities of color is of fundamental importance, since color is the basis for creating their works and expressing their ideas. When we talk about color, we talk about light, since without light there is no color to be seen.

The objects and environments around us are mostly colorful. Light is diffused through waves of different lengths, and each wave corresponds to a color.

Our eye only perceives a small fraction of the waves of light that exist in nature; the human eye only perceives a spectrum made up of seven colors: red, orange, yellow, green, blue, indigo, and violet.

Light waves have different lengths, and our perception of light depends on the length of the wave. A light wave with a length of around 750 nanometers (nm) may appear red. But if the light wave is 350 nm long, it will surely appear violet. If the light wave is between 350 and 750 nm, we will perceive one of the other colors.

10.1. HOW COLORS ARE PERCEIVED

It is said that the human eye distinguishes color based on the light, whether from the sun or artificial, which emits waves of lights of different wavelengths. The colors also change based on these lengths.

Think of the rainbow: you can clearly distinguish the seven colors that make it up because light waves generate them.

The different wavelengths also allow us to perceive the infinite colors of the chameleon in the image.

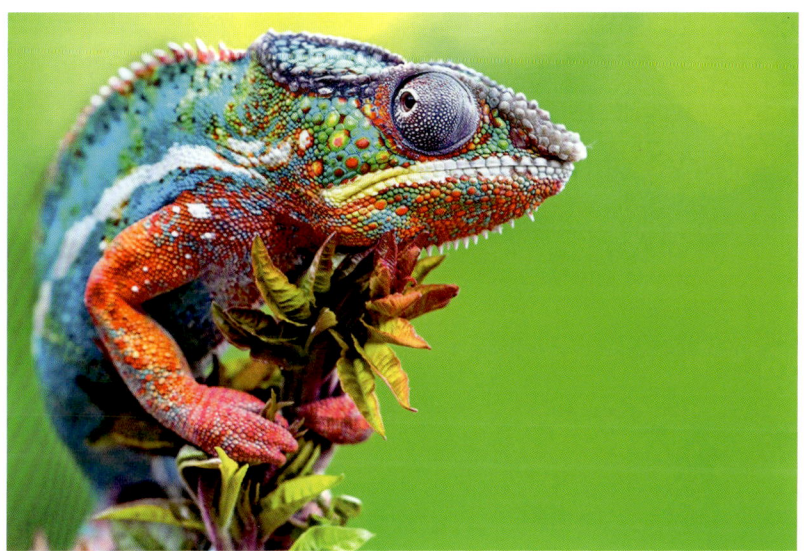

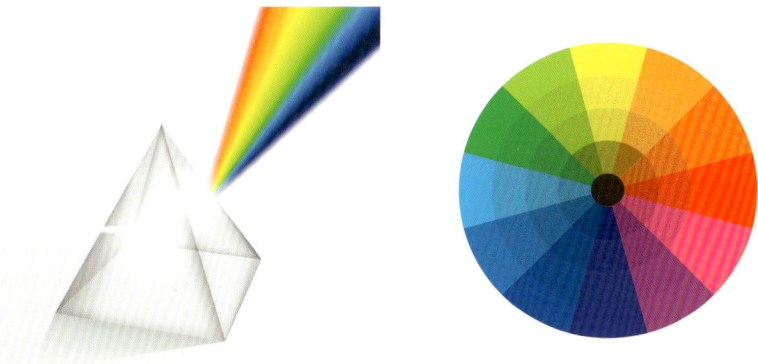

10.2. BLACK AND WHITE

It is wrong to consider black and white as colors by themselves.

Black is the color that completely absorbs light.

White is the color that reflects the most light, since it only absorbs a little bit of it. For a concrete example, think of a black car and a white car parked in a sunny parking lot: the black car will be hotter than the white car because it absorbs more waves of light.

Black is the absence of color, while white represents the sum of all colors.
So an object that reflects all wavelengths will appear white (white = sum of all colors); an object that absorbs all waves, without reflecting them appears black (black = absence of colors); an object that absorbs all waves except one has the color that corresponds to the single wave it does not absorb (for example, an object that does not absorb green appears green).

10.3. THE COLOR OF AN OBJECT

The color of a body is determined by the following factors:
- the actual color of the body;
- the color of its surrounding environment;
- the intensity of the light and its shadow;
- the color of the light;
- the type of light;
- the same color placed under a different light source takes on a different tone.

These two photos depict the same landscapes at different times of the day: the first is illuminated by the morning light, the second by a sunset.

In the first, the colors are generally cold, while in the second they are influenced by warm colors because of the light of the sunset.

To better understand the principles of sight, it is important to understand how light travels and how it behaves in the presence of an "obstacle".

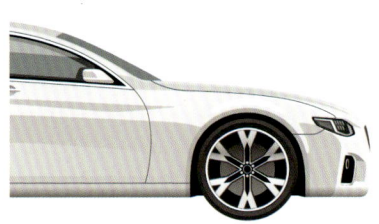
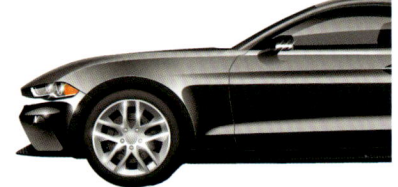

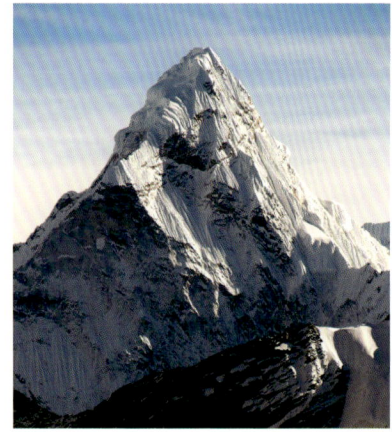
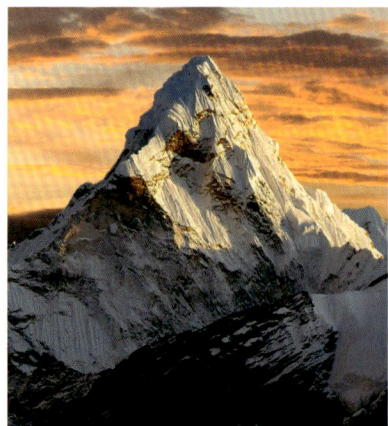

If it is unobstructed, light travels in a straight line. Just look at the shadows created by objects illuminated by a light source.

If the light sources are small, or seem small, the shadows will be more or less clear and their shape will reproduce the shape of the illuminated object. A pin light creates a perfectly clear shadow. Real-life light sources are generally larger, and this creates not only a shadow, but an area of semi-shadow whose size varies depending on the apparent dimensions of the light source and the distance between the object - the obstacle - and the surface on which the shadow is projected.

An object can be seen by the eye because the light that comes from it travels to the eye following a straight path. If this weren't the case, we would note, upon reaching out to grasp the object, that it wasn't where we saw it: light can deviate when it comes across an obstacle.

10.4. REFLECTION, DIFFUSION, REFRACTION, AND DISPERSION

When a beam of light coming from a light source hits a shiny surface, it "bounces back" in the opposite direction from whence it came. Another way of saying this is to say that incident light is reflected. This phenomenon is called light reflection (Fig. A).
Reflection follows two very precise laws:
- the angle of incidence is the same as the angle of reflection;
- the incident beam, the line running perpendicular to the point of incidence, and the reflected beam are all on the same plane, which is called the plane of incidence.

If instead of a mirror, however, we take an object with a rough surface, we won't see a beam of reflected light: instead we see diffused light. This phenomenon is called light diffusion (Fig. B).

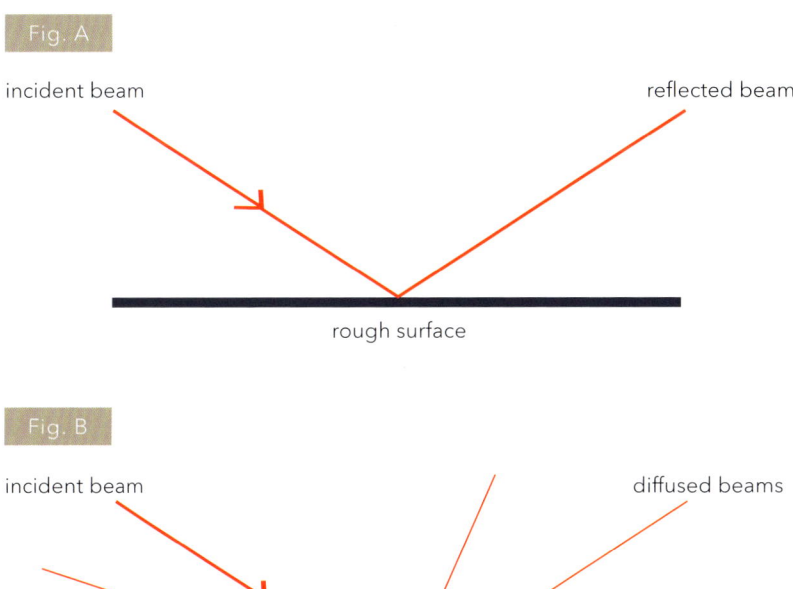

Fig. A

incident beam   reflected beam

rough surface

Fig. B

incident beam   diffused beams

diffused beams

rough surface

How does light behave when it is reflected by an object of macroscopic dimensions? If the surface of the object is smooth (for example, a mirror or a shiny metal surface), the reflection is mirror-like.

No real-life object perfectly reflects, perfectly diffuses, or perfect absorbs light; instead, these three phenomenons, reflection, diffusion, and absorption are present in varying degrees, at the same time. In particular, the amount of light reflected, whether mirrored or diffused, depends on the angle of incidence.

Refraction is the name of the phenomenon in which beams of light, passing from one means to another, deviate in their trajectory. When we look at a spoon immersed in a cup full of water, the spoon appears broken in two. This phenomenon is tied to that of refraction (Fig. C).

When a beam of white light undergoes refraction twice, upon entering and exiting a prism, it produces the phenomenon known as the "dispersion" of colors. If the prism's refraction index was constant for all colors, nothing in particular would happen. In reality, the refraction index changes (although slightly) from color to color.

Fig. C

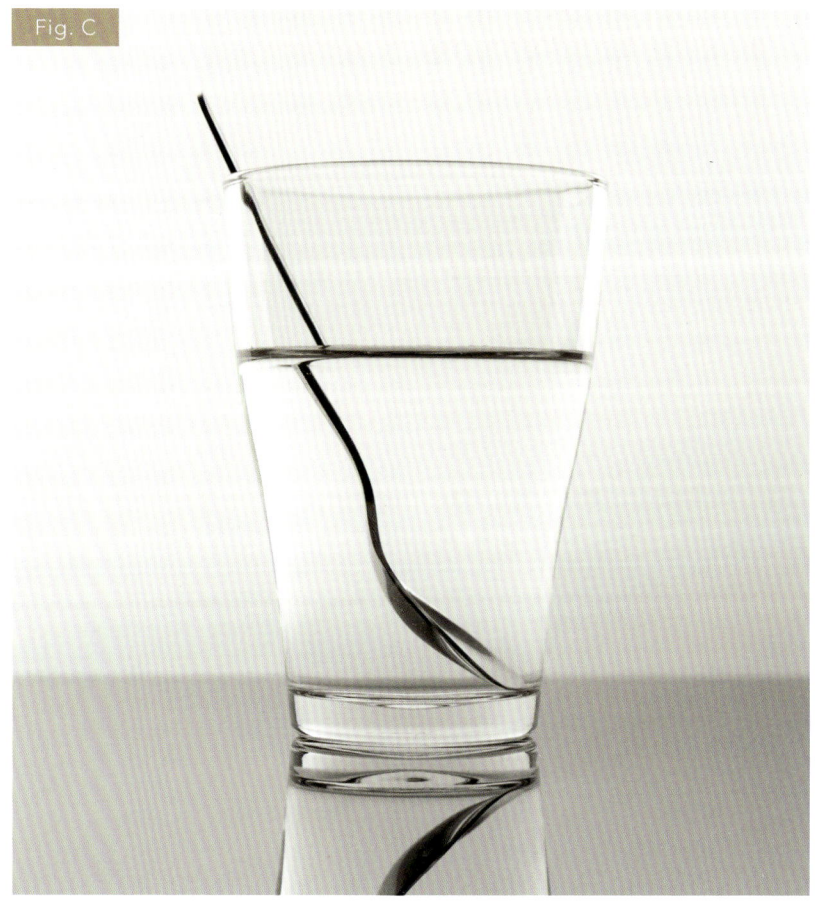

10.5. COLOR THEORY

Over the years, different researchers have focused on the science of pigment. Among these is Wilhelm Ostwald, who focused on a theory of subtractive color. The subtractive model can be verified by mixing pigments of different colors.

In Ostwald's theory, known as the "Ostwald Star", the three primary colors are yellow, magenta, and cyan, which will be referred to here more simply as YELLOW, RED, AND BLUE (Fig. A).
As shown in this figure, they are arranged along the points of an equilateral triangle (Fig. B).
Combining two primary colors, according to Ostwald, creates three other colors known as secondary colors (arranged at the points of another, upside-down, equilateral triangle). Adding blue and yellow creates green; red and yellow create orange, while blue and red create violet (Fig. C).
Ostwald continued by stating that combining a primary and secondary color resulted in a tertiary color, and so on. He also maintained that mixing equal parts of the three primary colors would result in a neutral brown (Fig. D).

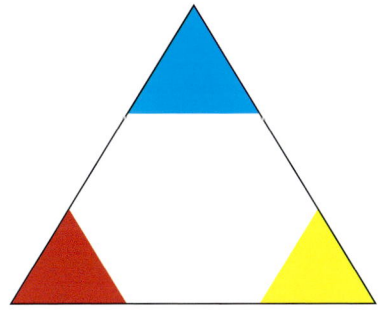

Fig. C

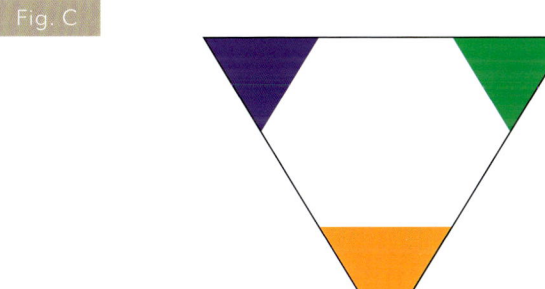

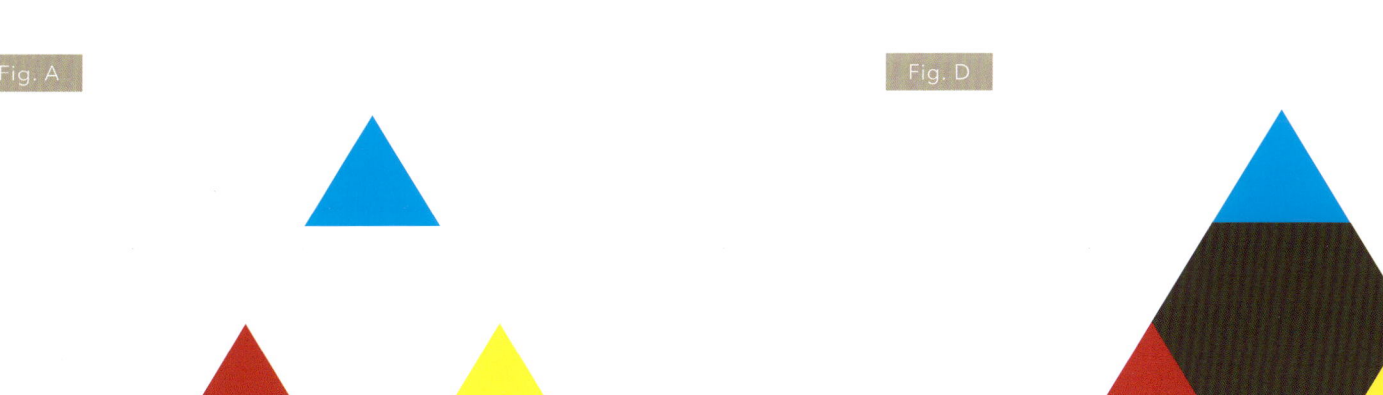

Neutral brown is also created by mixing the same quantities of secondary colors, since they are created by combining primary colors (Fig. E).

Black and white, which he defined as non-color colors, in addition to creating new colors, can be used to increase or decrease the luminosity of other colors, making them lighter or darker.

Fig. E

OSTWALD'S STAR

By combining the equilateral primary color triangle with the inverted secondary color triangle, we obtain the famous Ostwald Star (Fig. F). Unlike other color theories, this one offers an easy and quick way to understand the concepts of complementary colors and neutralization.

Two colors are said to be complementary when placing them next to each other makes them each seem enhanced and stronger. In Ostwald's Star, each tint's complementary color is located at the opposite vertex: red's complementary color is green, blue's complement is orange, and yellow's complement is purple.

Wearing a blue shirt with an orange tie, for example, sets off the colors of both garments, making them both seem brighter. In the same way, a tattoo artist who wants to highlight the blonde hair of a pin-up will place her against a background of purple flowers (Fig. G).

Two colors are said to neutralize each other if placing them on top of each other cancels them out. Referring back to Ostwald's Star, neutralizing colors are found diametrically opposed to each other, meaning they are also complementary colors. The difference is that while placing them next to each other makes them complementary, overlapping them makes them neutralize each other.

Fig. F

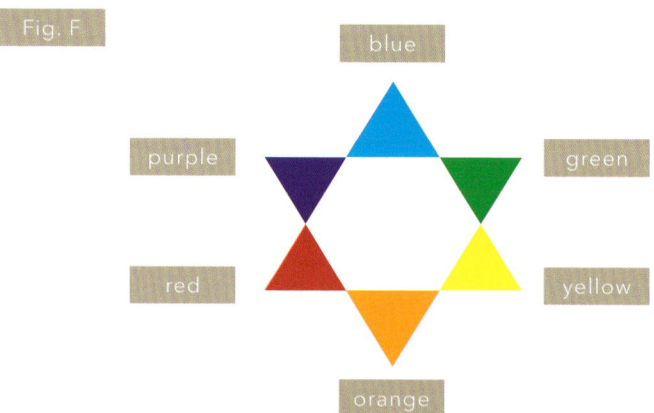

Fig. G

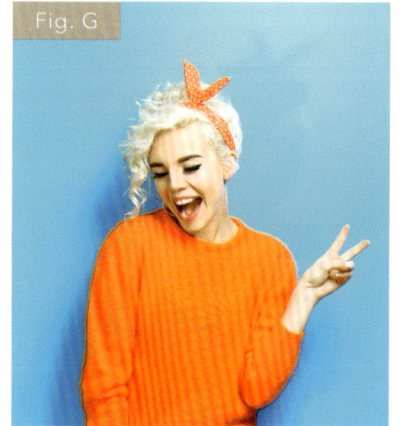

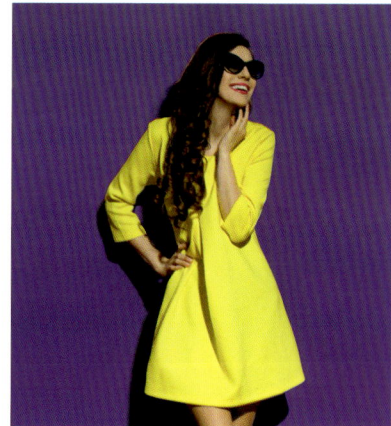

In fact, if you wanted to neutralize an unwanted red color to obtain a neutral brown, the color you would choose would be green, which is created by combining the primary colors blue and yellow.

In this way, the three primary colors would be combined to create brown (Fig. H).

One common task in permanent makeup is correcting prior work that was badly done in terms of color. A perfect understanding of this theory is necessary for solving these aesthetic problems (Fig. I).

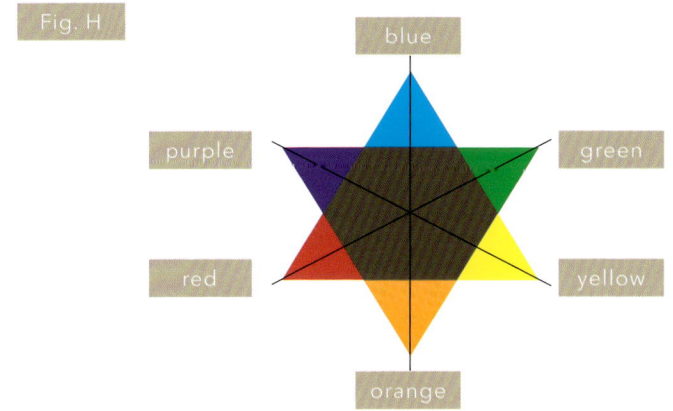

Fig. H

Fig. I

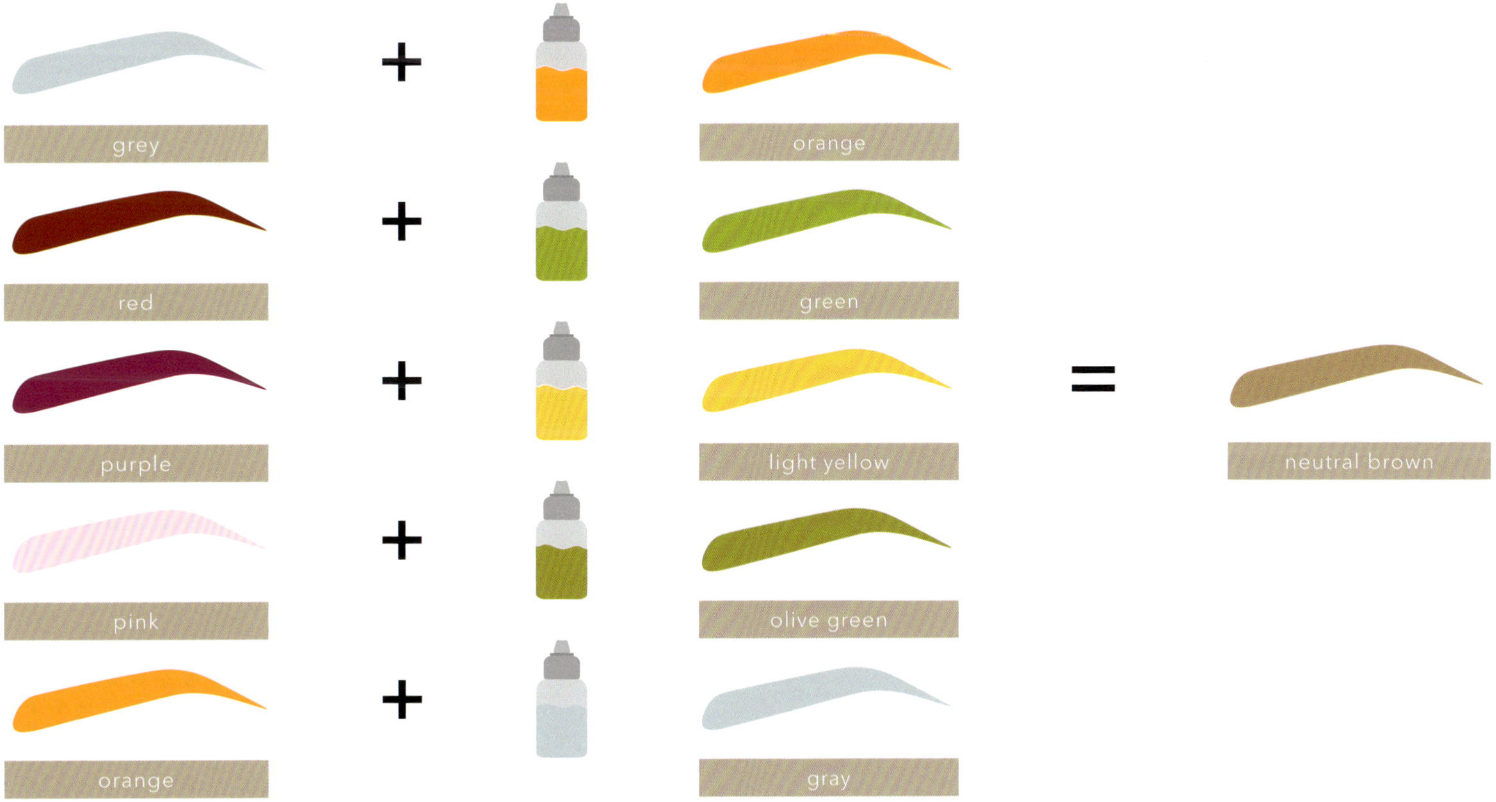

grey + orange =

red + green =

purple + light yellow = neutral brown

pink + olive green =

orange + gray =

TEMPERATURE

Don't undervalue an intrinsic feature of every color, which is that they transmit emotions! In fact, colors are also classified according to their "temperature" into "warm" and "cool" colors. Tracing a horizontal line divides Ostwald's Star into two parts: the upper part contains the cool colors, and the lower part contains the warm colors.

Warm colors are reminiscent of the light of the sun and fire: every shade of yellow, red, and orange, and on to the darkest tones of brown. Cool colors are the colors of ice, water, and the sky: green and blue shades.

This theory is extremely useful for professionals who apply color to a surface: for makeup artists who apply makeup to the skin, for example, to painters who apply acrylic to a canvas and so on. In dermopigmentation however, pigment isn't applied to a surface, in this case the skin, but is placed inside of it, more precisely in the dermis. For this reason, the principles of colorimetry are neither sufficient nor appropriate for permanent makeup. The science of pigment comes to the rescue for permanent makeup.

In the science of pigments, the primary colors are not blue, red, and yellow, but the following four colors:

- red
- black
- yellow
- white

Mixing these four colors creates a neutral brown, which can be made more or less intense based on the greater or lower percentage of each pigment.

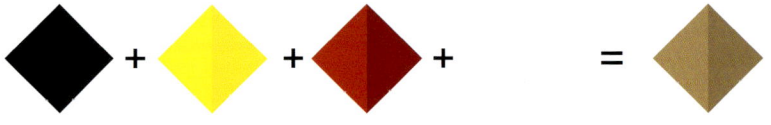

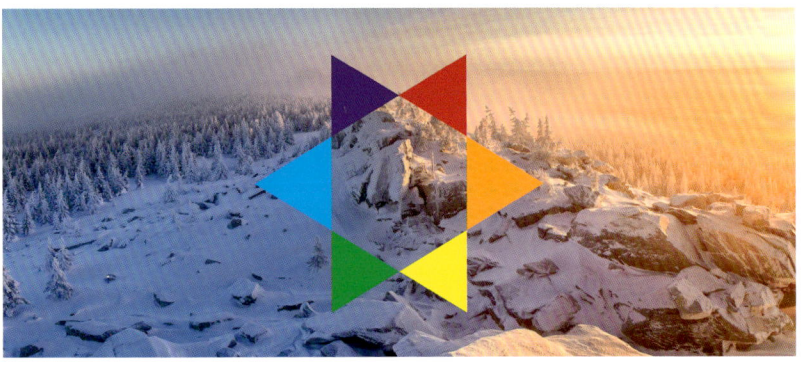

COLD COLORS

WARM COLORS

blue - purple - green

red - orange - yellow

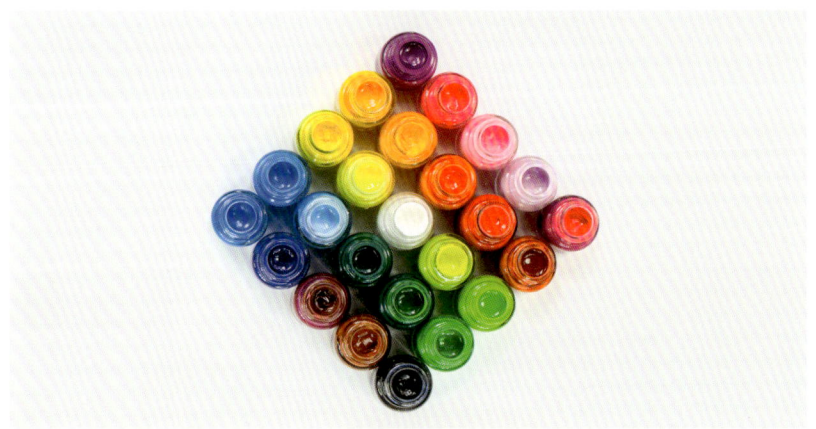

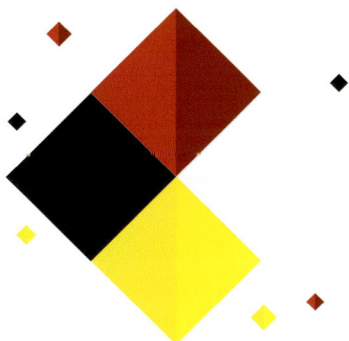

One obvious question is why there are four of them, and not three as in color theory. The answer is that pigment is inserted into the dermis, and therefore inside the skin, not applied to its surface. Accordingly, the skin's color is the result of a mix of four colors: red, black, white, and yellow.

The red color mainly comes from the blood. The hypodermis is irrigated by blood from the veins and arteries, while the dermis is irrigated only by small capillary vessels.

Combining black and white creates gray, which is the color of the stratum corneum, the outermost layer. A closer examination of pieces of exfoliated skin (for example, after burn) shows them to be gray: a basal cell loses a piece of its nucleus every day, until it turns into a corneal cell, a dead cell that is destined to be sloughed off through the skin's normal exfoliation.

The yellow color comes from melanin. Melanocytes are responsible for the production of melanin, which more specifically can be divided into eumelanin and pheomelanin. Eumelanin has a more true, yellowish color, while pheomelanin is brown in color. These two types of melanin are what differentiate, to different extents, the different skin type. Every skin color in the world is formed by

these four colors, in different proportions. Another reason for considering the science of pigment is that all of the pigments used in dermopigmentation are created by mixing different colored substances made from minerals, which are based on these four colors.

Just analyze the product sheets or color samples of every company in the world that produces pigments.

COMBINING COLORS

With these considerations in mind, we see why color theory does not apply to permanent makeup. According to Ostwald, black and white are not considered colors: in dermopigmentation, however, the opposite is true.

White and black are necessary pigments for creating all other pigments in nature. Like the three primary colors of color theory, combining the four colors of the science of pigments creates a neutral brown.

The difference is that mixing two of the four colors of the skin at a time does not create three secondary colors, but rather six bi-composed colors.

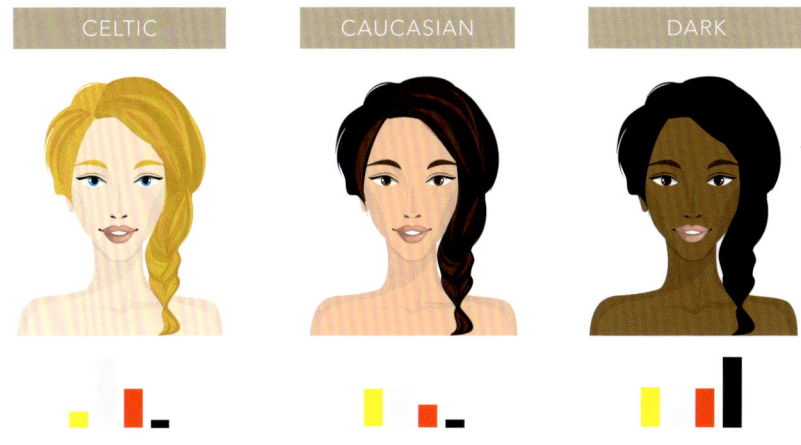

Black and yellow create olive green, black and white create gray, red and white form pink, black and red form a dark purple, red and yellow form orange, white and yellow form light yellow. Mixing three colors at a time creates 4 more colors known as three-part colors.

Black, yellow, and red create light chestnut; black, white, and yellow create green; black white, and red create light purple, and yellow, white, and red create orange.

And as explained above, mixing all four colors creates a four-part color: neutral brown.

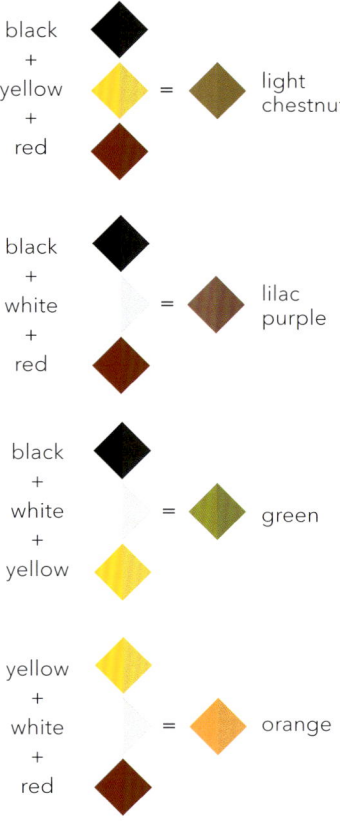

BI-COMPOSED

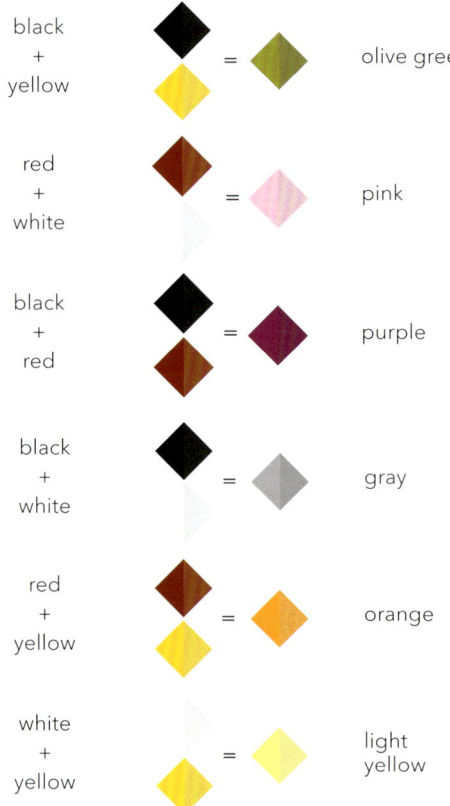

FOUR-PART

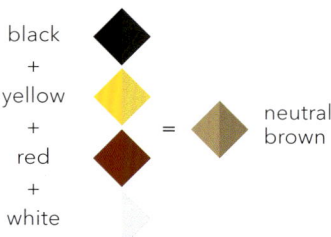

Mixing different proportions of the primary colors can create pigments with different temperatures. This diagram shows how lip colors can be made warmer or cooler based on differences in proportions, sometimes minimal, of primary colors, or by adding organic elements that add luminosity and shine. Any color can have different shades based on the different tonal values, while still maintaining the same temperature.

TEMPERATURE OF AMIEA EYEBROW AND LIP PIGMENTS

EYEBROW PIGMENTS

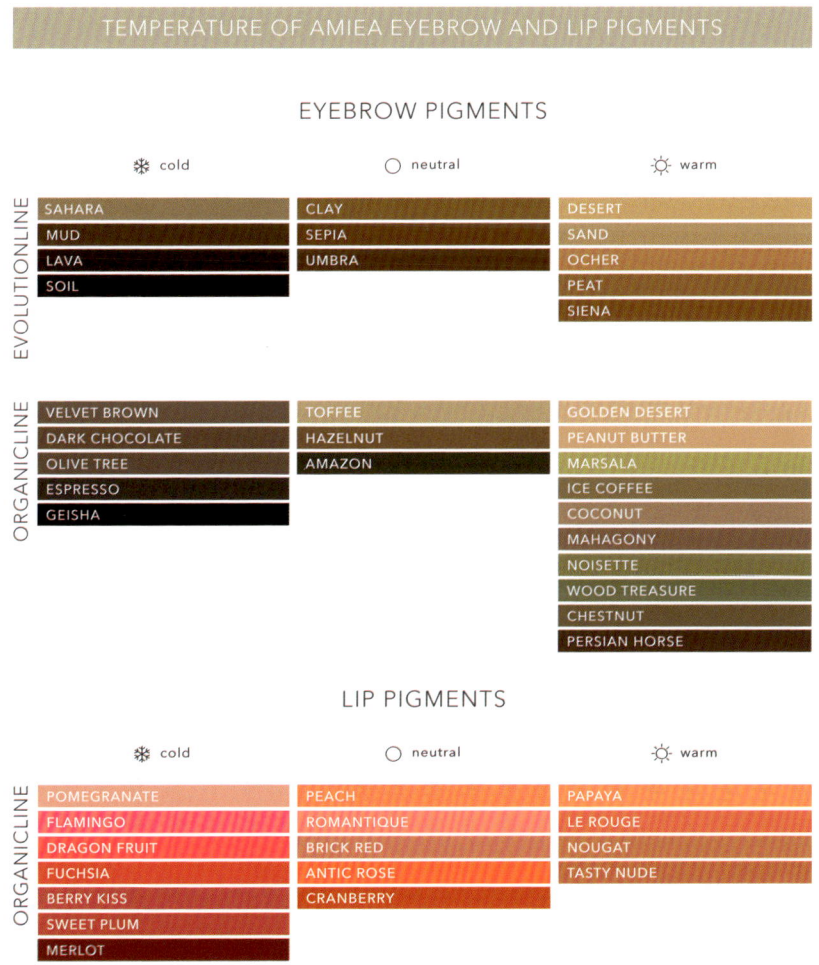

❄ cold   ○ neutral   ☀ warm

EVOLUTIONLINE

cold	neutral	warm
SAHARA	CLAY	DESERT
MUD	SEPIA	SAND
LAVA	UMBRA	OCHER
SOIL		PEAT
		SIENA

ORGANICLINE

cold	neutral	warm
VELVET BROWN	TOFFEE	GOLDEN DESERT
DARK CHOCOLATE	HAZELNUT	PEANUT BUTTER
OLIVE TREE	AMAZON	MARSALA
ESPRESSO		ICE COFFEE
GEISHA		COCONUT
		MAHAGONY
		NOISETTE
		WOOD TREASURE
		CHESTNUT
		PERSIAN HORSE

LIP PIGMENTS

❄ cold   ○ neutral   ☀ warm

ORGANICLINE

cold	neutral	warm
POMEGRANATE	PEACH	PAPAYA
FLAMINGO	ROMANTIQUE	LE ROUGE
DRAGON FRUIT	BRICK RED	NOUGAT
FUCHSIA	ANTIC ROSE	TASTY NUDE
BERRY KISS	CRANBERRY	
SWEET PLUM		
MERLOT		

11

THE CHEMISTRY OF PIGMENTS

An excellent micropigmentation professional should therefore have a perfect understanding of pigment theory while also understanding its chemical and physical basis. This includes the iron oxides, organic, and synthetic pigments within a product and how they affect its stability, duration, color changes, and structure.

Most pigments are synthetic. Both organic pigments and iron oxides, for example, carbon black, titanium dioxide, etc., are made in an industrial process. We do not use iron oxides from natural sources because of higher impurities.

From a purely chemical perspective, it is good to add green to the four colors of the skin since almost all preparations for eyebrows (except for very dark colors) use a small proportion of green. That's because green, or chromium oxide, neutralizes the red ferric oxide.

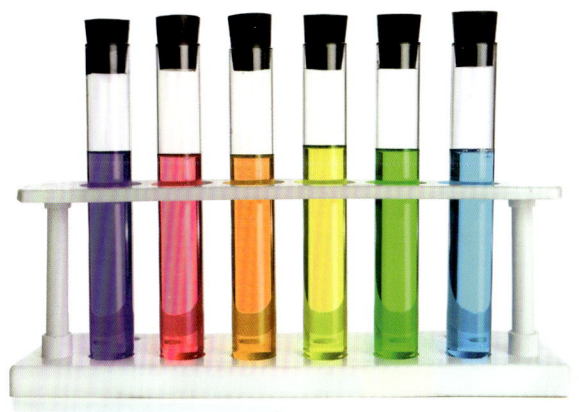

Here are the chemical sources of the colors:
- titanium dioxide makes WHITE;
- chromium oxide makes GREEN;
- ferric oxide makes YELLOW, RED, and BLACK depending on different states of oxidation and preparations. Ferric oxides comprise many inorganic pigments. Typically, Fe(II) pigments are black or dark gray, while Fe(III) are rusty red. More complex oxide compositions (hydroxides, hydrates, oxygen hydroxides) can have different color variations (yellows, reds, browns, and oranges).

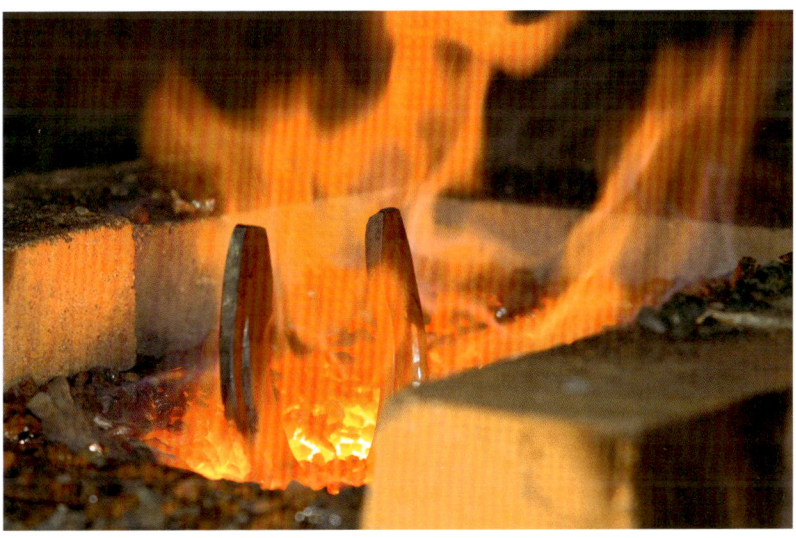

FERRIC OXIDE TRANSFORMED IN SPECIAL OVENS WITH TEMPERATURES REACHING 1,200° CELSIUS.

11.1. INORGANIC, ORGANIC, AND MIXED PIGMENTS

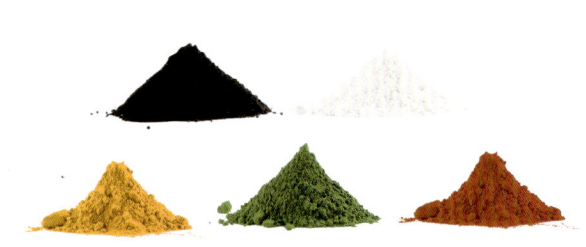

INORGANIC PIGMENTS
Black c. i. 77499; Red c. i. 77491; Yellow c. i. 77492; Green c.i. 77288; White c.i. 7789

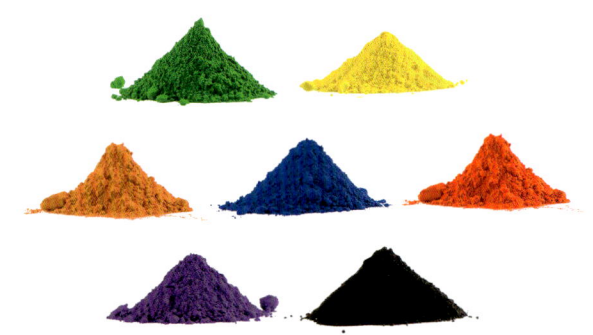

ORGANIC PIGMENTS
Black c.i. 77266; Yellow c.i. 56300; Red c.i. 65300 and c.i. 56110; Blue c.i. 69800

Colors are made up of a functional principle, an excipient, and an additive.

Because they are produced through precipitation or suspension, pigments are classified into:
- inorganic pigments;
- organic pigments.

The term inorganic means that the pigment is a mineral, usually an oxide or a sulphide of one or more metals, or of transition metals. The term organic means that the pigment is a molecule made up of carbon atoms combined with hydrogen, nitrogen, and oxygen atoms.

Both inorganic pigments and organic pigments can be either natural or synthetic:
- the term natural means that the pigment molecule is extracted from a mineral, plant, or animal source that exists in nature;
- the term synthetic means that the pigment molecule is assembled and also significantly modified using an industrial chemical process.

From this distinction, we can understand that there are both natural and synthetic inorganic pigments.
- natural inorganic pigments are metals or rare earths extracted from natural mineral deposits. With a few exceptions, these natural inorganic pigments are no longer used, since their extraction is expensive and does not produce satisfactory consistency in the colors;
- synthetic inorganic pigments, on the other hand, are industrially prepared raw minerals and make up 80% of pigment production worldwide.

In the same way, we can also distinguish between natural and synthetic organic pigments:
- natural organic pigments are extracted from plants or animal sources. With a few exceptions, these pigments are rarely used in PMU colors, because they are not safe enough;
- synthetic organic pigments are prepared from petroleum compounds, which mimic the chemistry of plant- and animal-based colors.

In permanent makeup, it is important to understand the technical characteristics of these two pigments: inorganic pigments are very opaque, but less luminous and brilliant. Just think of the color of a very dull, almost brownish red ferric oxide compared to an organic red that is very bright and brilliant. Organic pigments are less opaque, but very luminous, and are generally used for lip colors or for paramedical tattoos where brilliance is very important.

The latest generation of pigments is made from a mix of inorganic and organic substances, resulting in the following, hybrid characteristics:

	Inorganic pigments	Organic pigments	Organic and inorganic pigments
Results	Full-coverage	Transparent	Semi-transparent
	Opaque	Bright and intense	Semi-opaque
	Not very bright	Bright	Semi-bright
	Stable	Unstable	Semi-stable
	Not brilliant	Brilliant	Semi-brilliant

The effects of inorganic pigments are well known: once the most appropriate color for the client's skin is chosen, as well as the type of technique to be used and the correct pressure, and a profound understanding of the chemistry of the contents is present, it can safely be determined how the inorganic pigment will change over 6 months, a year, or longer.

The pigment's molecular structure is a key factor here.

For permanent makeup colors, it is best for the molecules to be less than 15 microns in size, so that they can be pushed into the skin more easily, and are less permanent.

Consider the immune system and especially the macrophage, whose process of phagocitation allows it to more easily digest and eliminate a molecule that is 7 microns large compared to one that is 40 microns large.

Imagine how Pacman can eat a ham sandwich in just a few minutes, while a loaf stuffed with 1kg of ham would take longer. The micronization of these molecules means the procedure won't last as long, but this shouldn't be seen as a negative: rather, it is a guarantee of how the colors and lines will behave over time.

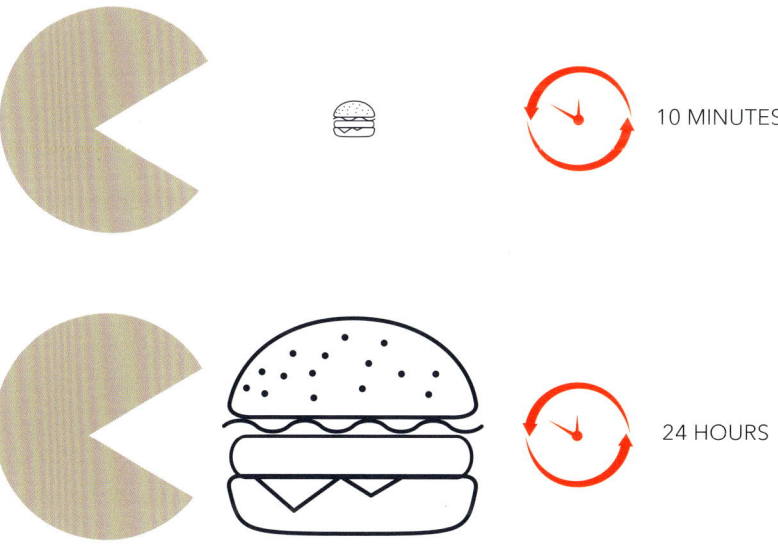

11.2. BIOABSORBATION OF PERMANENT MAKEUP PIGMENTS

Pigments will be swallowed by macrophages and will eventually disappear over an indefinite period of time.

Possible color changes over time:

· any pigment oxidizes upon contact with sunlight or artificial light, and will change color;
· structural changes: pigment inserted into the skin will expand, even if only very slightly, so that a very thin hair becomes much thicker over the course of a few months;
· anatomical changes: over the years, a face's elasticity changes as gravity pulls everything downwards, changing a shape that no longer suits this new anatomical state;
· color modifications: the need to change the color of a previous procedure, maybe because the client has aged or because fashion continuously evolves.

The speed at which the pigments are eliminated by the macrophages varies, and can't always be defined because there are so many variables, but depending on the conditions of the procedure this can take between 5 and 36 months. The duration depends on different factors: age (cellular regeneration takes place more quickly in young people), exposure to sunlight, individual scarring outcomes, the chosen application techniques and chemical composition of the pigment used.

11.3. PIGMENT STABILITY

• extremely stable:
 titanium dioxide

• very stable:
 red ferric oxide
 chromium oxide

• unstable:
 black ferric oxide
 yellow ferric oxide

different speed in bio absorbation

IMMEDIATELY AFTER MICROPIGMENTATION				
white	red	yellow	black	green

AFTER A FEW MONTHS				
white	red	yellow	black	green

Problems often arise from the color's ability to change over time. This is because some pigment molecules are more stable than others.

White (titanium dioxide TiO_2) is extremely stable.
Green (chromium oxide CrO_2) and red (ferric oxide Fe_2O_3) are very stable.
Black (ferric oxide Fe_3O_4) is stable.
Yellow (ferric oxide $Fe_2O_3 * H_2O$) is not stable.

It is very important to understand this, as it will help us understand why sometimes, 6/8 months after inserting a chestnut brown pigment the color changes and takes on undesirable red or gray tones.

Here is an example that will make this clear. Take a medium chestnut brown.

Composition: 1 ball of white, 2 balls of red, 4 balls of yellow, 3 balls of black, and 1 ball of green.

Phagocytosis process: the macrophage begins eating the pigments, starting with the least stable: the first two to disappear will be the two yellow balls, followed by the two black balls; the red and the green will disappear more or less at the same time, then the black and yellow, and white goes last. If the molecules aren't compensated for within a pigment to maintain a stable equilibrium, the color will change. And even though certain pigments are created with the intention of being warmer or cooler, it is up to the professional to understand these characteristics and use them appropriately.

11.4. DESCRIBING THE PIGMENT

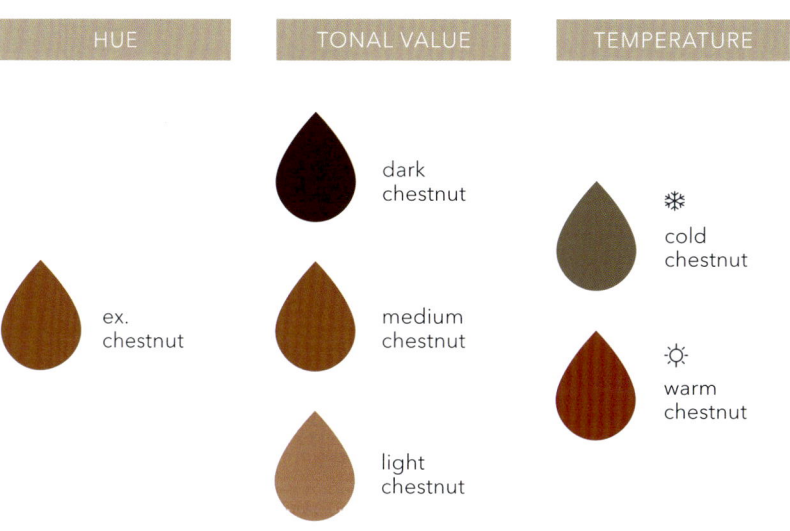

A pigment can be described using different characteristics to allow a shared means for dermopigmentation professionals to communicate clearly.

- Color or hue gives the pigment its name by describing the combination of the four primary colors.
- Tonal value is the different gradient of the hue. The tonal value changes luminosity using white or black. Adding white lightens the color, while adding black darkens it.
- Temperature: colors can be warm or cool. In the skin, a warm color has a higher proportion of red, while a cool color has more gray or yellow.

11.5. CHOOSING THE PIGMENT

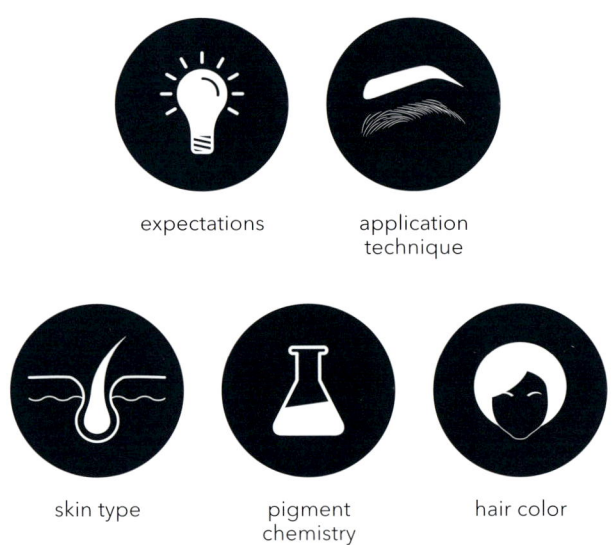

expectations   application technique

skin type   pigment chemistry   hair color

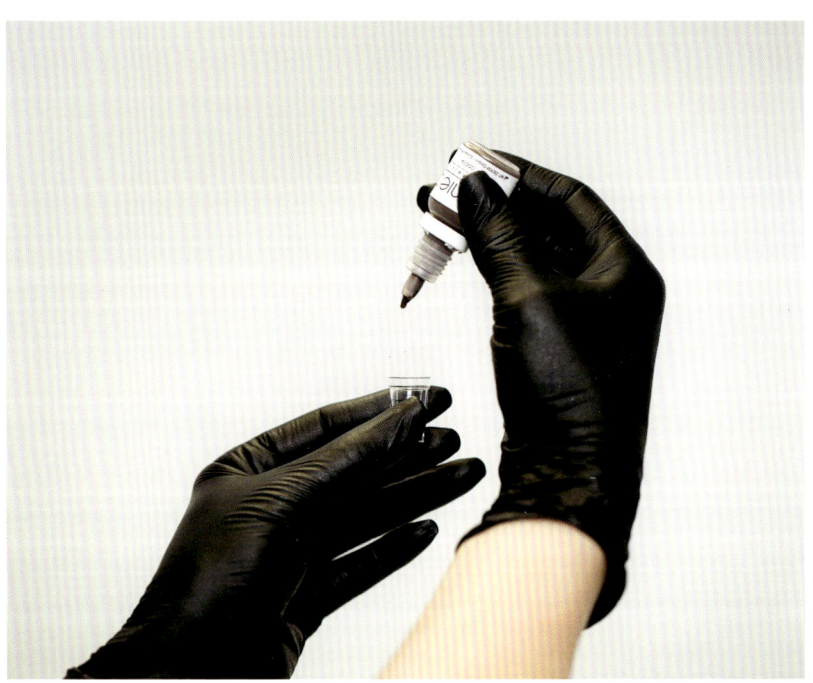

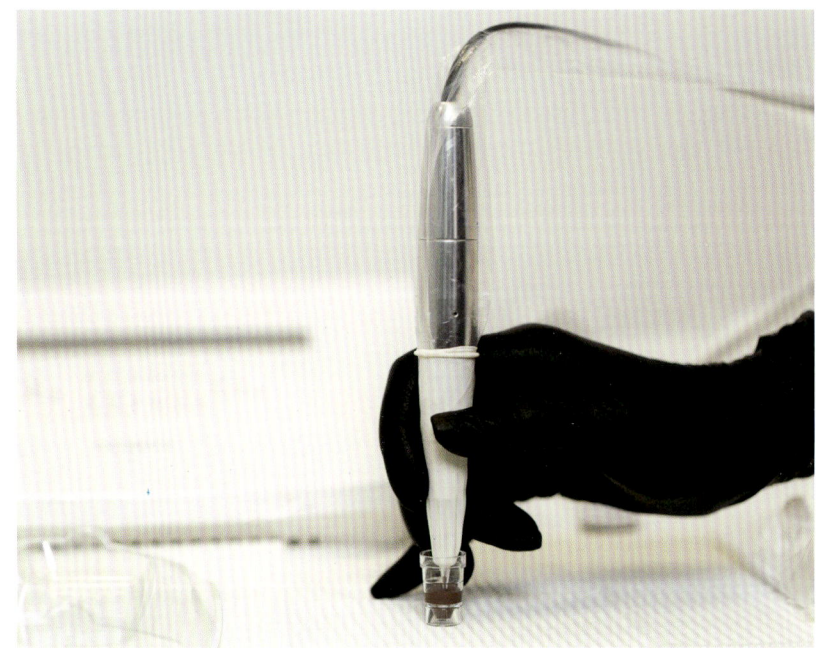

Different factors influence the choice of color:

- The client's wishes and preference.
- The application technique (depending on the application technique, the color can be more or less intense at the end of the procedure. A lighter application will always be more transparent than an opaque application that saturates the area more fully).
- Chemical composition of the pigment.
- Skin type (phototype, temperature, oily or dry).
- Natural hair/eyebrow color (for eyebrows, for example, the perception of the color can change or be influenced by the amount of hairs themselves).

Once you have chosen your pigment based on the information above, pour it into mono-use, ideally sterile containers. If you are mixing several colors, a mixer allows the colorant substances to be combined effectively and make them ready for use. At this point, turn on the handpiece and let it suck up pigment. Pay careful attention to prevent the needle from touching the bottom of the container, which may dull the needle tip and lead to imprecise lines during dermopigmentation.

FIND THE RIGHT COLOR ONLINE

Discover our Online Color Finder for your client's most personalized range of colors.

www.color.amiea.com

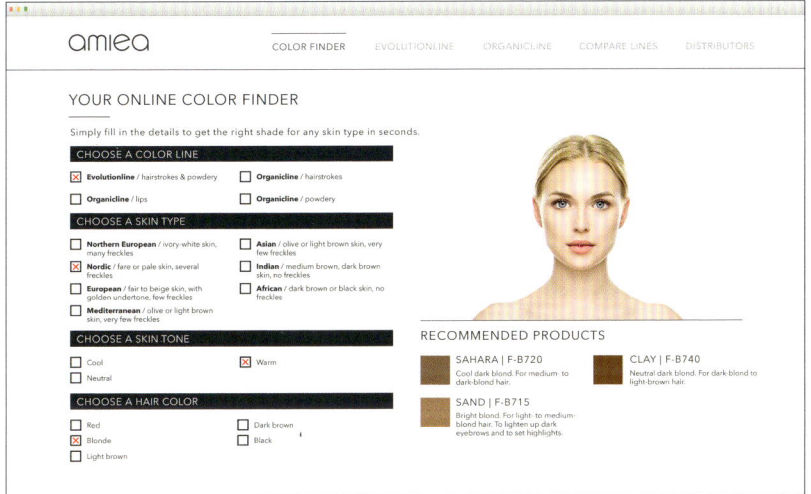

SELECT THE PERFECT COLOR

Find the right tone for the most personalized result with our Color Guide. Determine each client's skin type and skin tone. On the back of the color cards you'll find an additional description of your target tone and the suitable application areas. In the mixture section, you'll find out which pigments the color consists of and their quantity.

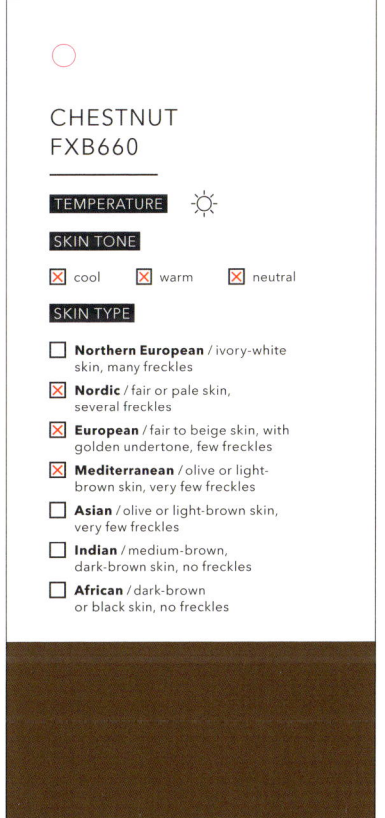

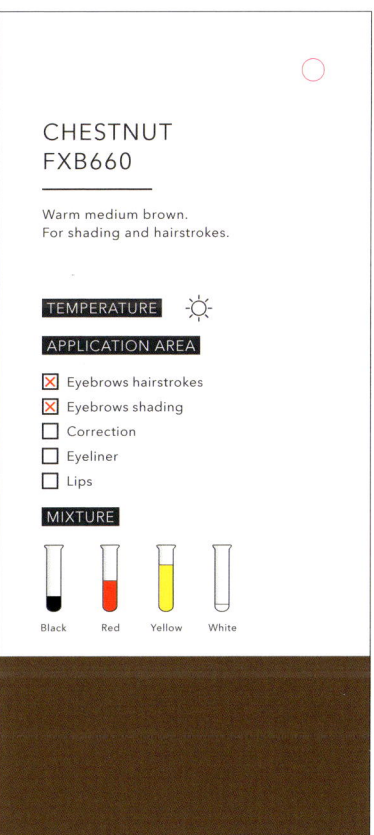

12

AN EFFECTIVE CONSULTATION

12.1 TECHNICAL AND COMMERCIAL ACTIVITIES

Today, taking care of our bodies has taken on great importance in our society. The power of the media and economic opportunities mean that self-care and caring for one's appearance are no longer self-absorbed behaviors or a frivolous practice reserved for a few elites.

We focus on improving our image to feel better about ourselves, to feel more confident in interpersonal relations, or just to make ourselves happy.

Even gender barriers have come down; solutions that used to be mainly aimed at an entirely female clientele are now available to both men and women, who share equally in this general process of self-improvement regardless of age, social class, or profession.

It is clear that any discourse on dermopigmentation centers around the client, since it concerns their appearance and the weight of their decision. In fact, the entire aesthetic process starts with the potential client.

All of the debates concerning the various aspects of dermo-pigmentation can be analyzed, explored, and resolved, without omitting any detail.

In fact, even in developing countries, the trends in face and body care have been steadily moving towards this kind of aesthetic procedure.

Women, who used to be the only target group for dermo-pigmentation, are now treated alongside men, who are now much more open to aesthetic solutions and also constitute potential clients. In the past, dermopigmentation only appealed to a certain group of people, mostly women aged 40 to 50, but these days we see two main age groups: the first, between 20 and 40 years old and including both men and women, seeks dermopigmentation for reasons based on fashion or cultural identity, rather than for any aesthetic necessity; the second group, between 50 and 80 years old, seeks to recover a more youthful appearance, with more defined and pronounced facial (or body) features.

12.2. THE RESULT

As demand increases, permanent makeup must respond to the many questions of clients who expect safe, correct, and long-lasting results. Safe results mean that the professional guarantees all of the preventative measures used to protect the client's health. Dermopigmentation and tattoo procedures, in fact, carry health risks as they can transmit diseases or can cause undesirable effects such as nasty scars and bacterial infections.

Correct results achieve harmony between the client's original appearance and the new appearance created through the procedure. In other words, aesthetic changes should be used to correct, not overthrow, the fundamental aspects of their appearance. Long-lasting results mean the procedure's effects don't fade quickly. This perspective emphasizes the quality of the products used in micropigmentation. That means making sure there are no harmful substances in the products we use, to avoid any possible health risks.

In addition to results, which generally represent the clients' most pressing expectations, there are two other fundamental elements to consider.

The first concerns the professional, who should possess all of the requirements for working in the field of dermopigmentation. Although they are not doctors, they should hold official documentation certifying and attesting to their professional level. Other fundamental elements concern the place in which the appointments take place and the equipment used for the procedures. This means the professional, the place, and the products used all become factors which the client considers in making their choice, and guarantee a safe and satisfactory aesthetic procedure.

12.3. MOTIVES

Every client makes an appointment for different reasons, and their requests should be considered with the utmost attention. Professionals should learn to get to know their clients, and to "grasp" their personality.

Of course, during the observation phase, the professional will certainly notice the emotions that characterize the client, and reveal their confusions or fear or make up their personality. The professional will listen attentively to the client's questions and understand if their expectations match what the procedures can offer. It will then be very easy to offer the client all of the necessary technical explanations and reassurances needed to convince them to undergo the procedure.

For the sake of argument, and speaking purely theoretically, we can define some types of clients based on their motivations, creating a comprehensive, varied framework to help us better understand each client's personality and provide the most appropriate and suitable answers to different problems.

The most common reasons for which clients consider dermo-pigmentation are the following:
1. wanting a more polished appearance for the professional and business enviroment;
2. wanting to appear flawless for upcoming events;
3. for convenience, to save time spent applying makeup every day and to always feel put-together;
4. because of difficulty applying makeup, and especially, because of problems caused by vision problems or tremors, for example among older people;
5. to feel confident, correcting defects that compromise their self-image (nipple areolae, alopecia, etc.);

6. for social status;
7. to appear younger;
8. to achieve a change quickly, which with minimal re-touching (every 12/24 months) can effectively guarantee the desired results.

Understanding the reasons behind our clients' choices allows professionals to satisfy their expectations, after first explaining that dermopigmentation does not replace makeup, but provides a guideline to make daily makeup application easier.

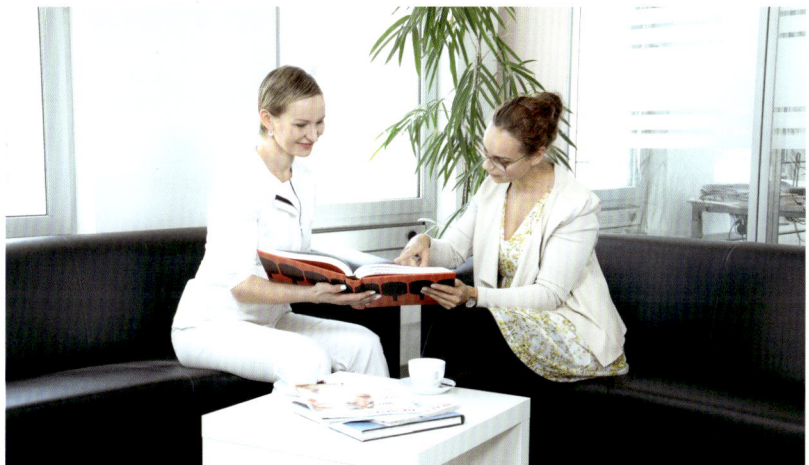

12.4. THE CLIENT-PROFESSIONAL RELATIONSHIP: THE IMPORTANCE OF THE CONSULTATION

The client agrees to undergo the procedure, even though it may be expensive, because the cost is spread out over the time that the procedure itself lasts.

These considerations form the basis from which to approach the client-professional relationship, touching on all of the fundamental aspects tied to the procedure. Thus, the consultation and its goals, extensive knowledge of the products and instruments, the hygienic rules, and being able to see the results already achieved are all prerequisites for the first appointment. A good consultation is the basis for being able to connect with the client.

Make sure to set precise goals, so that they are not disregarded. First, the professional will need to fully understand the client's goals – what it is they want to achieve, where, and how – and see if their expectations match what the professional can offer. In some cases, it may be best to turn down a job, if for various reasons you won't be able to achieve it, rather than accept it and have poor results turn into bad publicity for you. The second goal is, of course, to convince the client, and the third goal is to get good publicity out of each job.

We all have two ears and one mouth: therefore, especially in this initial phase, you should listen more than you talk.

12.5. ASKING THE RIGHT QUESTIONS

A discussion with the client is the best way to get to know them better, but it also serves to put them at ease by allowing them to talk about themselves, and gain the necessary trust in the professional.

It's best to always start consultations with questions:

- how can I help you?
  This is a crucial question because it makes it clear that the professional has already seen the problem and is ready to resolve it. This leads the client to see their own problem as something clear, to be solved immediately;

- why have you decided to have permanent makeup applied?
  You need to identify the reasons that have led them to this point, assess the emotional aspect, and verify their intentions.

- what do you know about permanent makeup?
  The professional should check what the client already knows about what they are about to do: in most cases, they will first have to dispel myths, then create the appropriate basis for acquiring new knowledge.

- why did you choose me?
  This question has a purely commercial basis. Based on the client's answer, you can gain important information about your own publicity system: which channels to use and which ones best transmit information.

12.6. TECHNICAL AND COMMERCIAL ASPECTS

These answers help the professional acquire a comprehensive understanding of the client, assess their emotional factors, find out if they have received incorrect information, if they are interested in the technical aspect, and if they are worried about costs or afraid of the pain associated with their selected procedure. At this point, the professional can begin to explain how to the procedure is performed, displaying confidence and providing all of the necessary information. The professional should also maintain a certain distance using expressions like, "If you decide to have the procedure done..." because it is important for the client to understand that their decision to choose our practice is important to us, but not crucial.

12.7. HEALTH AND HYGIENE

Start by discussing health and hygiene, without sparing any detail on the subject of single-use tools: a correct and professional procedure is important.

In some countries only sterile single-use markers are allowed for this purpose. Highlight the use of certified, bio-compatible colors, and begin to explain how everything that will come into contact with the client during the procedure will be carefully covered with hygienic materials, from the cart to the disinfectant. The goal is remind the client of any procedures they've had done in practices that did not take these precautions, and for them to decide who to trust (us) after realizing these dangers.

12.8. TALKING ABOUT YOUR PRACTICE

At this point, talk about your work philosophy, analyzing in detail the technical aspects you highlight in your own method of working. Above all, explain to the client that your first goal is to work in a way that emphasizes natural-looking results.

The most beautiful makeup is the kind you don't see, that looks natural; makeup is intended to deceive, and the deception lies in its ability to look as though it has always been part of the client's appearance. Makeup tricks the eye, and offers us a different perception of the ourselves, without overtaking physical features, reference colors, and our general self-image.

By using a selection of images depicting the "before" and "after" of a procedure, you can better explain the intervention and why one solution was chosen over another. Proceed by assessing which color to choose in relation to the client's complexion, eyes, eyebrows, and the type of makeup they wear daily. An aesthetic proposal should fit the client's taste: more proposals make the choice easier because they offer useful means of comparison for reaching a final result. Take enough time on the proposals; after all, this is a phase that is still reversible, and in which everything is up for discussion. A series of appropriate proposals can often prevent misunderstandings later. Explain to the client that the sketch phase will establish the results agreed upon, not with simple drawing ("sketch") that risks being compromised during the procedure, but by marking out an area so that the results will be as close as possible to what was agreed. The chosen technique will be applied within this reference area.

12.9. IS THE PROCEDURE PAINFUL?

At this point, it is important to address the "pain" factor that worries many people who choose to undergo permanent makeup or tattoo procedures. The client is reassured by the professional's confidence: they will feel no pain, since numbing products will be used; all they will feel is slight discomfort. It is important to follow the regulation in your own country and use only products authorized for permanent makeup artists.

12.10. TIME FRAMES

To complete the preliminary consultation with all necessary information, the professional can also explain the time needed for each procedure. Paradoxically, the sketching phase takes more time than the procedure, but, as has been emphasized many times, careful use of sketching tools forms the basis for the final result. The procedure will take about two hours, while how long the results last depends on different factors. One of these is age: cellular regeneration takes place more quickly among young people than among those over fifty.

Other factors include sun exposure, levels of scarring, which vary from person to person, as well as the chosen technique. Permanent makeup is a unique combination of the procedure itself and the choice of colors and shapes, from the first procedure to refreshers. These parts cannot be split up for the results to meet expectations.

After about a month, the initial result won't be final: a second session may be required to perfect the procedure. In the meantime, the makeup may have undergone various color and structural changes; these should not cause alarm as they are the result of cellular turnover, which inevitably changes the appearance of the work. In any case, within a period of eight months/one year, a second session is required to refresh the work. We don't call this a touch-up because it is not about correcting errors, but reviewing the color, which may have changed in tone. It is important that this refresher takes place within the above time frame for the shape to remain intact, and so that the intervention only has to deal with color fading. Make sure to mention that the cost of this revision equals 50% of the cost of the initial procedure.

12.11. PRICES

So far, we have not discussed prices, and this is crucial. The work that is to be done, proving our own abilities and deciding on the most suitable choices for the person in front of us, as well as the need to reassure the client are the most important elements, and should be prioritized.

As for the purely commercial aspect, it is for each one of us to consider their own situation, without undervaluing the services provided by offering prices that are too low, nor inflating fees without being able to guarantee services of a certain level.

Using a single, flat rate for all permanent makeup procedures, however, could seem unprofessional and leave the client frustrated. How much permanent makeup costs depends on different technical and anatomical factors: it depends on the area being worked on, the presence of obvious defects that need to be corrected, which of the many techniques will be used, the time the procedure takes, and the tools used.

The price is therefore framed as a range, which of course includes both a minimum and maximum price. The range can vary depending on the type of procedure, and is often used to help convince the client. Think of seeing a luxury window display of one of the hottest brands: the window itself displays two purses, one of which you immediately fall in love with.

There's only one price tag however, and it shows two prices: 3,000.00 € and 1,000.00 €, without offering a precise description to let us know which of the purse corresponds to which price. The higher price inevitably gives us "sticker shock", meaning it is the kind of price that scares us in any negotiation. We then decide to go into the store to ask for more information, and the

salesperson tells us that the purse in the window costs 1,000.00 €. The immediate psychological reaction is the thought that we have saved 2,000.00 €, and the bag, although pricy, seems like a very good deal. That is why a range is a good way to inform clients about the price: together, by reaching an intermediate price together, the client will know that they have not paid the maximum, and will trust in the agreement.

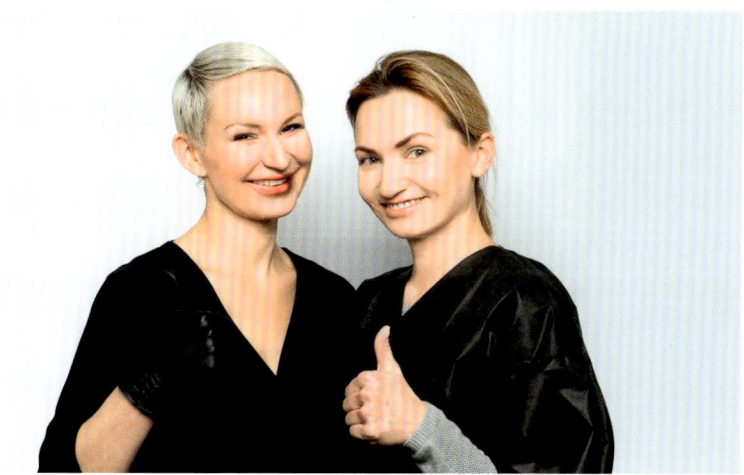

12.12. HOW TO MAKE AN APPOINTMENT

This is why you should not obtain all of the information needed for a procedure over the phone: you need to have an in-depth understanding of the more personal aspects (including financial), of the client in front of you: so that you can interact with them, assess their reactions, and listen to their reasons for coming this far. Before the client leaves, provide them with written information that summarizes all that you have discussed during the consultation.

This includes three pieces of information in particular:
• commercial information (the classic "business card");
• pre-treatment reminder information;
• post-treatment technical information.

At this point, there are two possibilities: the first is that the client leaves, and thinks the procedure over a little more. Don't underestimate the very likely possibility that they have or will compare offers at various practices: in which case it is obvious that they must retain the information they receive. The second possibility is that they are already convinced, and want to make an appointment right away. In this situation, don't be carried away by the desire to seal the deal.

Have the client wait a little bit, so that they understand that you have many requests, and that your practice is busy fulfilling them all as quickly as possible. It is important that "as soon as possible" does not mean "immediately".

Here is a simple example. Imagine a busy restaurant in the heart of a big city, and another one, which is on the same street and benefits from the same foot traffic, but looks empty: which restaurant would you choose if you wanted to be sure of a good meal? Surely, the one that is empty creates distrust, leading customers to choose the more popular one, even if it means that they have to wait. The guarantee is given by the other people who have already made the more thoughtful choice.

The same idea holds for the practice, which therefore needs to share the qualities of the busy restaurant in the city center: the client will feel more confident in their choice by knowing that many others have chosen this practice over others. That means, "We'll call you if a spot opens…" often is the phrase with the most impact.

12.13. THE IMPORTANCE OF A DEPOSIT

This is always a thorny topic when discussing the cost of the procedure. The client must understand that the deposit requested by the professional is indispensable for a number of reasons:

1. The preparatory phase, from the appointment to the sketch, requires a lot of skill and knowledge on the part of the professional, involving both their expertise and materials;
2. to guarantee that the client shows up to their appointment;
3. to protect the client and guarantee the seriousness and rigor of the professional and their office.

It should be made clear that the deposit is not an expense that is added to the final cost, but which will be deducted from the final cost. It is paid in order to guarantee attendance on the agreed date: it is useful to add that it will be withheld if the client, for any reason, decides not to keep the appointment and does not provide 24 hours notice.

12.14. THE APPOINTMENT

The professional's last task is to eliminate any remaining confusion or fears, and to reiterate all the information in order to reassure the client. Many of the objections to dermopigmentation come from a series of reluctances regarding the pain, the inability to change one's mind about the color once it has been applied, the risk of infection, the lack of guarantee about maintaining the same results over time, and last, but not least, the suspicion that the investment in the procedure – in terms of money – will not pay off. All of these concerns reveal a real sense of fear regarding micropigmentation, which the professional must cleverly dispel.

This is not the time to obscure any truths: first, acknowledge that while dermopigmentation is extremely natural, it will be visible. But this visibility should be a point of pride for the client, since their new appearance will comprise a valuable aesthetic change. The second truth concerns pain: this factor depends on each person's sensitivity; in any case (and this is unequivocal) the pain is very much bearable. Finally, any fear of having treatments performed on the eye area can be dispelled by showing them the exact positions used during the procedure, the exercises that relax the area, and the minimal danger of the needle.

At this point, the client becomes convinced of the feasibility of the procedure, and will be invited to undergo the preparatory phases that involve sketching their new image. This process highlights all of the details that will make their appearance more beautiful and harmonious. The eyebrows, eyes, or lips will be studied in order to correct any defects; physiological transformations that took place over time (such as new wrinkles due to aging) will be considered; the correct, but never exaggerated, changes will be agreed upon; the most appropriate and suitable colors will be chosen.

The client will see the tools, the place where the procedure will be performed, and above all, will learn about all of the guarantees of sterilization, the risks, and the hygienic procedures that precede and follow the procedure. There are different kinds of uncertainties surrounding permanent makeup: some big questions and many minor ones.

The biggest question is a given, and has to do with objective difficulties regarding the practice of micropigmentation; more minor questions have to do with possible problems that could arise. An expert professional can not only answer these questions correctly, but guarantees results that correctly respond to any future questions.

12.15. HOW TO PROMOTE YOUR BUSINESS

Today's micropigmentation professionals are characterized by their technical abilities, deep knowledge, and excellent communication skills. There are countless professionals who are technically very advanced, but are completely unknown because they don't know how to advertise and promote their abilities. They are probably professionals who rely exclusively on word of mouth, which does generate promotion, but has much slower results than systems like email marketing, blogs, SEO, SEA, and SMM.

Email marketing is a type of direct marketing which uses emails to share commercial (and other) messages with the public, using newsletters or stand-alone messages that are rich in content.
A blog is a particular kind of website in which content is viewed chronologically, in text or post form. A company's blog notably increases its reputation and SEO, generating more traffic to its website.

SEO (Search Engine Optimization) is the sum of all activities aimed at increasing a website's visibility so that it is positioned at the top of search engines' lists of "organic" results.

In contrast, SEA (Search Engine Advertising) uses "paid" campaigns on search engines to improve a site's position or to advertise events, products, and services. SMM (Social Media Marketing) promotes the company's activities through social media channels, using the different advertising tools offered by each platform.

A company's investment in promotions should, however, always be accompanied by an editorial calendar that allows the publication of this content to be managed in an effective and organized way, defining what, when, and how to post on these different channels.

A well-planned editorial calendar allows you to:
- better manage your presence on search engines and social media
- create content that fits your business target
- coordinate marketing activities
- reduce stress regarding this content, since material will be ready well ahead of time (photos, videos, banners, texts, mailings)
- monitor the results of these activities

Promoting your own activity also means performing perfect procedures, taking high-quality photos, correcting potential imperfections in brightness and adjusting color, producing technical and advertising videos, identifying the most appropriate social media channels for your company's marketing needs, working efficiently, making contacts, and providing perfect consultations.

Taken together, these guarantee permanent makeup that is performed and shared correctly.

These steps are not always executed completely autonomously; rather, they require technical support in the form of photographers or social media managers, who need to have a deep understanding of dermopigmentation in order to understand their target audience and the tastes of the intended clients.

Content is definitely an indispensable tool, both in traditional and digital marketing. It is surely worth investing in your own work with specific training courses that grant you the necessary knowledge, techniques, and tools to attain your goals.

Another way to increase visibility is to create joint ventures with other professionals, like hairdressers, doctors, and aestheticians, in order to gain productive publicity which clients tend to trust. This would require considering informational brochures illustrating all of the health and hygiene conditions, as well as the techniques and offers, and show some examples of permanent makeup for the eyebrows, lips, and eyes. The agreement could be provisional, based on well-performed procedures, or simply entail reciprocal client referrals.

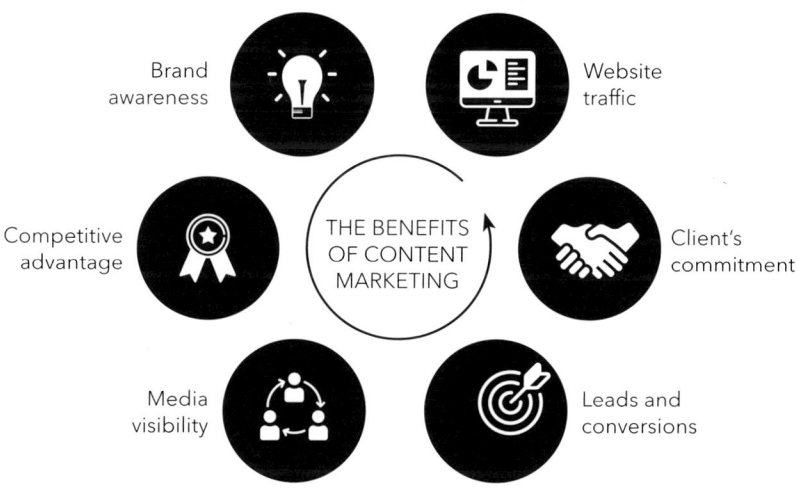

12.16 THE AMIEA PRO APP AND ITS BENEFITS

The amiea app has been developed to connect you with your fellow artists and trainers and to make your life easier by automating your client and procedure documentation:

• Post your photos to your Facebook and Instagram account directly from the app.

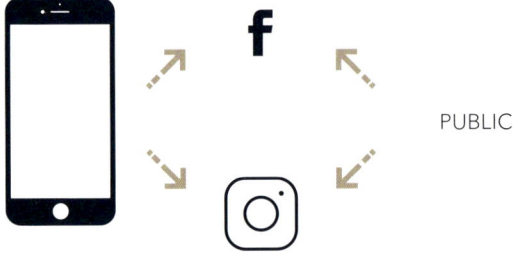

PUBLIC

• Store all your client and procedure data (photos, addresses, photographed consent form, utilized colors, procedure notes and much more) in one safe place. Whenever you need access to that data, you will have it available with just very few clicks. For a follow-up treatment, for example, retrieve past photos and information on the color utilized instantly and simply on your smartphone or tablet.

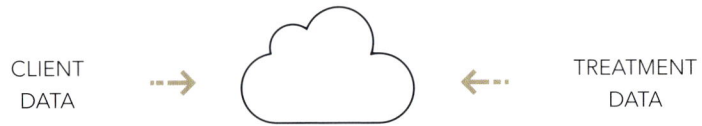

CLIENT
DATA

TREATMENT
DATA

• Easily create a profile for new clients with procedures and a photo gallery.

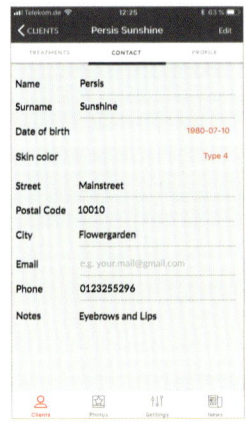 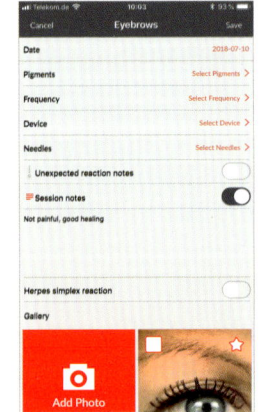 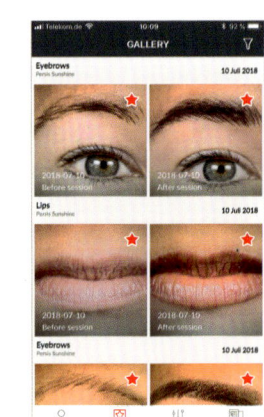

13

PERMANENT MAKEUP
AND APPLICATION TECHNIQUES

Here are the essential steps for obtaining the desired results:

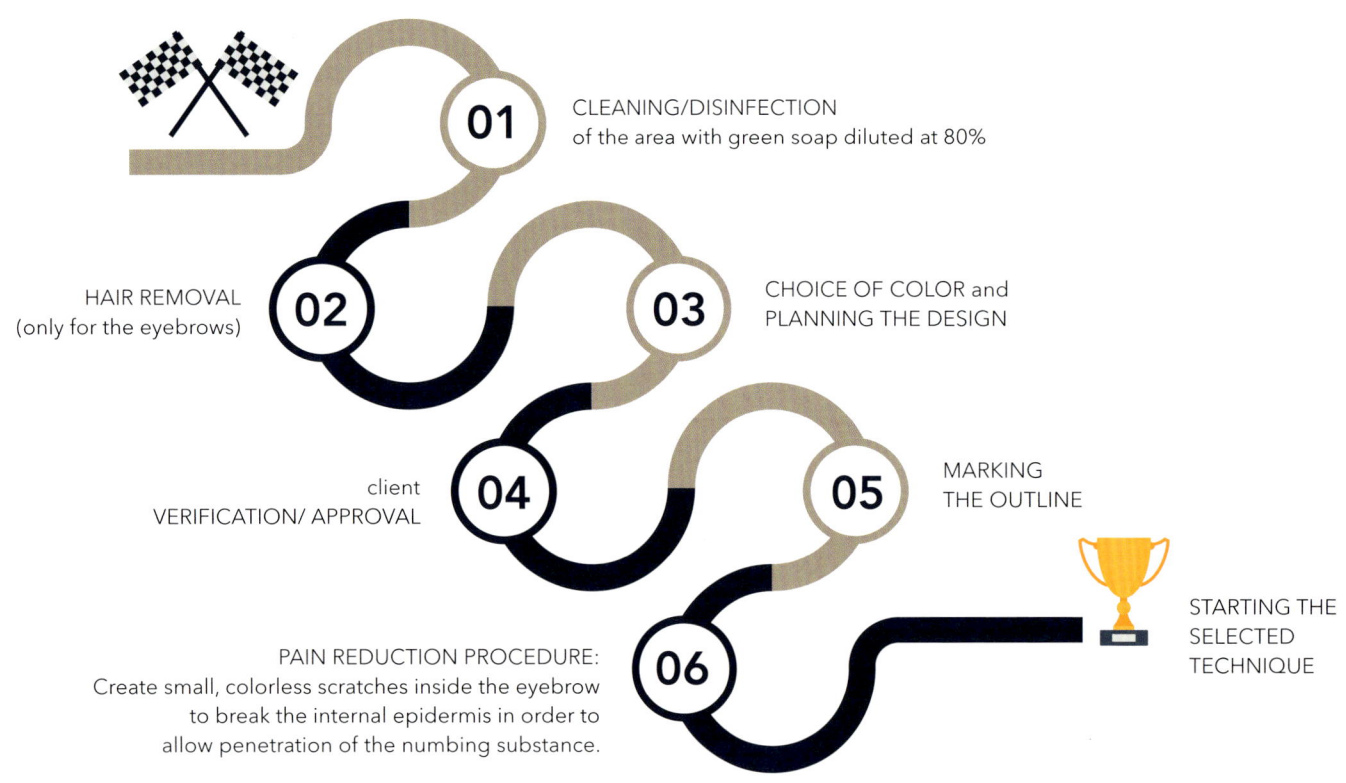

01 CLEANING/DISINFECTION
of the area with green soap diluted at 80%

HAIR REMOVAL
(only for the eyebrows) **02**

03 CHOICE OF COLOR and
PLANNING THE DESIGN

client
VERIFICATION/ APPROVAL **04**

05 MARKING
THE OUTLINE

PAIN REDUCTION PROCEDURE:
Create small, colorless scratches inside the eyebrow
to break the internal epidermis in order to
allow penetration of the numbing substance. **06**

STARTING THE
SELECTED
TECHNIQUE

13.1.

EYEBROWS
STEP BY STEP

PARAMETERS

The icons below indicate the parameters necessary for performing the procedure correctly and safely. The many different movements, hand speed, and the different angles of the handpiece will be described, as well as the frequency at which to set the console, and the needles and pigments to be used in each step.

● = Movement

● = Hand speed

● = Angle

● = Frequency

● = Needle

● = Pigment

13.1.1. MARKING THE OUTLINE

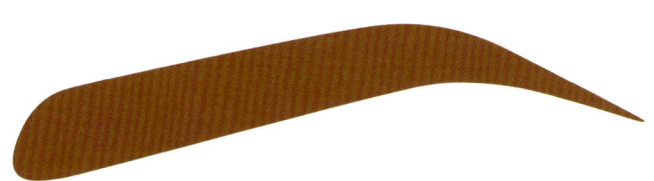

Once the client has approved the visagistic proposal, it is time to set the sketch with a reference outline on the epidermis, which is very useful for ensuring that professionals never lose sight of the initial sketch, and for the client be sure that the results agreed upon will be obtained.

The outline is marked out on the skin using a very thin needle. Based on the professional's level of confidence, training, and experience, this can be done in one of three ways.

SMALL HAIRS AROUND THE OUTLINE

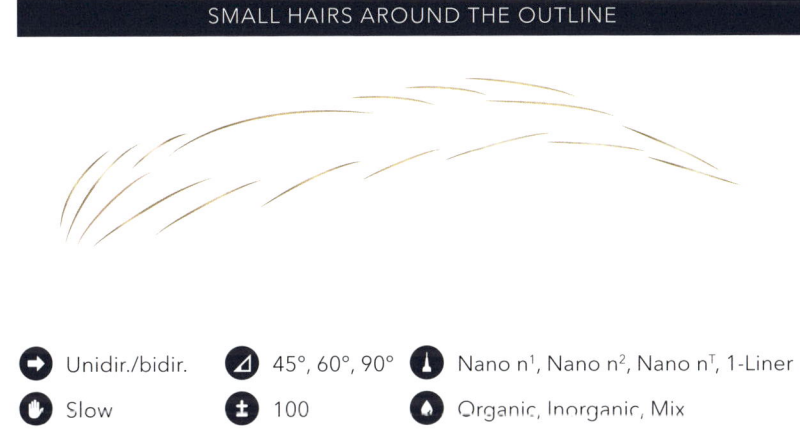

➡ Unidir./bidir.　　◢ 45°, 60°, 90°　　⬘ Nano n¹, Nano n², Nano nᵀ, 1-Liner

✋ Slow　　± 100　　◉ Organic, Inorganic, Mix

Drawing hairs from the start: in the sketch phase, you will draw all of the ascending, descending, or mixed hairs along the entire outline you have drawn. This option is recommended for very confident professionals who don't need to create an outline within which to work.

REMEMBER

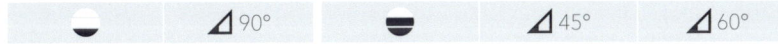

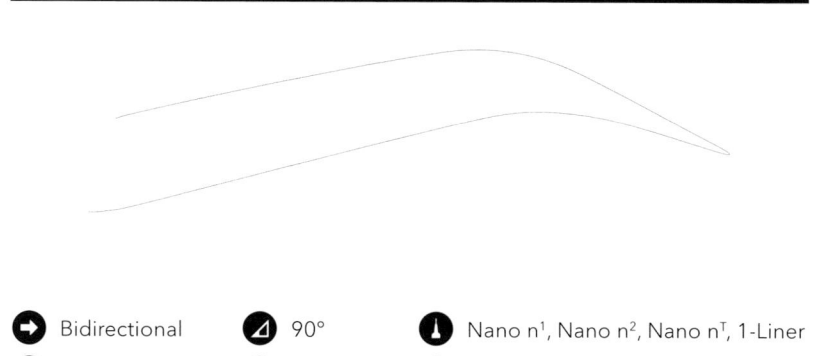

DOTTED OUTLINE

- ➡ Light Dots
- ⬇ Fast
- ◢ 90°
- ± 100
- ⬇ Nano n[1], Nano n[2], Nano n[T], 1-Liner
- ◌ Organic, Inorganic, Mix

Creating small dots along the outline with very gentle pressure, so that they disappear within 2/3 days through skin exfoliation. This is recommended for professionals who want to take precautions, and don't feel skilled enough to try the first option.

DASHED OUTLINE

- ➡ Bidirectional
- ⬇ Fast
- ◢ 90°
- ± 100
- ⬇ Nano n[1], Nano n[2], Nano n[T], 1-Liner
- ◌ Organic, Inorganic, Mix

Create dashes using a bidirectional movement to create a linear outline, ensuring absolute precision when creating the hairs within its borders. The base of the body will not be dermopigmented, to avoid creating lines that are too harsh in case of any errors. This is recommended for professionals without much experience, or when the eyebrow already has a large amount of hairs. Thick eyebrows could obscure the dots if a dotted outline is used, therefore leading to the risk of not following the agreed-upon shape.

13.1.2. NATURAL TECHNIQUES

Permanent makeup applied to the eyebrows can have more or less defined results, which is why it can be divided into three main categories:

- NATURAL: it is difficult for viewers to differentiate between real hairs and hairs that are drawn. This means also creating light defects, or small areas of sparseness.
- DEFINED: more like makeup, as when the entire arch of the eyebrow is filled in using a makeup pencil. This eyebrow is definitely more defined and perfect, but also noticeably more fake.
- MIXED: the natural hair technique is combined with a more defined part. This is recommended for more indecisive people, who want a precise effect without completely forgoing the natural look.

Natural eyebrows mean using a hair-by-hair technique which improves the color of the eyebrows or makes them appear more dense using small lines of pigment.

In the Nineties, small vertical lines were drawn over natural eyebrows, which, compared to a full-bleed color application, looked very realistic. Today, this technique is considered unnatural and old-school. Over time, we have learned more about how hairs grow in, and now emphasize curved hairs: in general, hairs don't always grow straight, instead, in a domino effect, each hair rests on the next one, meaning the hairs don't have the exact same placement from the body to the tail.

Think of a diver, a diving board, and a pool. Before diving, the diver stands erect. As he prepares to dive, he changes the posture of his body, modifying its angle and, throwing his hands out front, continues to change the angle of his body until he enters the water. Keep the diver's technique in mind for the eyebrow. In each eyebrow, the hairs start out straight, but progressively start to bend until they reach the tail.

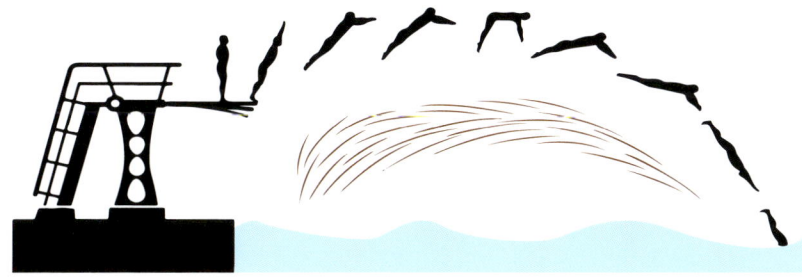

Today, we can say that depending on ethnicity, gender, and anatomy, there is not one universal direction and placement in which hairs grow. Just think about drawings from Asian countries, where body hair is mostly descending, completely different from that of Europeans. Over the years, these observations and our continued analysis of them has allowed us to define 3 types of layouts in the arch of the brow:

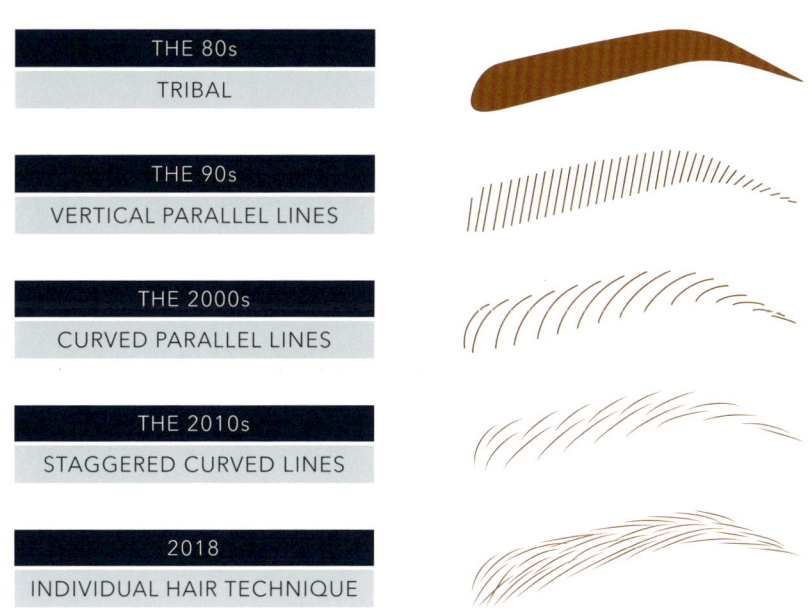

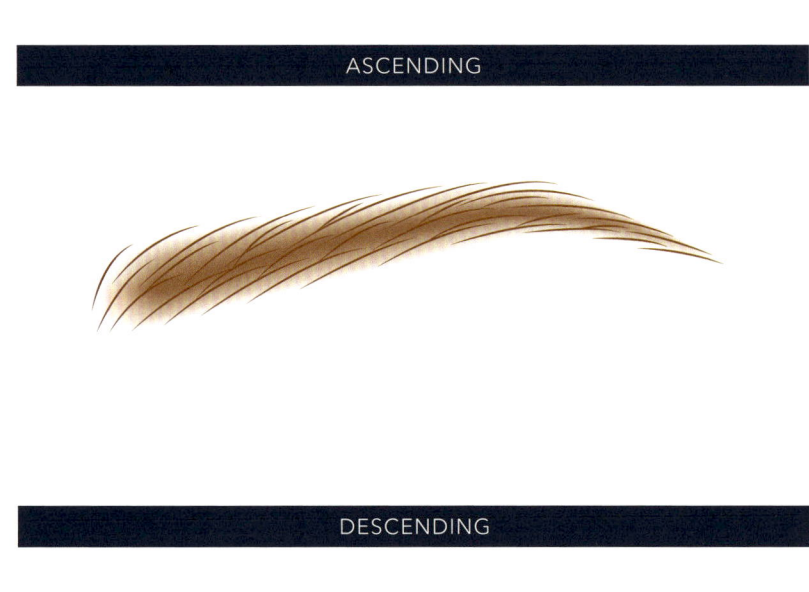
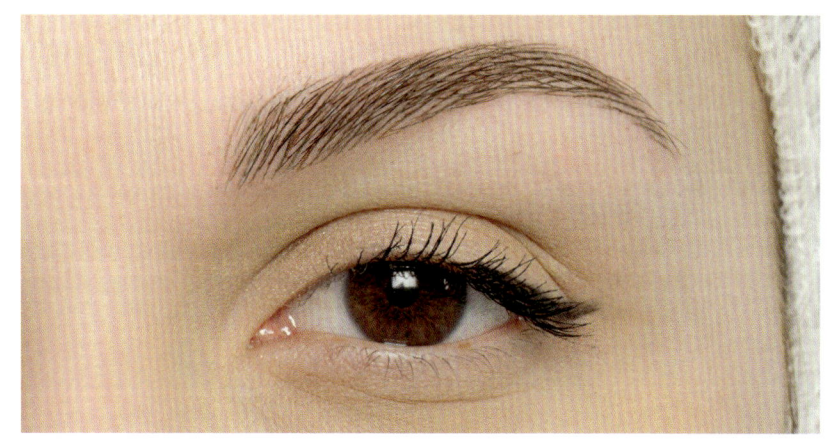

DESCENDING

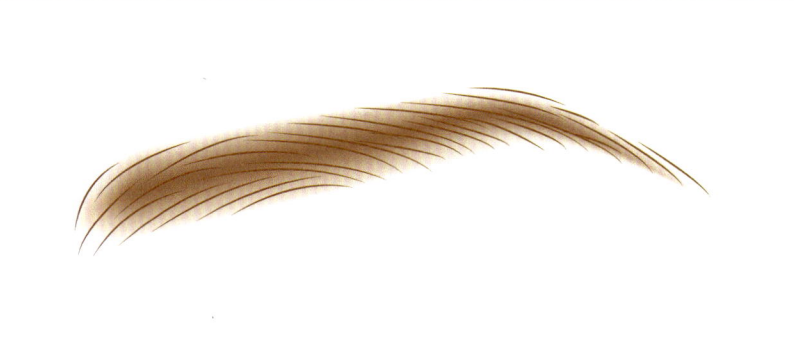
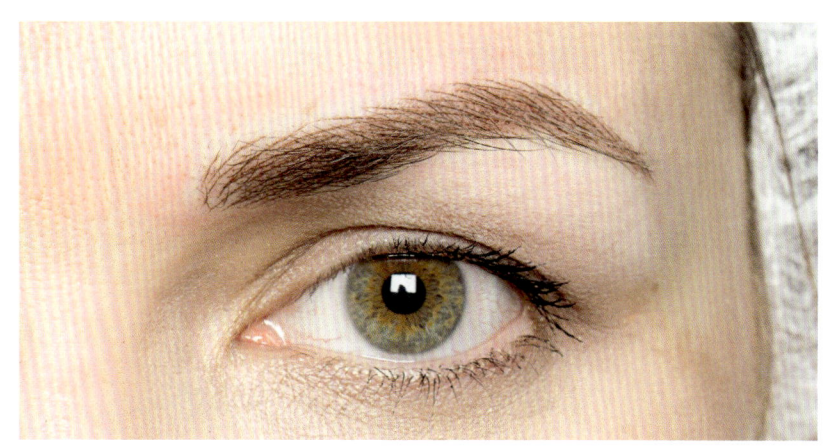

ASCENDING AND DESCENDING

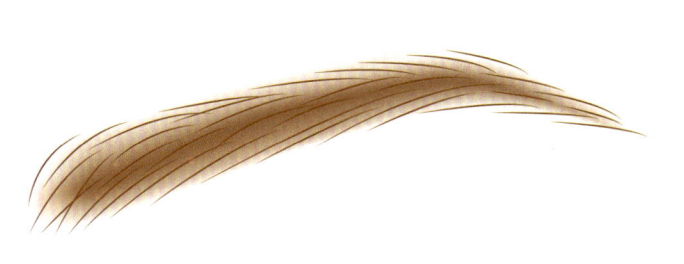
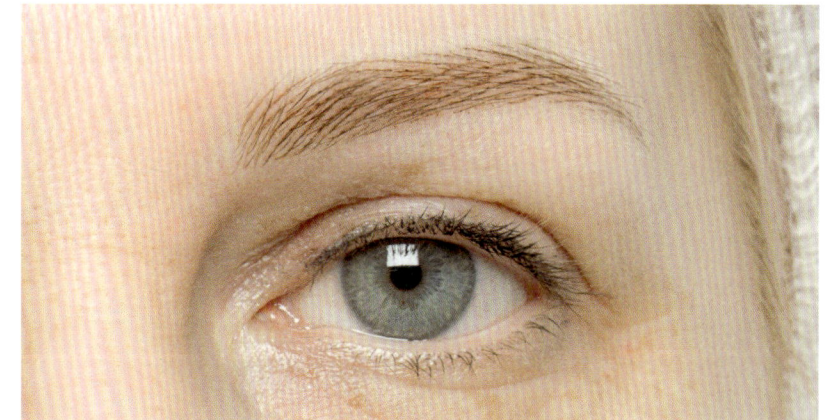

13.1.2.1. ASCENDING HAIRS

1 INITIAL SITUATION

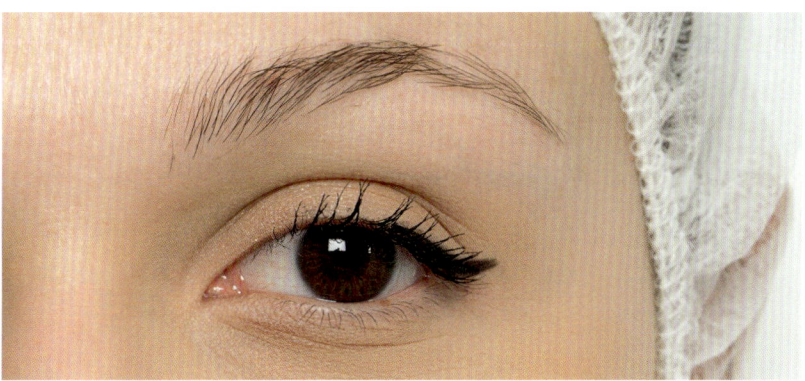

Before applying permanent makeup, the eyebrow area must be hygienically prepared.

3 HAIR REMOVAL

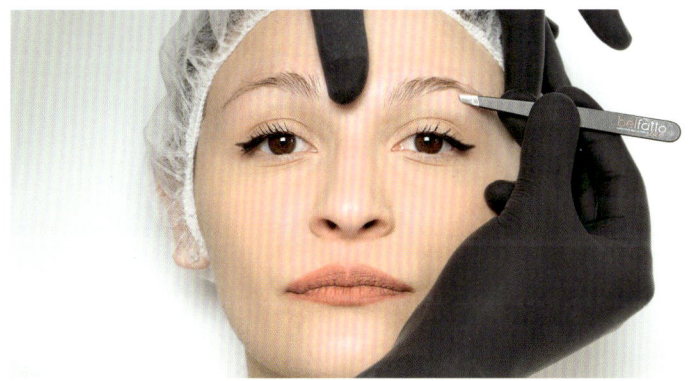

This step is done with tweezers instead of traumatic hair removal methods such as waxing or shaving, making sure to sterilize the tweezers in an autoclave to avoid cross-contamination between clients. First, we remove the hairs that clearly lie outside of our sketch; a second, more precise hair removal phase takes place after drawing in our new eyebrow, to perfect it.

2 CLEANING

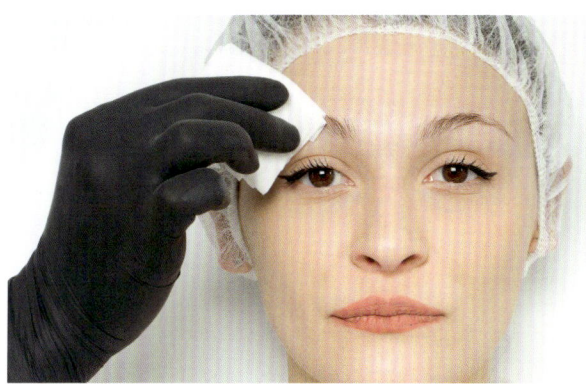

The first phase involves deep-cleaning the area to remove any previously applied makeup or cosmetic products, and to eliminate any potential non-pathogenic microorganisms. We recommend not re-using the dirty part of the wipe.

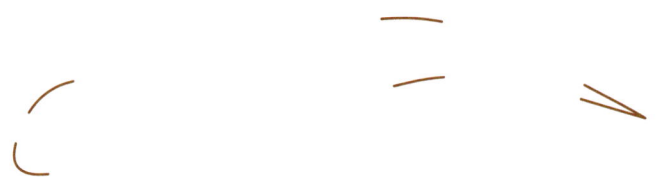

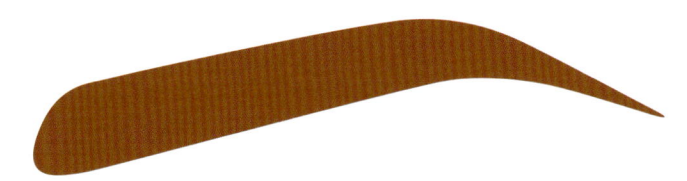

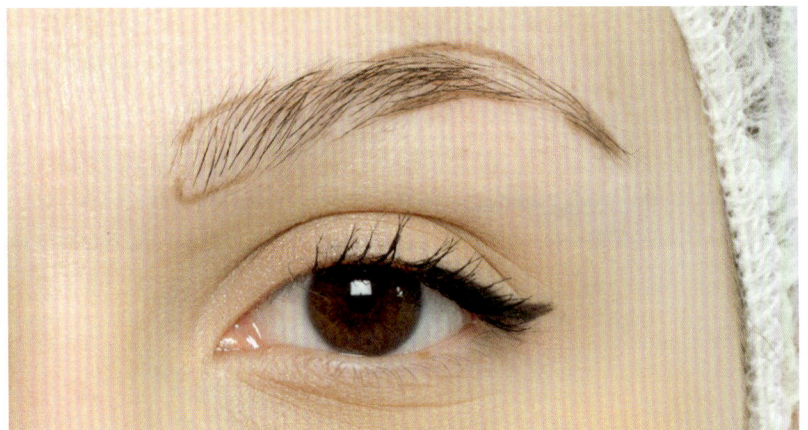

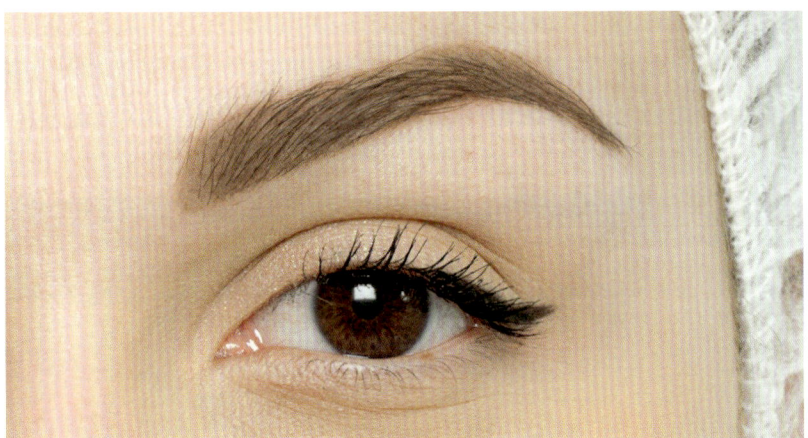

Before beginning any sketch, you should have a clear vision of what you want to achieve for the client, and never leave anything up to improvisation. There are five specific reference points that will help you achieve the desired results as accurately and quickly as possible. The first two points serve to lay out the base of the body and its thickness, while the other two indicate the height of the brow and the width of the vertex, and the last point determines the length and thickness of the tail.

Once these five points are determined and drawn in, all you need to do is connect them and fill in the ouline in order to see the chosen shape, and if necessary, make corrections and adjustments.

6 VERTICAL GUIDELINE

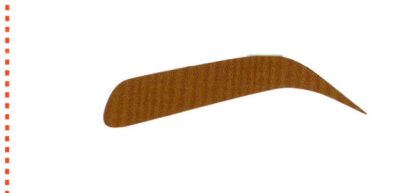

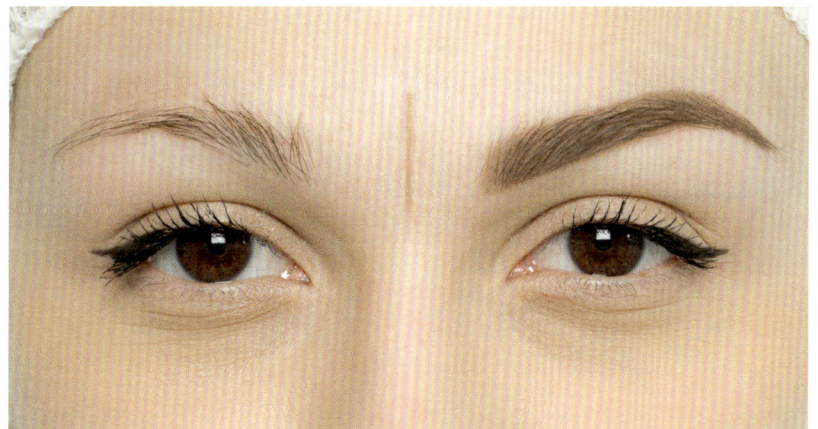

Using a sketching tool and the pigment chosen for the procedure, trace a vertical line at the center of the face, using the forehead, eyes, and nose as reference points. This guideline will be useful for verifying that the distance between the two eyebrows is correct and centered according to the part of the face in question.

⚠ ATTENTION

In some countries only sterile, single-use markers are allowed for this purpose.

7 FIRST HORIZONTAL GUIDELINE

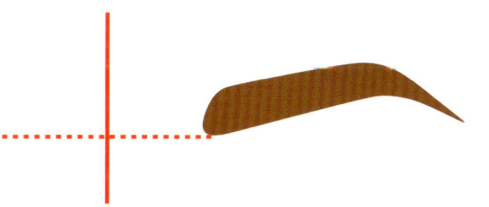

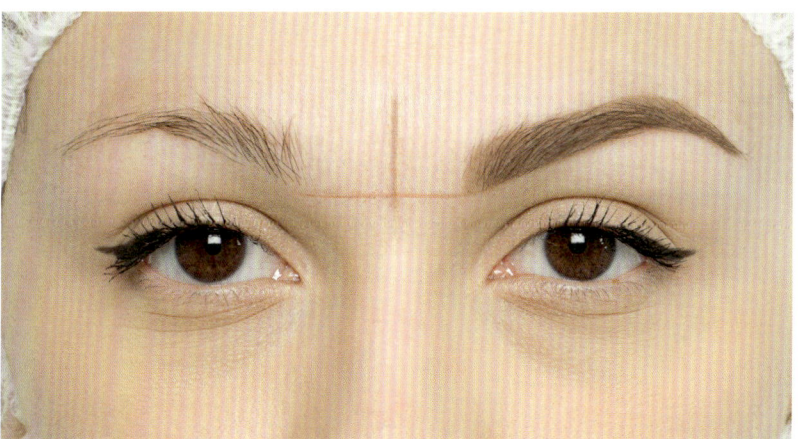

Next, we establish the first horizontal guideline, which is a line that runs parallel to the ground; it starts from the previously drawn eyebrow and leads to the point chosen for the beginning of the second eyebrow. The first horizontal guideline serves to ensure that the eyebrows are placed at the correct height compared to the eyes.

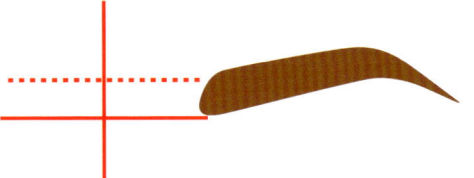

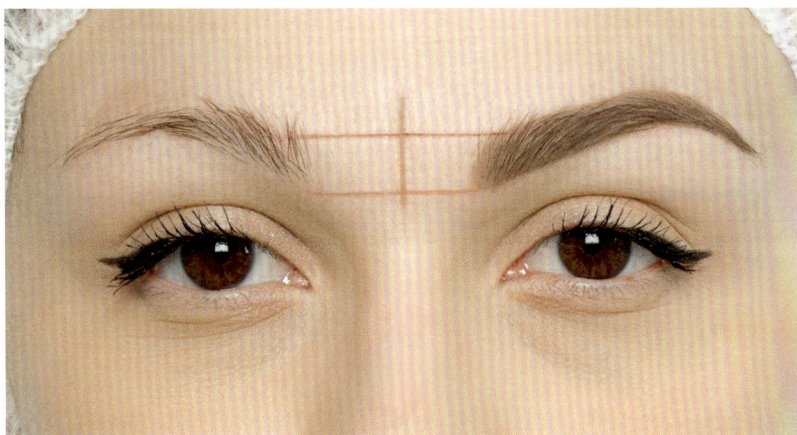

The second, upper horizontal reference point indicates the maximum height of the base of the body of the eyebrow and therefore the width of the base of the eyebrow.

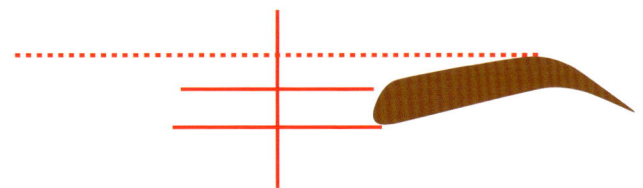

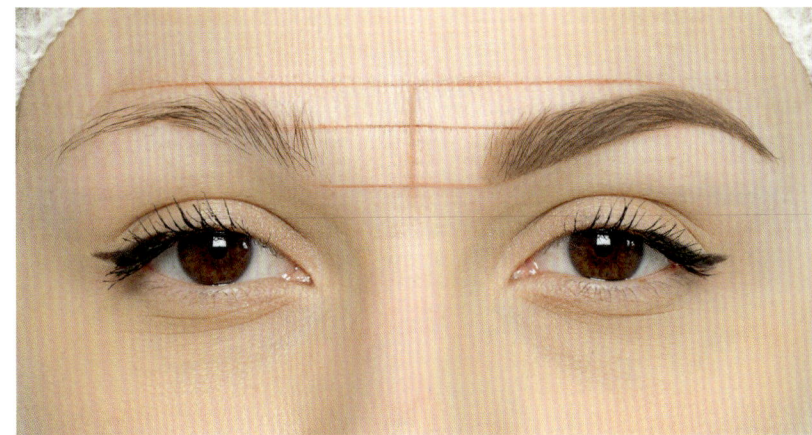

The third horizontal guideline concerns the vertex: a line that runs parallel to the floor and connects the brow arches and determines the highest point of the entire eyebrow.

The vertex is one of the most important parts in characterizing a face's non-verbal expression, which is why the original intentions should be considered very carefully.

10 FIRST OBLIQUE GUIDELINE

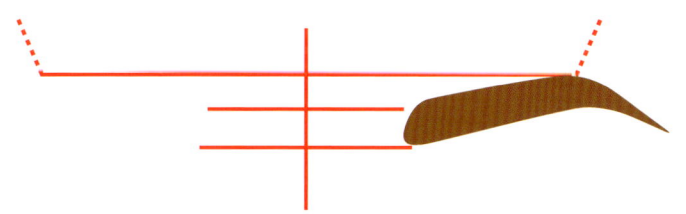

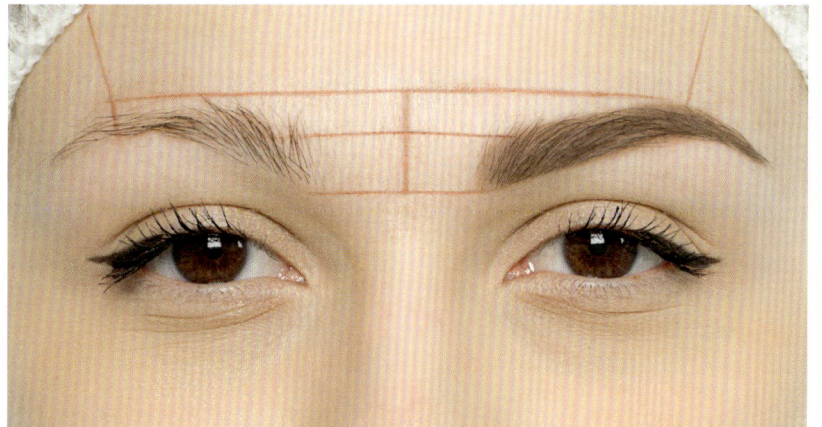

11 SECOND OBLIQUE GUIDELINE

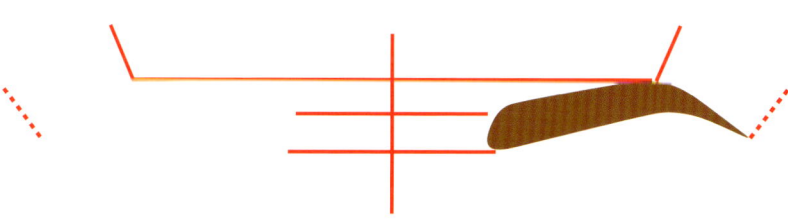

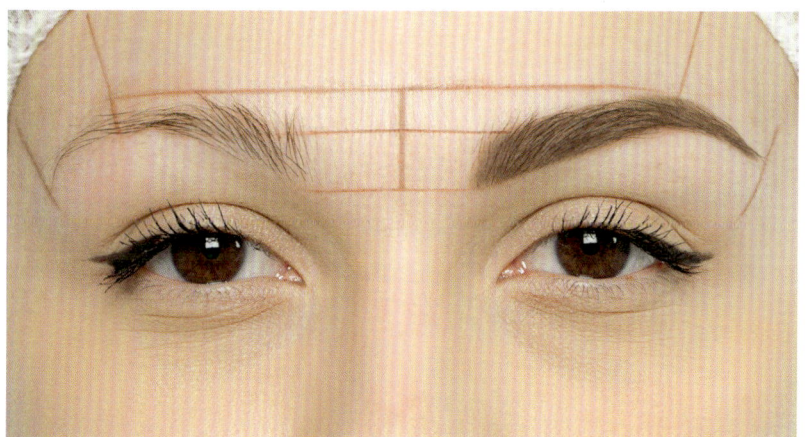

Now it is time to determine the innermost or outermost position of the vertex. Not just its height. The best way to prevent the client from continuously moving their eyes is to firmly place a finger in front of their face, at a distance of about 40 cm, and ask them to stare at it to align the center of the pupil. Only then should you begin tracing an imaginary oblique line that starts from the wing of the nose, passes through the center of the pupil, and therefore indicates the correct placement of the vertex. Repeat the same process for the other eye.

The second oblique guideline determines the length of the tail of the eyebrow. Starting from the wing of the nose once again, trace a second imaginary line, which this time passes through the outer corner of the eye, indicating the maximum length of the tail.

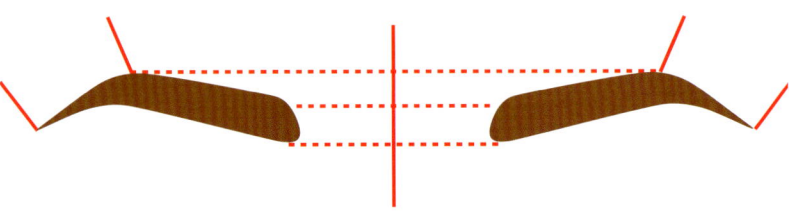

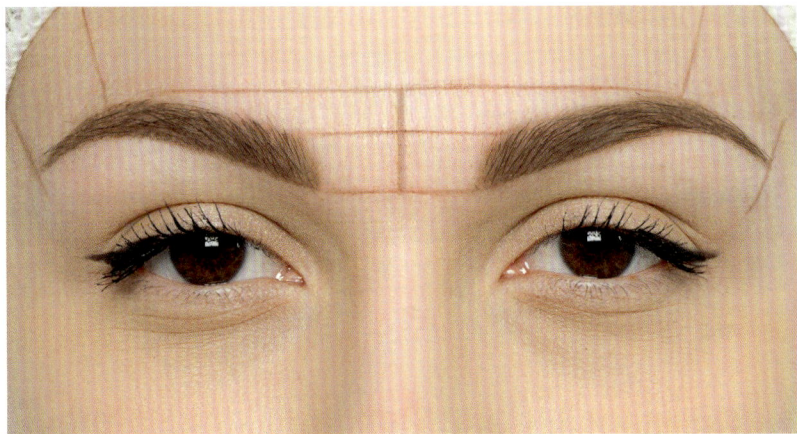

Once this is done, we'll have a grid within which we can quickly position the second eyebrow.

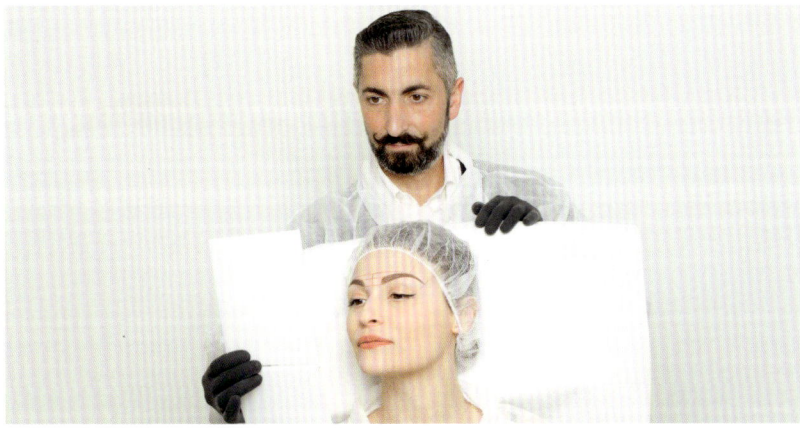

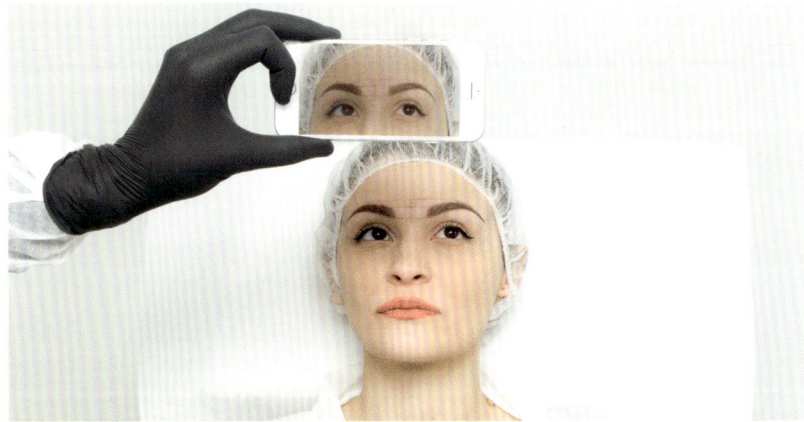

Using these reference points creates a symmetrical and accurate sketch, which should be checked, first through a direct, frontal observation of the client, then through an indirect observation made using two fundamental tools: the mirror and the camera (or a cell phone, if more convenient). This will guarantee the quality of the final results.

14 SKETCH

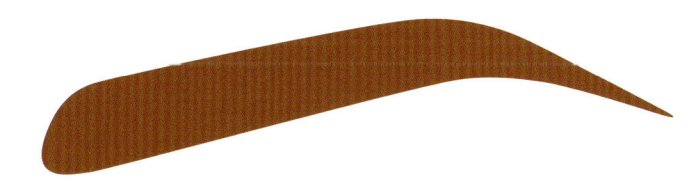

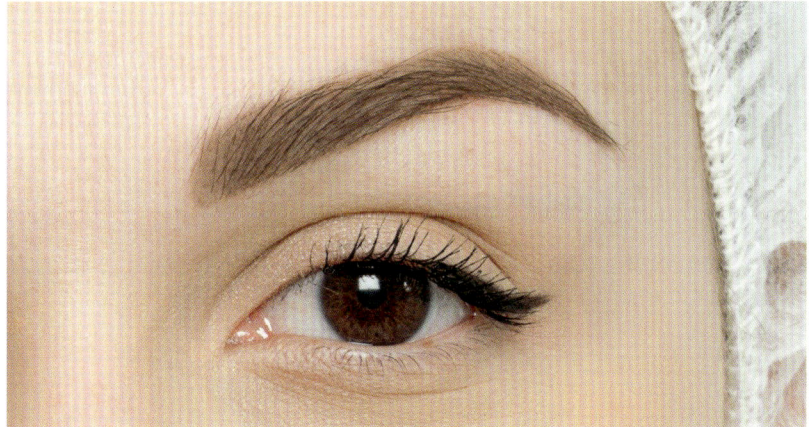

After having created a careful sketch, proceed by marking out the outline.

15 MARKING THE OUTLINE

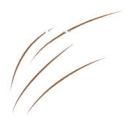

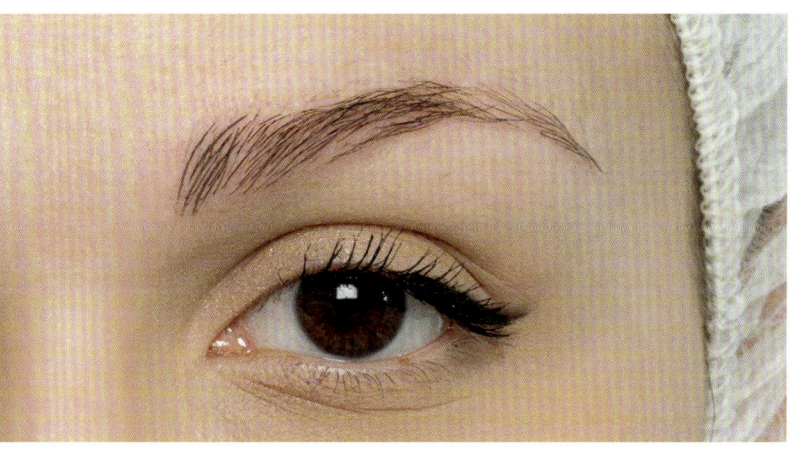

➡ Unidir./bidir.	◩ 90°	🌡 Nano n¹, Nano n², Nano nᵀ, 1-Liner
✋ Slow	± 120	💧 Organic, Inorganic, Mix

We recommend doing the first 4 hairs as shown in the diagram, in order to avoid an overly harsh effect at the base of the eyebrow.

REMEMBER
Hairstrokes with 1 point configurations

	◢ 90°		◢ 45°	60°

Hairstrokes with 3-slope

	◢ 60°

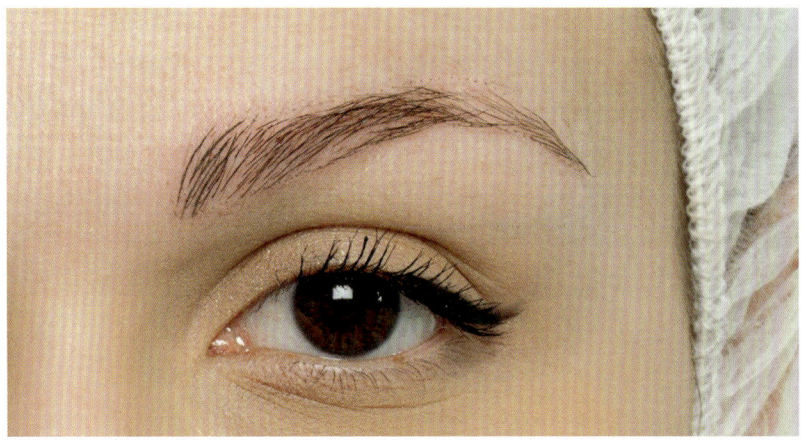

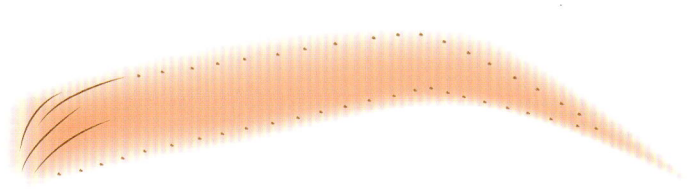

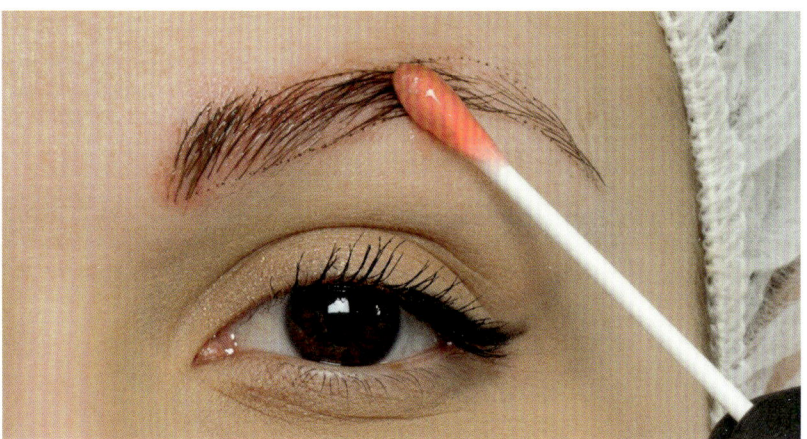

→ Dots   ◢ 90°   Nano n[1], Nano n[2], Nano n[T], 1-Liner

↻ Fast   ± 120   Organic, Inorganic, Mix

You can continue with the dotted or dashed effect, depending on your level of training or experience. We recommend tracing the outline dots very lightly, so that no traces remain visible after 30 days.

In countries where the law permits it, apply a numbing solution; this not only inhibits pain but also decongests the area, preventing bleeding which could dilute the color. Wait 1–3 minutes and wipe off if necessary. The sketched skin area will turn into a lighter color due to the vasoconstrictive properties of the solution, which makes the design even more visible.

18 LOWER ASCENDING HAIRS

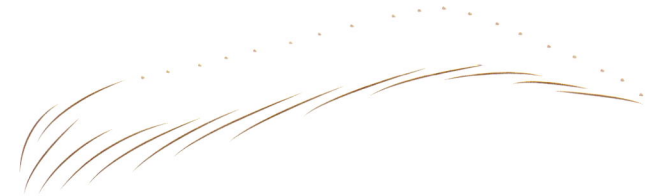

Drawing extremely curved hairs prevents you from adding more, while making them extremely straight would create a very unnatural effect.

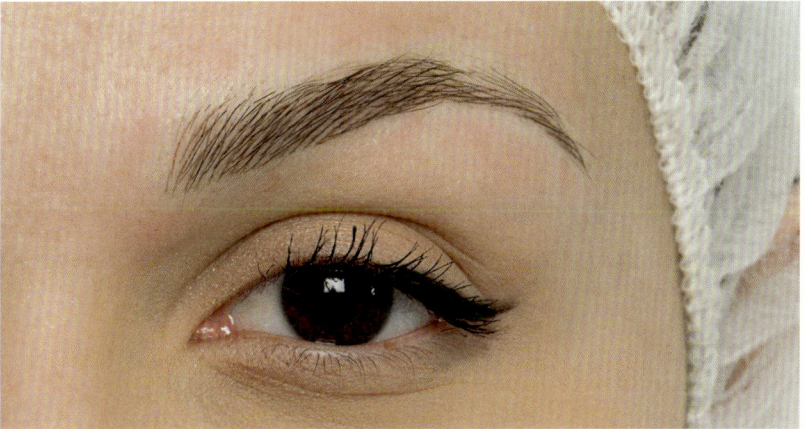

 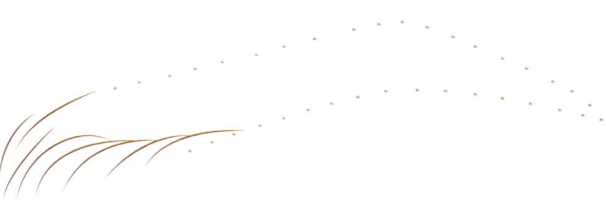

 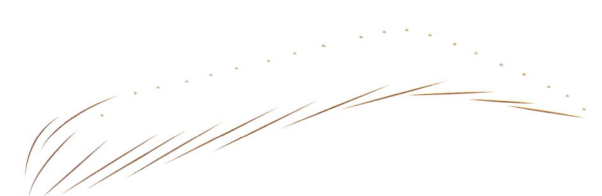

➡ Unidir./bidir.   ◹ 45°, 60°, 90°   ⬇ Nano n¹, Nano n², Nano nᵀ, 1-Liner

✋ Slow   ± 120   ⬤ Organic, Inorganic, Mix

For the ascending technique, after drawing the outline, you will create the lower part of the ascending hairs. These are drawn with a unidirectional movement: the first hairs will definitely be taller, and as you approach the vertex and tail of the brow, they begin to dip down. It is important that the hairs maintain a certain consistency.

During the first session, it is recommended that you not exceed a distance of half a millimeter. The hairs should neither be too curved nor too straight, but rather have a mostly linear shape with a slight curve.

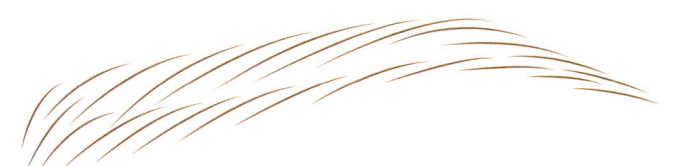

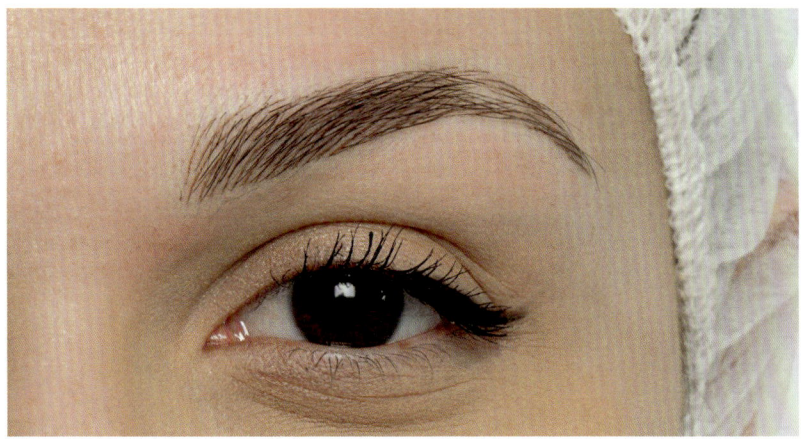

➡ Unidir./bidir.	◢ 45°, 60°, 90°	🌡 Nano n¹, Nano n², Nano nᵀ, 1-Liner
✋ Slow	± 120	💧 Organic, Inorganic, Mix

Proceed to the upper ascending hairs. They start at the center of the brow and reach the upper part of the sketch. In this case, the hairs will also be spaced out about half a millimeter apart, and as shown in the image, they will be neither extremely straight nor extremely curved.

REMEMBER
Hairstrokes with 1 point configurations

⬭	◢ 90°	⬬	◢ 45°	◢ 60°

Hairstrokes with 3-slope

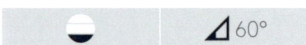

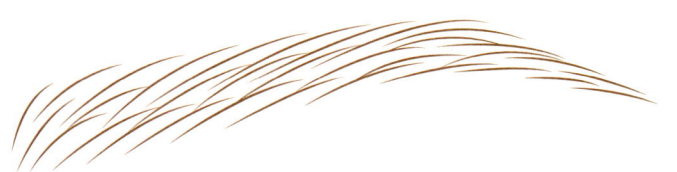

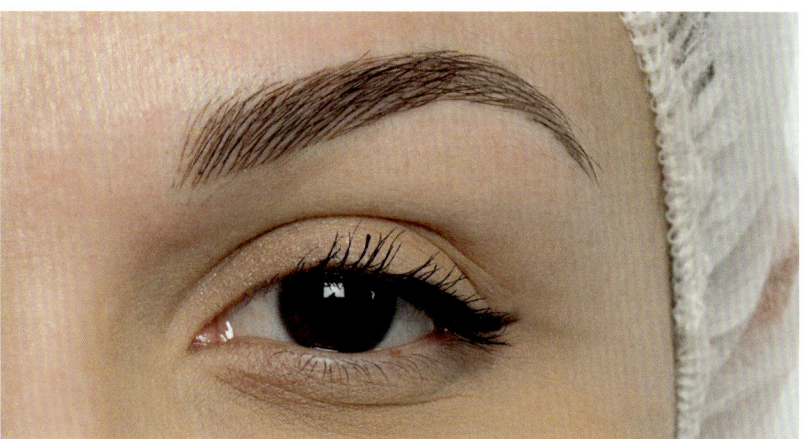

➡ Unidir./bidir.	◢ 45°, 60°, 90°	🌡 Nano n¹, Nano n², Nano nᵀ, 1-Liner
✋ Slow	± 120/140	💧 Organic, Inorganic, Mix

Continue with the density hairs, which always grow upwards. They will start from the lower hairs and fill in the center part of the eyebrow, with a more horizontal angle, without ever reaching the external outline.

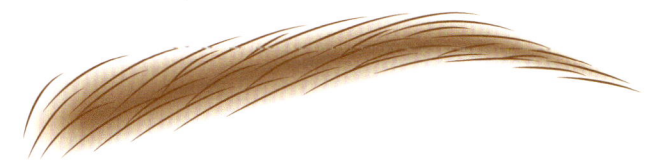

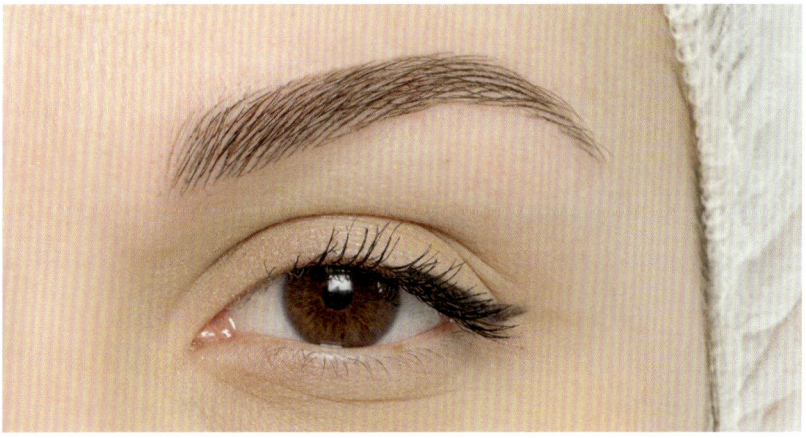

⮕ Zigzag bidir.   ◿ 90°   🌡 Nano n^1, Nano n^2, 1-Liner

👆 Fast   ± 100   💧 Organic, Inorganic, Mix

If necessary, you could also add shading for more density. This is done when the eyebrow hairs are sparse: the central shading, done with bidirectional motions between the hairs for the most natural and three-dimensional look, should never be saturated enough to obscure or cover over the hairs that are already drawn in.

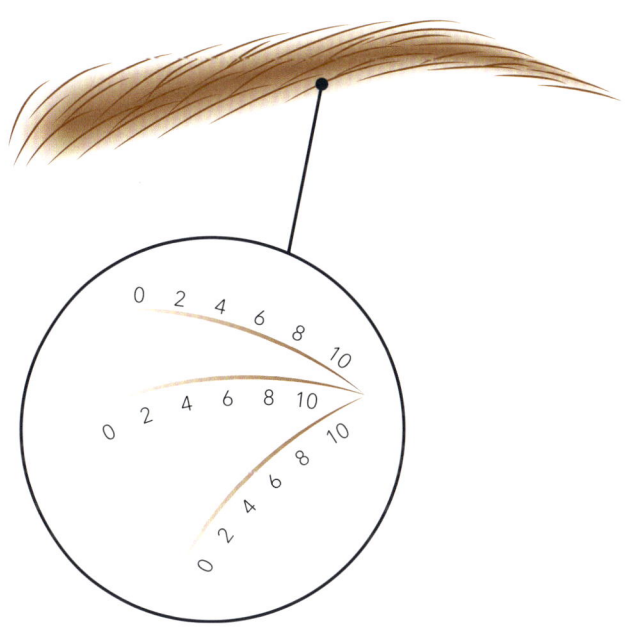

To correctly create shading for density, use a rapid, bidirectional motion that follows the previously drawn hairs, in order to define them even more. Starting from the center of the eyebrow, the shading will be entirely in between the hairs, filling in only the central part in order to achieve a much darker line, which slowly fades out as it extends towards the external outline. The number 10 indicates the darker central color, while the number sequence 8-6-4… indicates that the color gradually lightens until it reaches 0, which is the very light shading around the external outline of the eyebrow.

EYEBROWS

LIPS

EYES

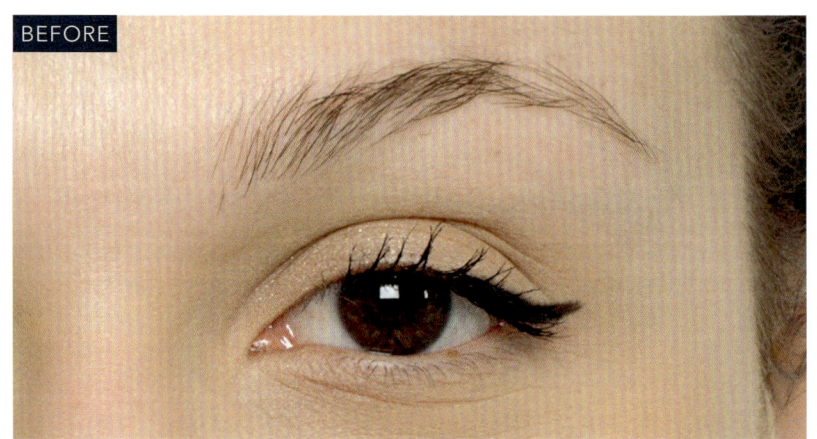

BEFORE

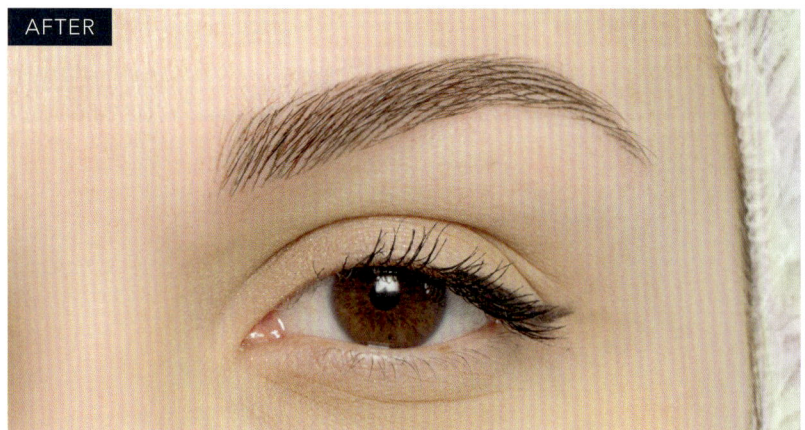

AFTER

Permanent makeup will appear darker at the end of the appointment than in the actual final result. In fact, within 40 days, following cellular mitosis, the color will lighten and appear more natural.

13.1.2.2. DESCENDING HAIRS

1 INITIAL SITUATION

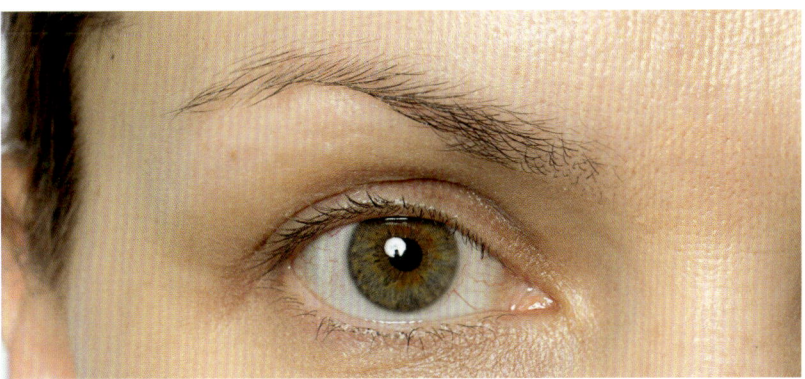

Before applying permanent makeup, the eyebrow ridge must be hygienically prepared.

3 HAIR REMOVAL

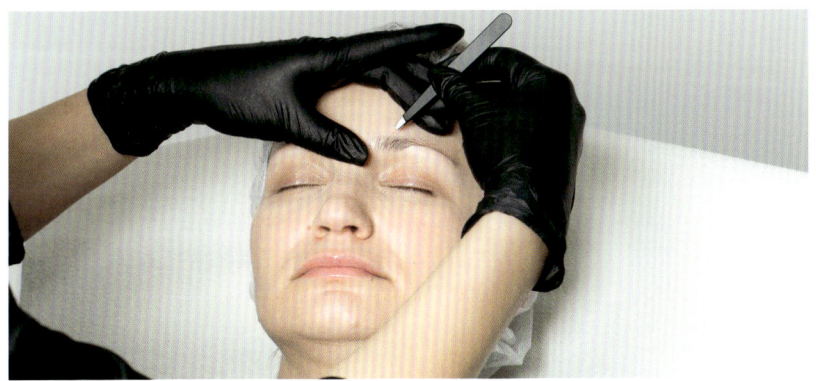

This step is done with tweezers instead of traumatic hair removal methods such as waxing or shaving, making sure to sterilize the tweezers in an autoclave to avoid cross-contamination between clients. First, we remove the hairs that clearly lie outside of our sketch; a second, more precise hair removal phase takes place after sketching in our new eyebrow, to perfect it.

2 CLEANING

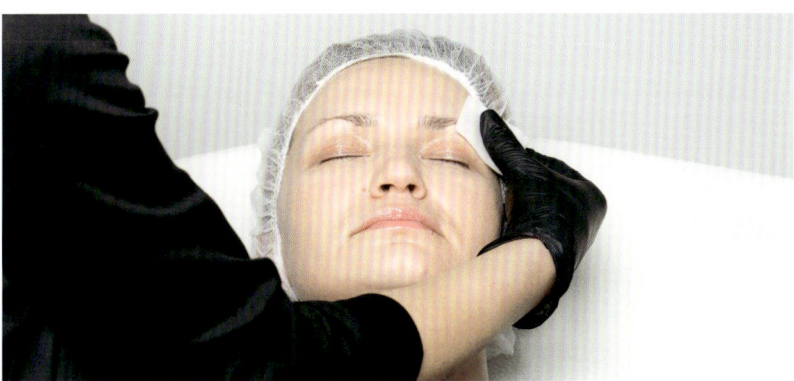

The first phase involves deep-cleaning the area to remove any previously applied makeup or cosmetic products, and to eliminate any potential non-pathogenic microorganisms. We recommend not re-using the dirty part of the wipe.

Treatment steps and pictures by Elena Nikora.

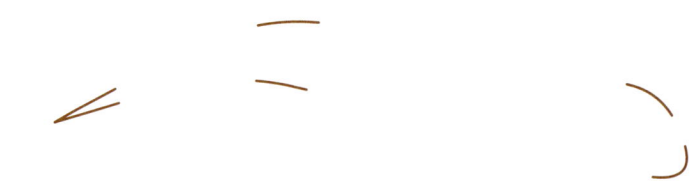

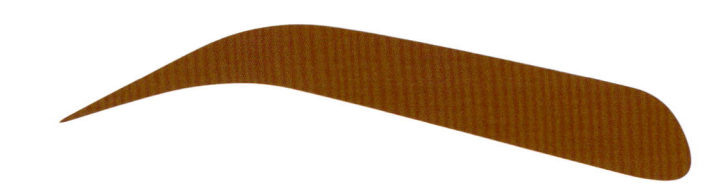

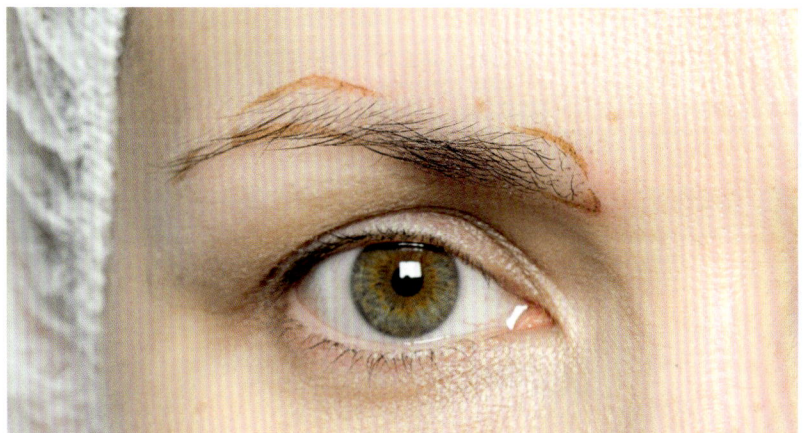

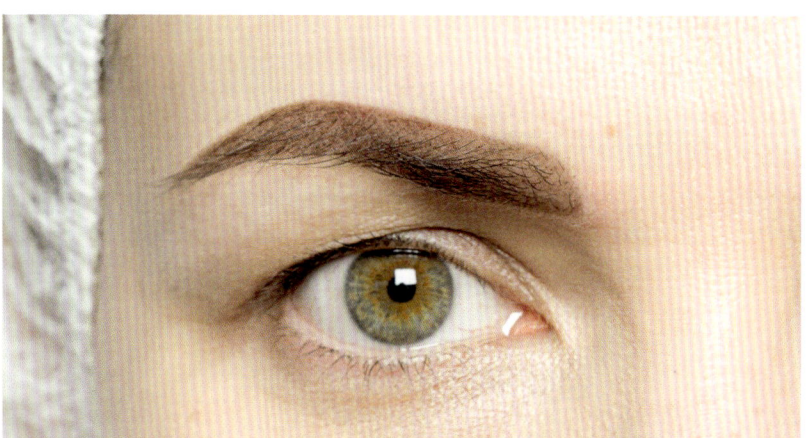

Before beginning any sketch, you should have a clear vision of what you want to achieve for the client, and never leave anything up to improvisation. There are five specific reference points that will help you achieve the desired results as accurately and quickly as possible. The first two points serve to lay out the base of the body and its thickness, while the other two indicate the height of the brow and the width of the vertex, and the last point determines the length and thickness of the tail.

Once these five points are determined and drawn in, all you need to do is connect them and fill in the outline in order to see the chosen shape, and if necessary, make corrections and adjustments.

6 VERTICAL GUIDELINE

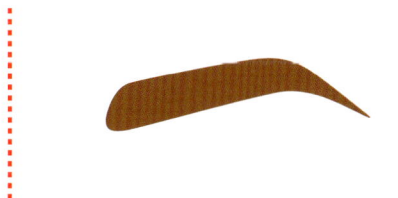

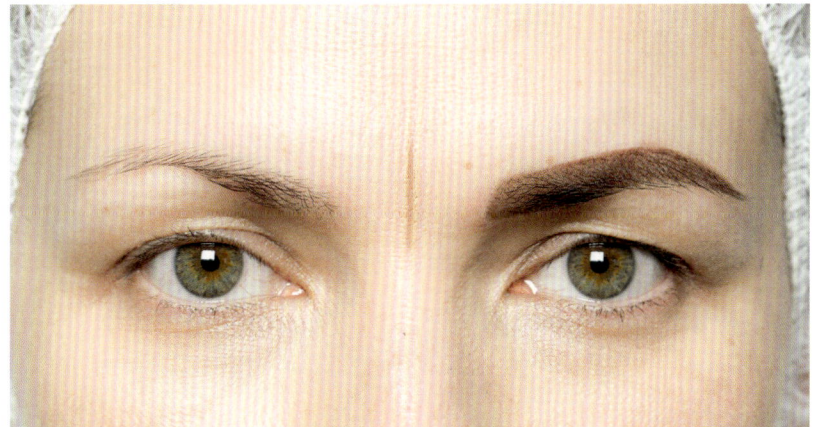

Using a sketching tool and the pigment chosen for the procedure, trace a vertical line at the center of the face, using the forehead, eyes, and nose as reference points. The guideline will be useful for verifying that the distance between the two eyebrows is correct and centered according to the part of the face in question.

⚠ ATTENTION

In some countries only sterile, single-use markers are allowed for this purpose.

7 FIRST HORIZONTAL GUIDELINE

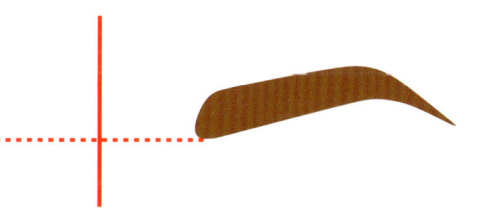

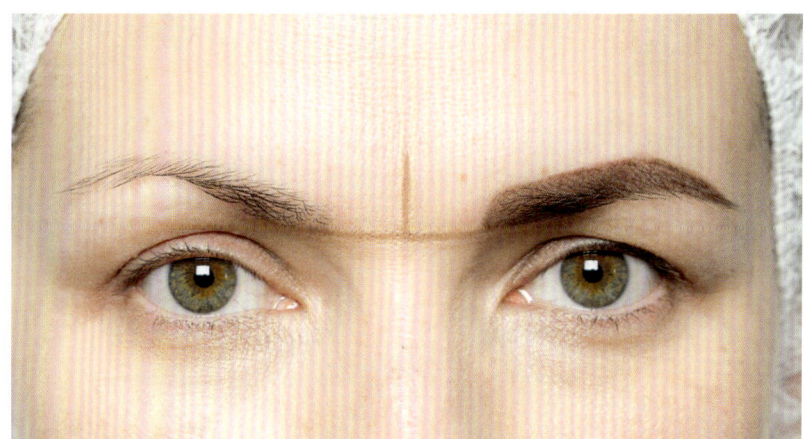

Next, we establish the first horizontal guideline, which is a line that runs parallel to the ground; it starts from the previously drawn eyebrow and leads to the point chosen for the beginning of the second eyebrow. The first horizontal guideline serves to ensure that the eyebrows are placed at the correct height compared to the eyes.

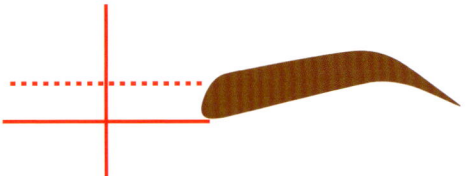

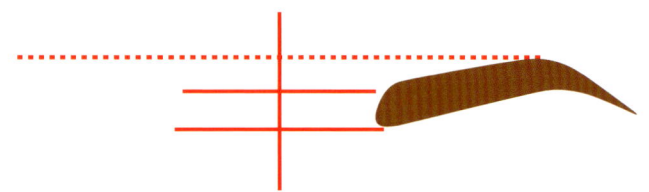

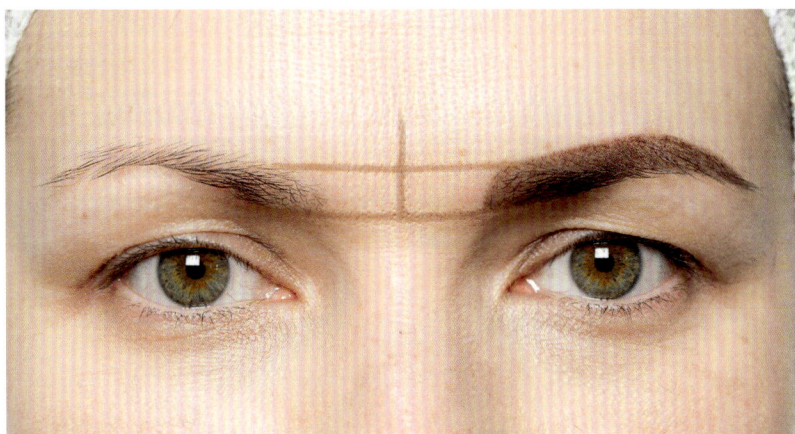

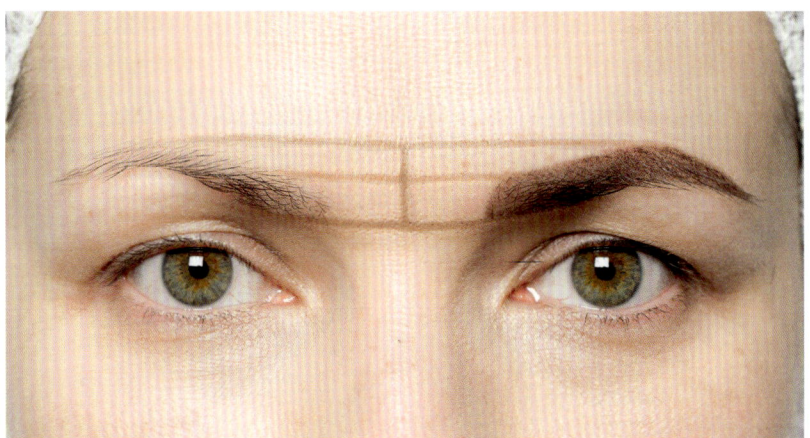

The second, upper horizontal reference point indicates the maximum height of the base of the body of the eyebrow and therefore the width of the base of the eyebrow.

The third horizontal guideline concerns the vertex: a line that runs parallel to the floor and connects the brow arches and determines the highest point of the entire eyebrow. The vertex is one of the most important parts in characterizing a face's non-verbal expression, which is why the original intentions should be considered very carefully.

10 FIRST OBLIQUE GUIDELINE

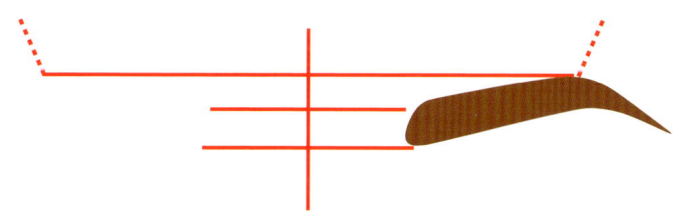

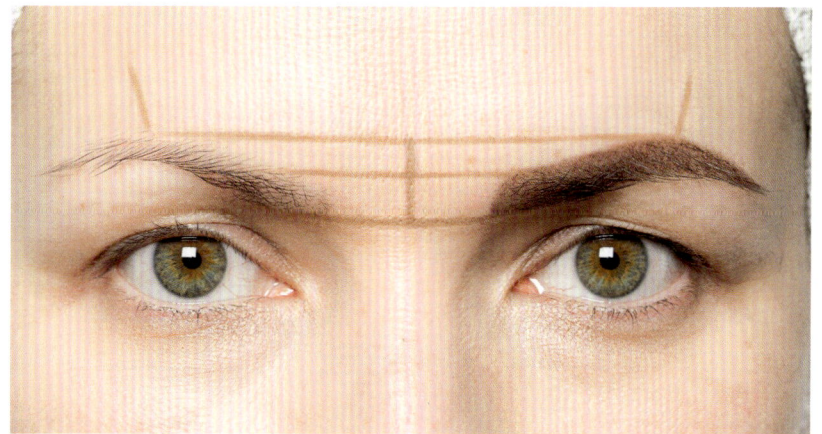

11 SECOND OBLIQUE GUIDELINE

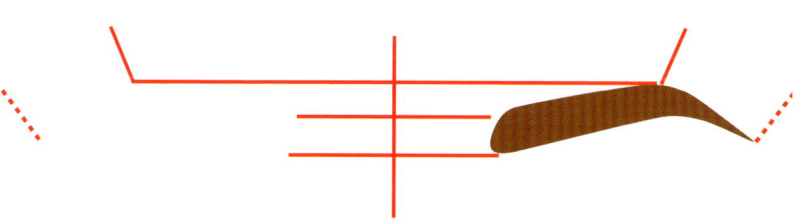

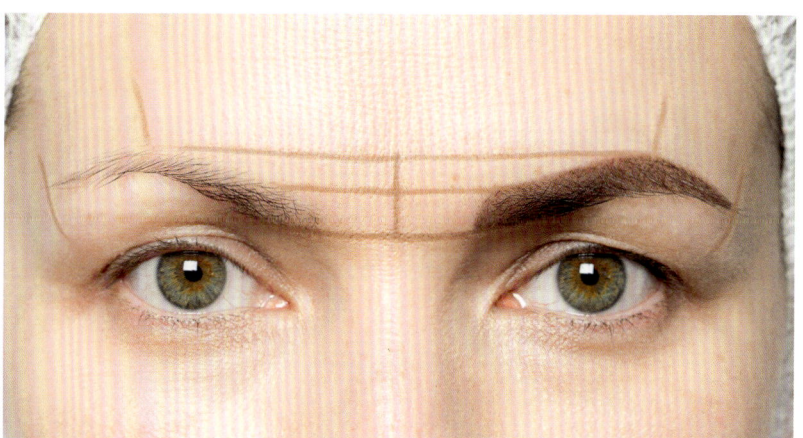

Now it is time to determine the innermost or outermost position of the vertex. Not just its height. The best way to prevent the client from continuously moving their eyes is to firmly place a finger in front of their face, at a distance of about 40 cm, and ask them to stare at it to align the center of the pupil. Only then should you begin tracing an imaginary oblique line that starts from the wing of the nose, passes through the center of the pupil, and therefore indicates the correct placement of the vertex. Repeat the same process for the other eye.

The second oblique guideline determines the length of the tail of the eyebrow. Starting from the wing of the nose once again, trace a second imaginary line, which this time passes through the outer corner of the eye, indicating the maximum length of the tail.

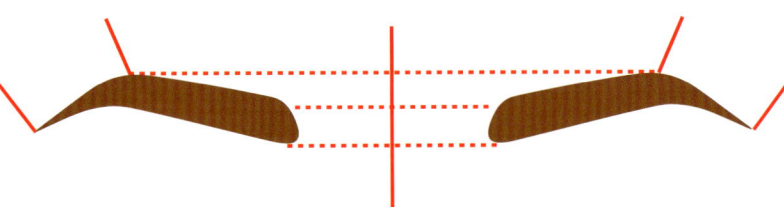

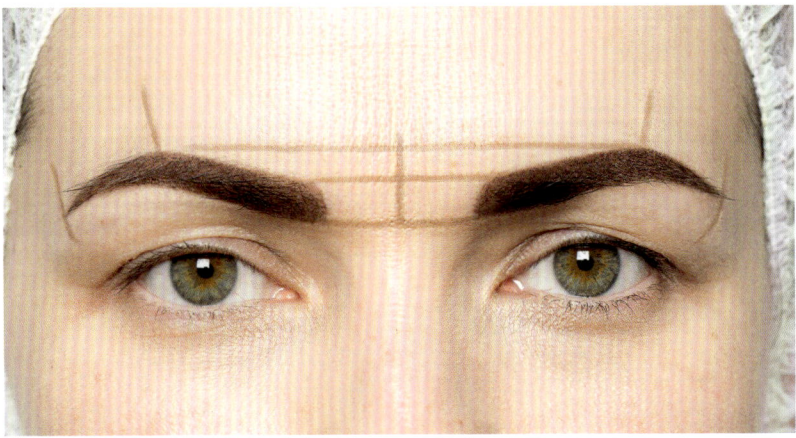

Once this is done, we'll have a grid within which we can quickly position the second eyebrow.

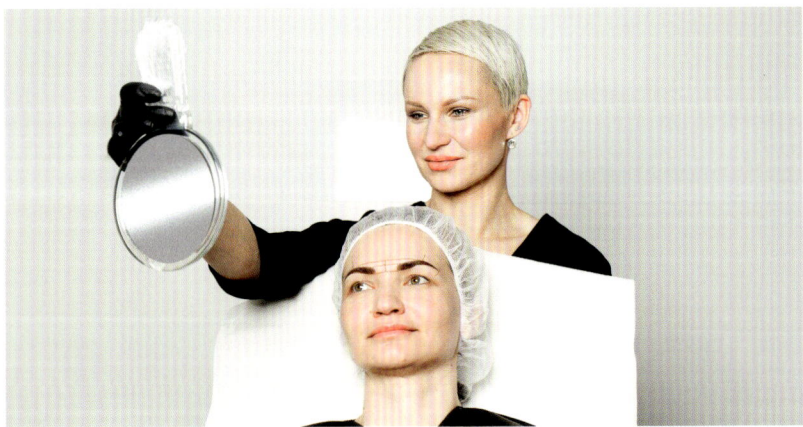

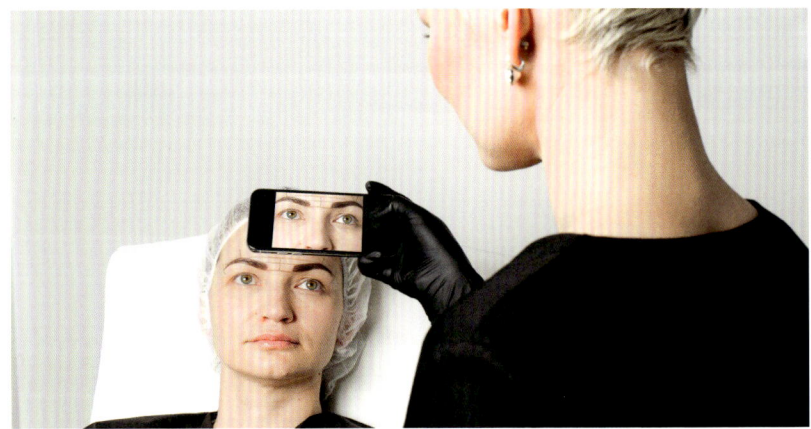

Using these reference points creates a symmetrical and accurate sketch, which should be checked, first through a direct, frontal observation of the client, then through an indirect observation made using two fundamental tools: the mirror and the camera (or a cell phone, if more convenient). This will guarantee the quality of the final results.

14 SKETCH

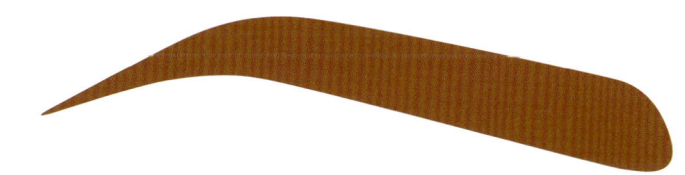

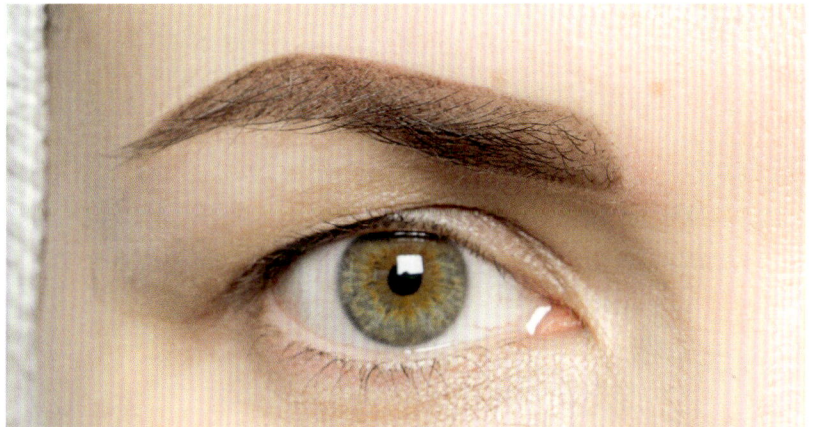

After having created a careful sketch, proceed by marking out the outline.

15 MARKING THE OUTLINE

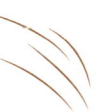

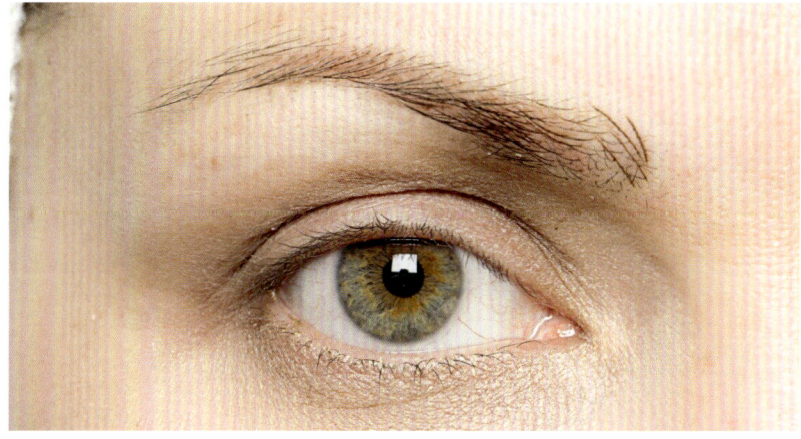

 Unidir./bidir.   90°   Nano n¹, Nano n², Nano nᵀ, 1-Liner

Slow   ± 120   Organic, Inorganic, Mix

We recommend doing the first 4 hairs as shown in the diagram, in order to avoid an overly harsh effect at the base of the eyebrow.

REMEMBER
Hairstrokes with 1 point configurations

| | ◢ 90° | | ◢ 45° | ◢ 60° |

Hairstrokes with 3-slope

| | ◢ 60° |

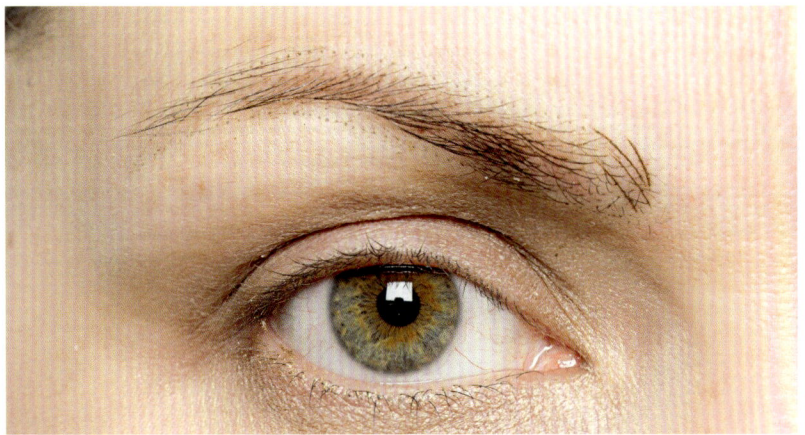

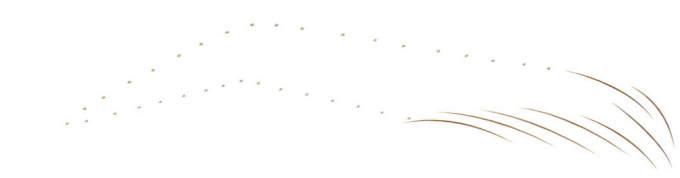

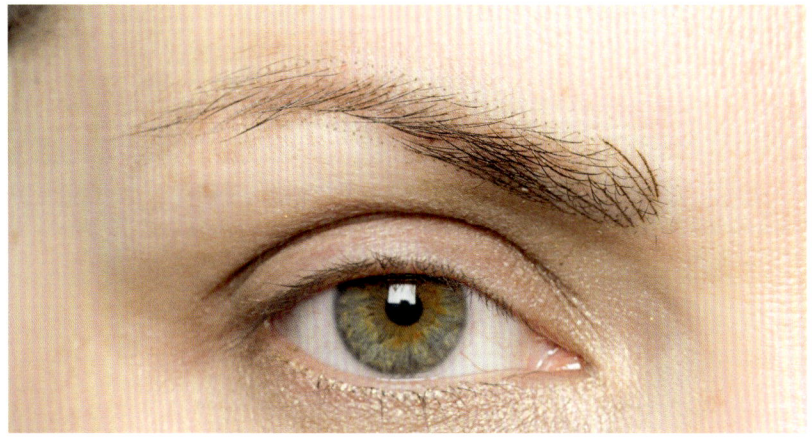

➡ Dots	◢ 90°	🖊 Nano n[1], Nano n[2], Nano n[T]
🕐 Fast	± 120	💧 Organic, Inorganic, Mix

➡ Unidir./bidir.	◢ 45°, 60°, 90°	🖊 Nano n[1], Nano n[2], Nano n[T], 1-Liner
🕐 Slow	± 120/140	💧 Organic, Inorganic, Mix

Continue with the dotted or dashed technique, depending on the professional's level of training and experience. We recommend tracing the outline dots very lightly, so that no traces remain visible after 30 days.

In countries where the law permits it, apply a numbing solution; this not only inhibits pain but also decongests the area, preventing bleeding which could dilute the color. Wait 1-3 minutes and wipe off if necessary. The sketched skin area will turn into a lighter color due to the vasoconstrictive properties of the solution, which makes the design even more visible.

Immediately afterwards, draw a series of very horizontal ascending hairs, which will serve to connect the ascending and descending hairs.

REMEMBER
Hairstrokes with 1 point configurations

⬤	◢ 90°	⬤	◢ 45°	◢ 60°

Hairstrokes with 3-slope

⬤	◢ 60°

18 UPPER DESCENDING HAIRS

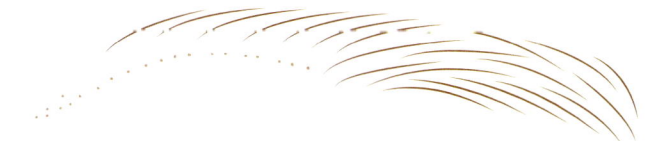

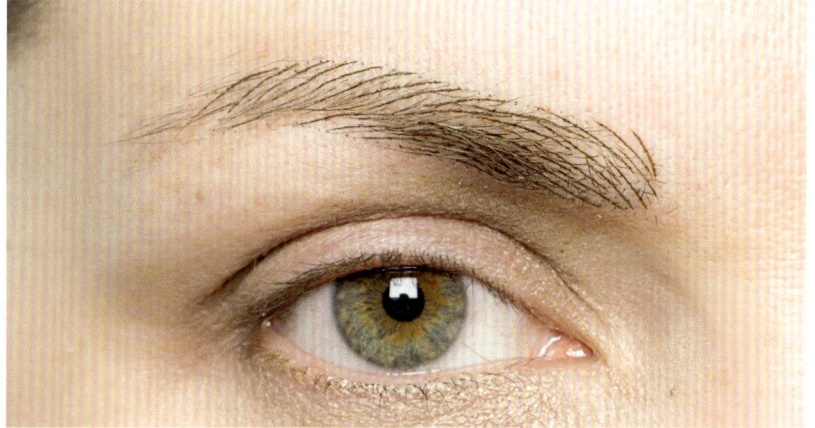

➡ Unidir./bidir. ◢ 45°, 60°, 90° ⬇ Nano n[1], Nano n[2], Nano n[T], 1-Liner
✋ Slow ± 120/140 💧 Organic, Inorganic, Mix

The upper descending hairs will rest on the base of these connecting hairs. We recommend creating these hairs starting from the center of the eyebrow and moving towards the upper area in order to avoid making the extremity overly thick.

18 LOWER DESCENDING HAIRS

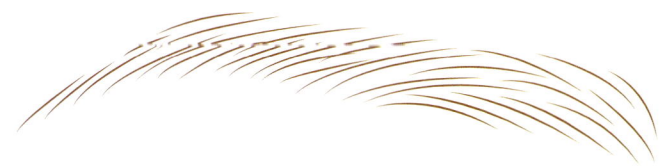

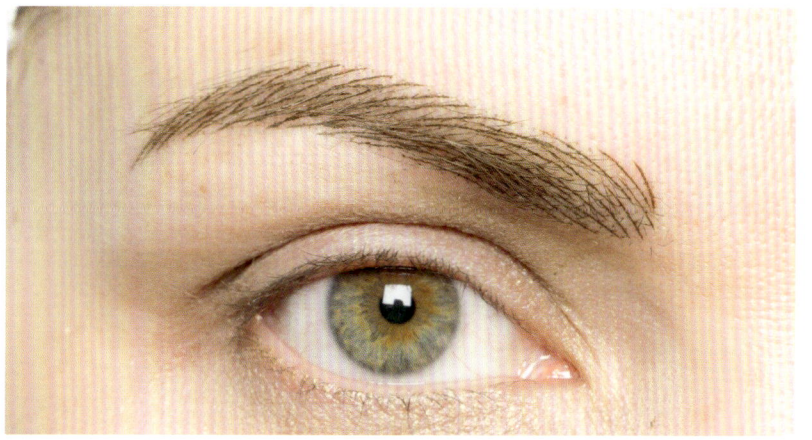

➡ Unidir./bidir. ◢ 45°, 60°, 90° ⬇ Nano n[1], Nano n[2], Nano n[T], 1-Liner
✋ Slow ± 120/140 💧 Organic, Inorganic, Mix

Now it is time to insert the lower descending hairs, which start from the center of the eyebrow and end in the tail, creating continuity with the tails drawn before. It is not common to find hairs that extend a long the entire length: usually they are divided up. Therefore, two or three hairs should be added if the eyebrow is thicker.

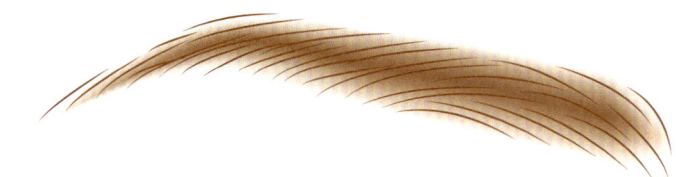

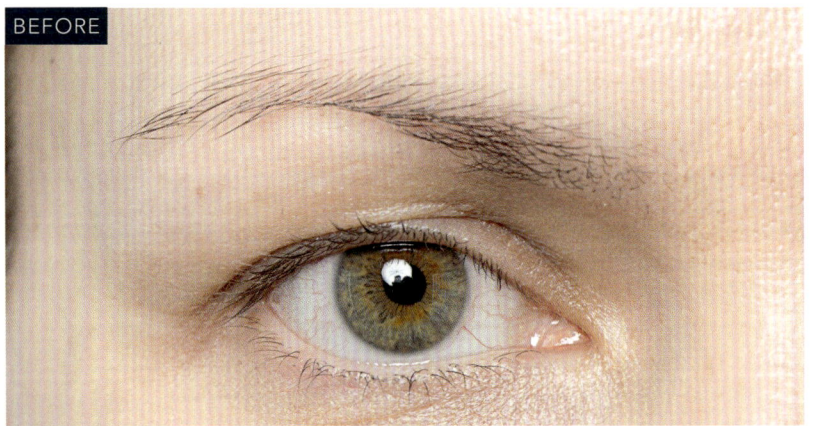

BEFORE

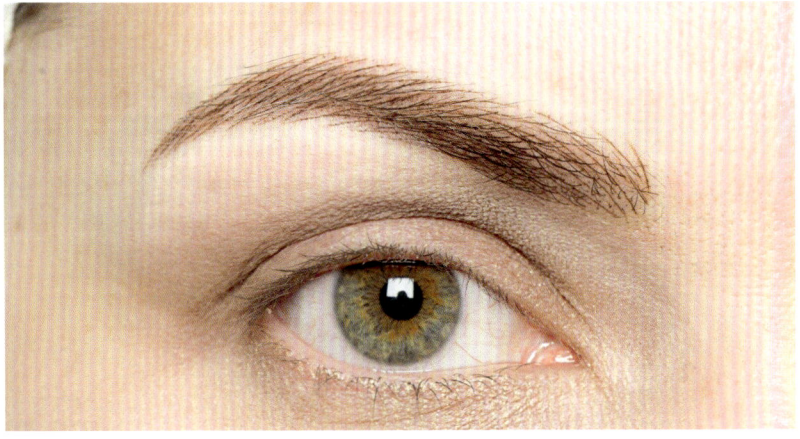

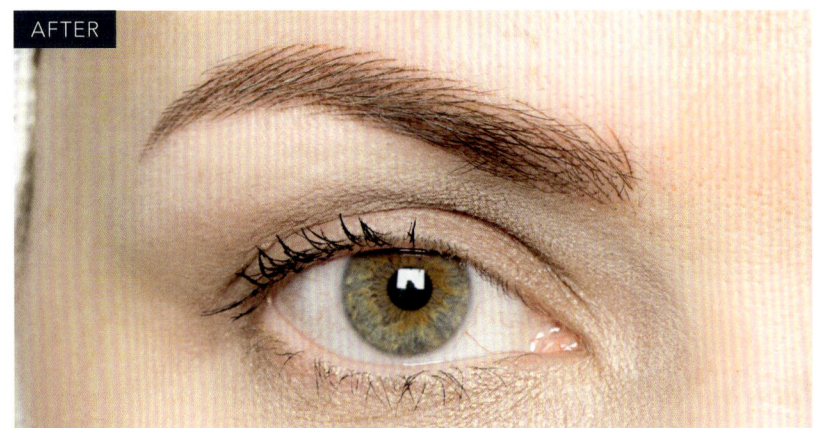

AFTER

➡ Zigzag bidir.   ◿ 90°   🌡 Nano n¹, Nano n², Nano nᵀ, 1-Liner

✋ Fast   ± 100   💧 Organic, Inorganic, Mix

Proceed with the central shading using bidirectional movements between the hairs: it is good to reiterate that the center part should be made darker, and it should lighten and fade out towards the upper and lower outlines, to obtain the same level of density.

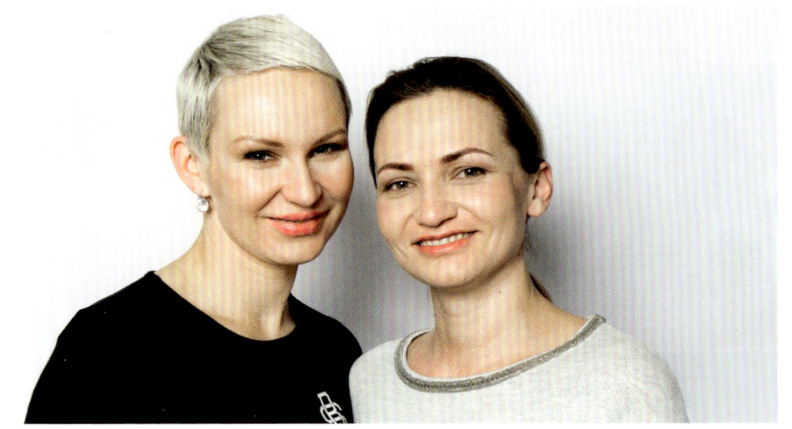

13.1.2.3. ASCENDING AND DESCENDING HAIRS

1 INITIAL SITUATION

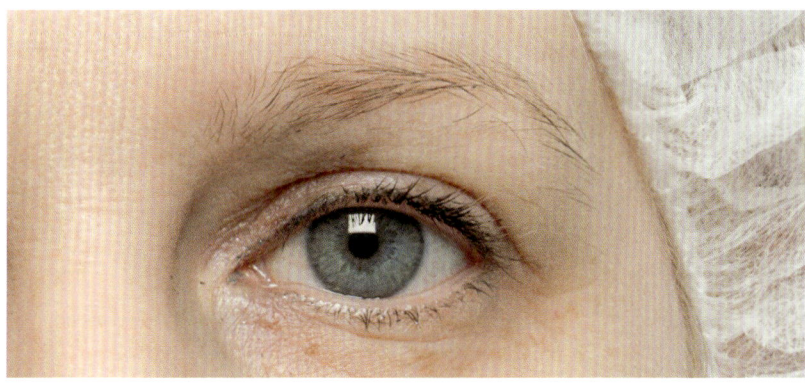

Before applying permanent makeup, the eyebrow ridge must be hygienically prepared.

2 CLEANING

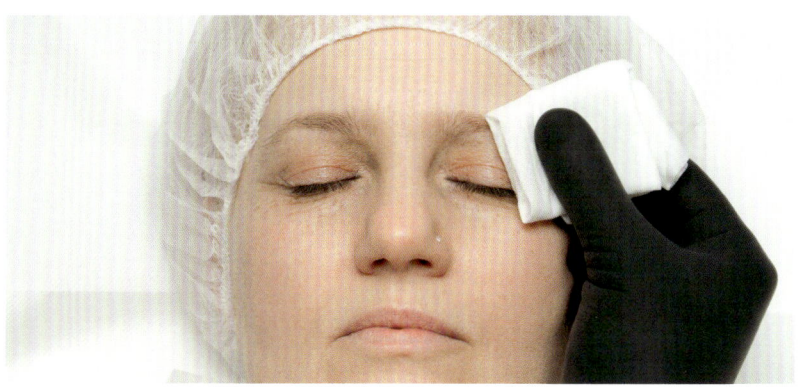

The first phase involves deep-cleaning the area to remove any previously applied makeup or cosmetic products, and to eliminate any potential non-pathogenic microorganisms. We recommend not re-using the dirty part of the wipe.

3 HAIR REMOVAL

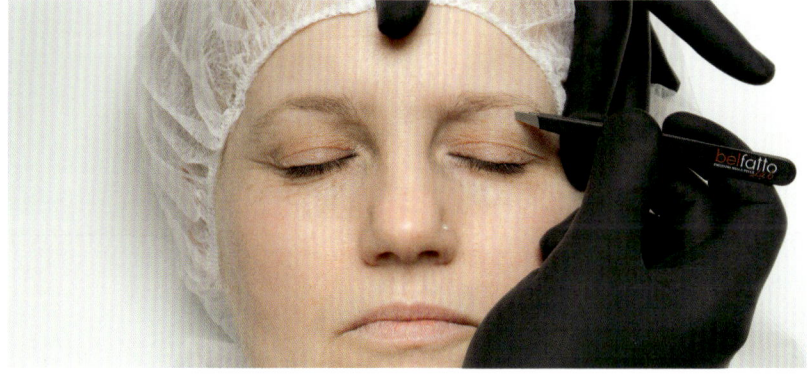

This step is done with tweezers instead of traumatic hair removal methods such as waxing or shaving, making sure to sterilize the tweezers in an autoclave to avoid cross-contamination between clients. First, we remove the hairs that clearly lie outside of our sketch; a second, more precise hair removal phase takes place after drawing in our new eyebrow, to perfect it.

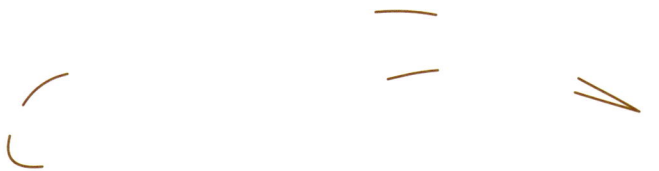

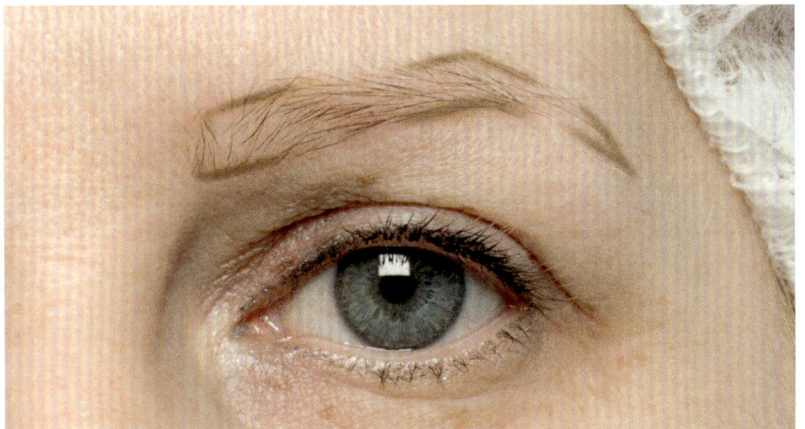

Before beginning any sketch, you should have a clear vision of what you want to achieve for the client, and never leave anything up to improvisation. There are five specific reference points that will help you achieve the desired results as accurately and quickly as possible. The first two points serve to lay out the base of the body and its thickness, while the other two indicate the height of the brow and the width of the vertex, and the last point determines the length and thickness of the tail.

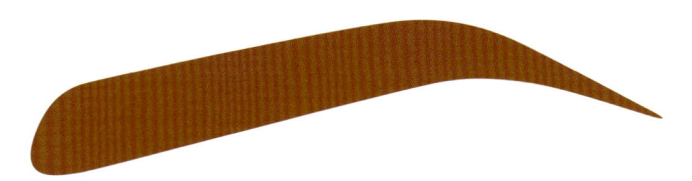

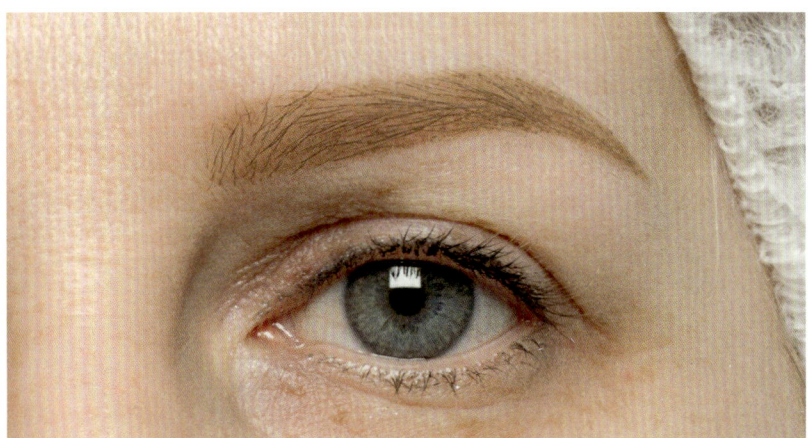

Once these five points are determined and drawn in, all you need to do is connect them and fill in the outline in order to see the chosen shape, and if necessary, make corrections and adjustments.

6 VERTICAL GUIDELINE

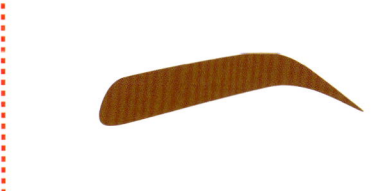

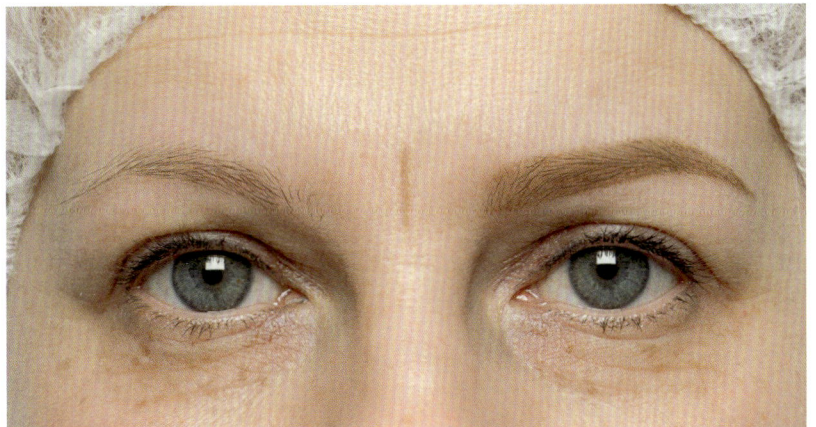

Using a sketching tool and the pigment chosen for the procedure, trace a vertical line at the center of the face, using the forehead, eyes, and nose as reference points. This guideline will be useful for verifying that the distance between the two eyebrows is correct and centered according to the part of the face in question.

⚠ ATTENTION

In some countries only sterile, single-use markers are allowed for this purpose.

7 FIRST HORIZONTAL GUIDELINE

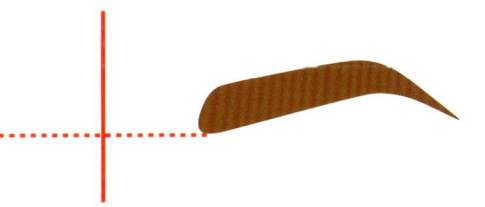

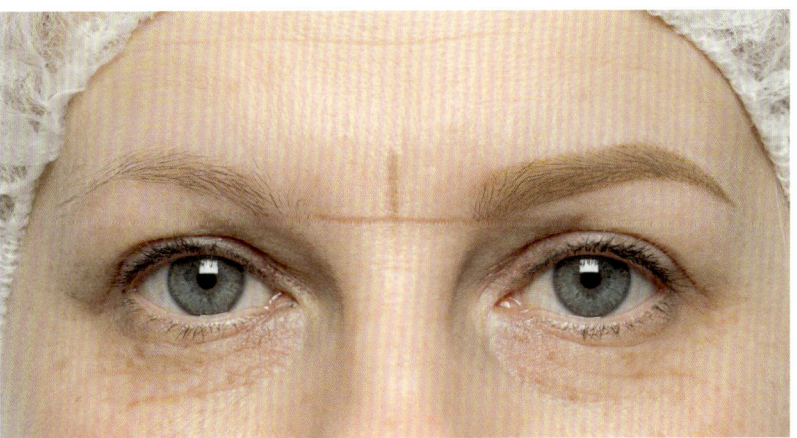

Next, we establish the first horizontal guideline, which is a line that runs parallel to the ground; it starts from the previously drawn eyebrow and leads to the point chosen for the beginning of the second eyebrow. The first horizontal guideline serves to ensure that the eyebrows are placed at the correct height compared to the eyes.

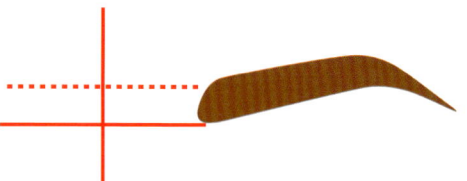

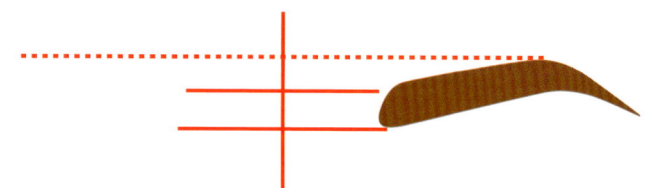

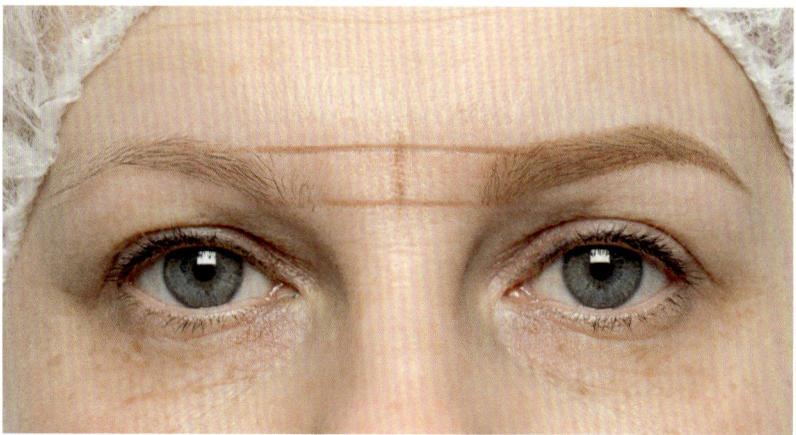

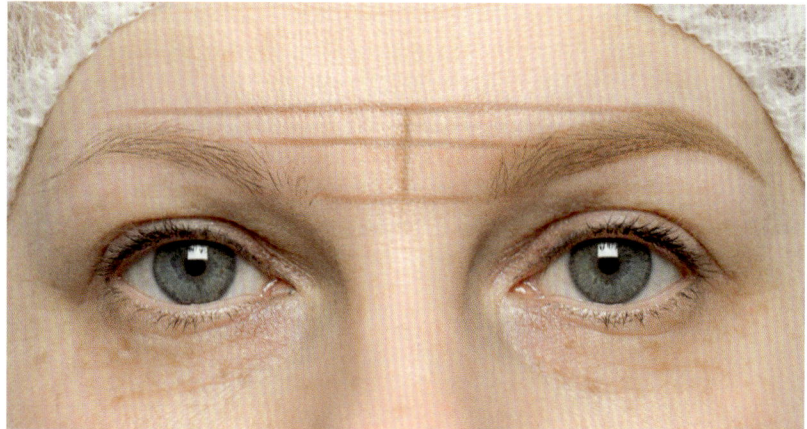

The second, upper horizontal reference point indicates the maximum height of the base of the body of the eyebrow and therefore the width of the base of the eyebrow.

The third horizontal guideline concerns the vertex: a line that runs parallel to the floor and connects the brow arches and determines the highest point of the entire eyebrow. The vertex is one of the most important parts in characterizing a face's non-verbal expression, which is why the original intentions should be considered very carefully.

10 FIRST OBLIQUE GUIDELINE

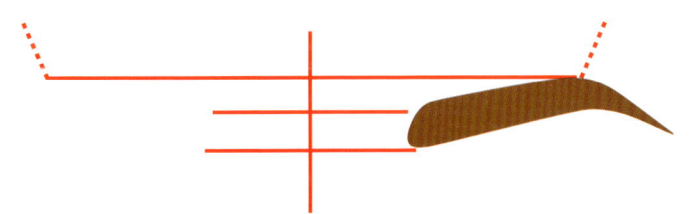

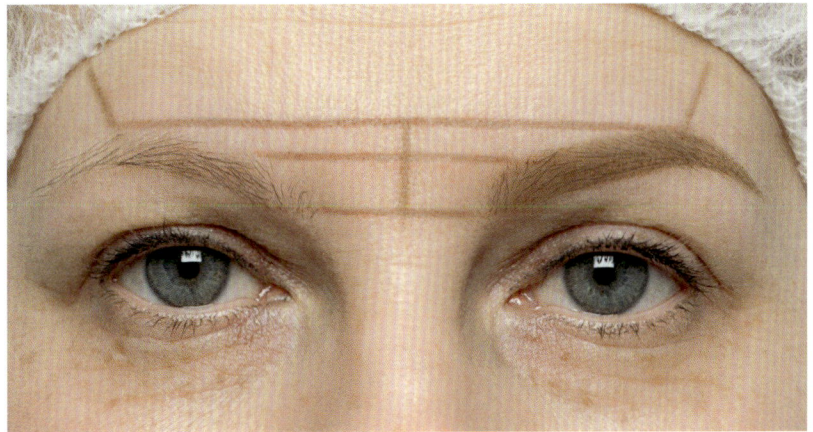

Now it is time to determine the innermost or outermost position of the vertex. Not just its height. The best way to prevent the client from continuously moving their eyes is to firmly place a finger in front of their face, at a distance of about 40 cm, and ask them to stare at it to align the center of the pupil. Only then should you begin tracing an imaginary oblique line that starts from the wing of the nose, passes through the center of the pupil, and therefore indicates the correct placement of the vertex. Repeat the same process for the other eye.

11 SECOND OBLIQUE GUIDELINE

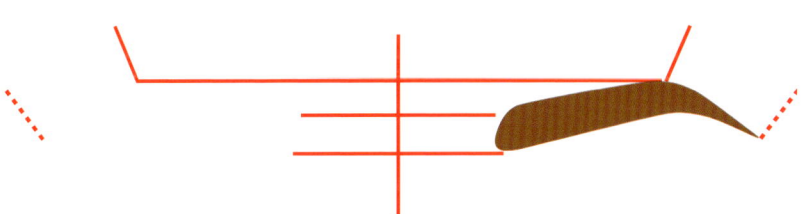

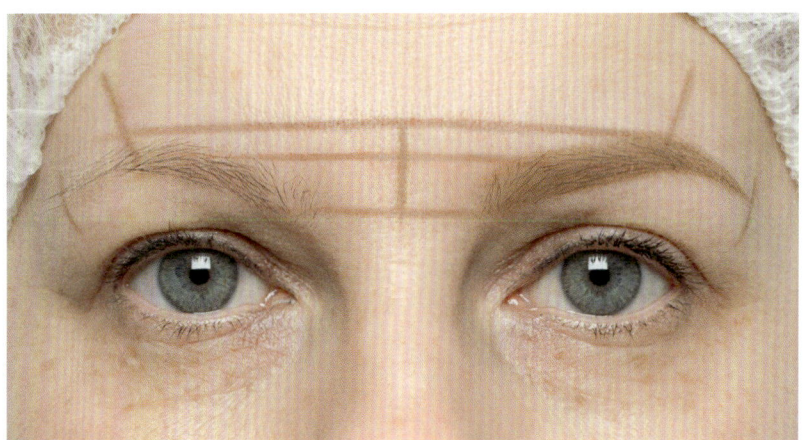

The second oblique guideline determines the length of the tail of the eyebrow. Starting from the wing of the nose once again, trace a second imaginary line, which this time passes through the exterior angle of the eye, indicating the maximum length of the tail.

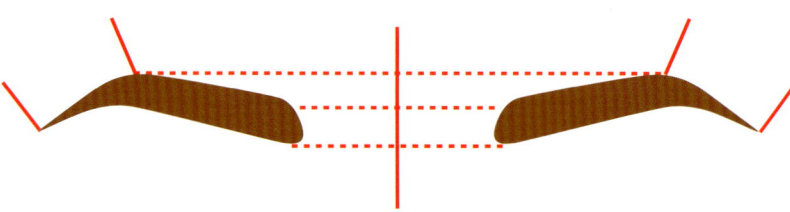

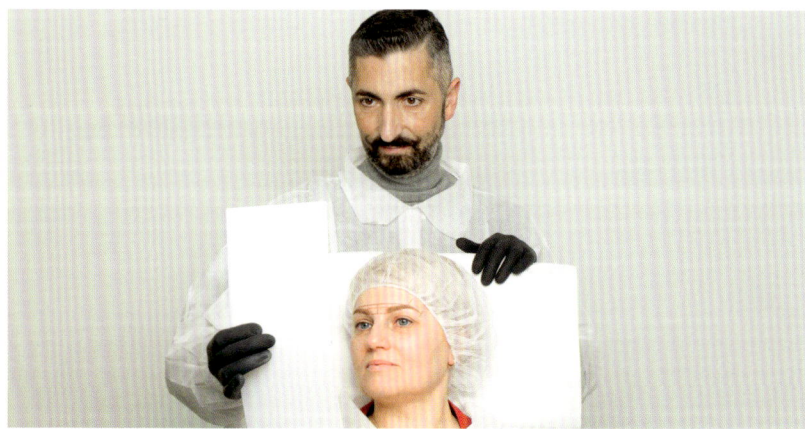

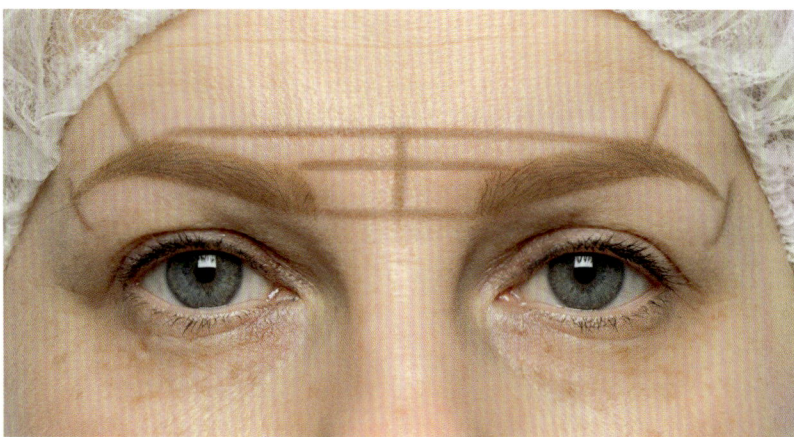

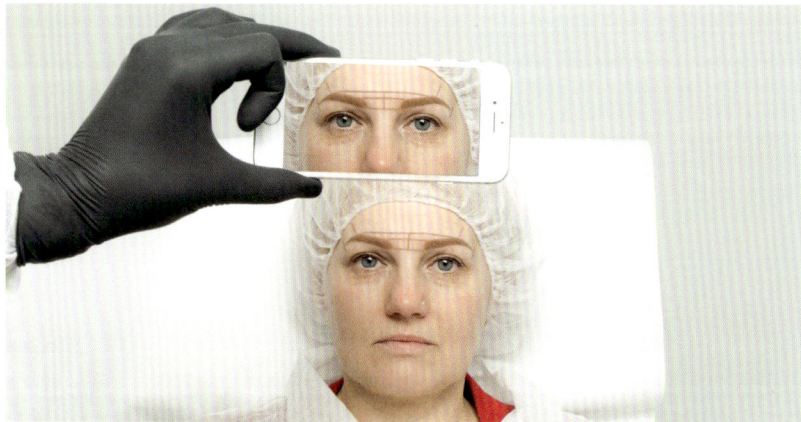

Once this is done, we'll have a grid within which we can quickly position the second eyebrow.

Using these reference points creates a symmetrical and accurate sketch, which should be checked, first through a direct, frontal observation of the client, then through an indirect observation made using two fundamental tools: the mirror and the camera (or a cell phone, if more convenient). This will guarantee the quality of the final results.

14 SKETCH

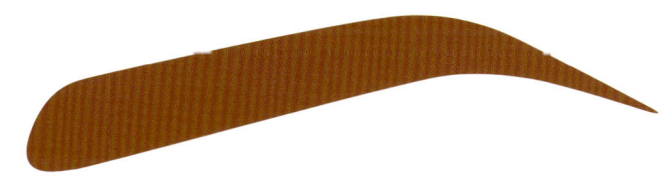

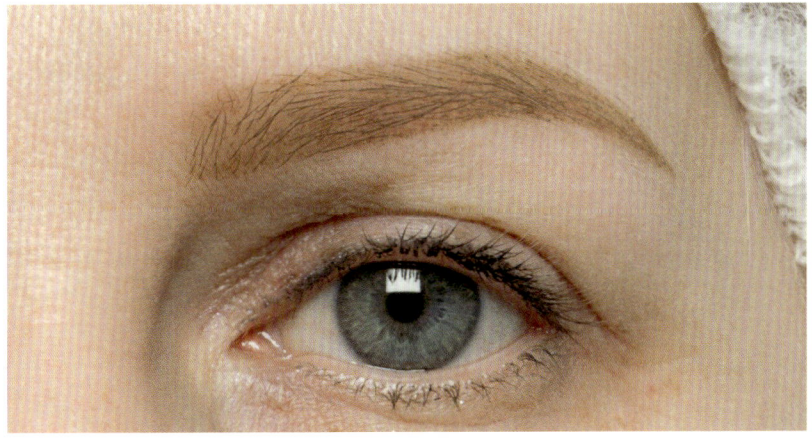

After having created a careful sketch, proceed by marking out the outline.

15 MARKING THE OUTLINE

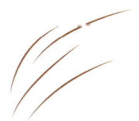

➡ Unidir./bidir.	◢ 90°	🌡 Nano n[1], Nano n[2], Nano n[T]
✋ Slow	± 120	💧 Organic, Inorganic, Mix

Start with the first 4 hairs at the base of the eyebrow to avoid an overly defined effect.

REMEMBER
Hairstrokes with 1 point configurations

◐	◢ 90°	◓	◢ 45°	◢ 60°

Hairstrokes with 3-slope

◐	◢ 60°

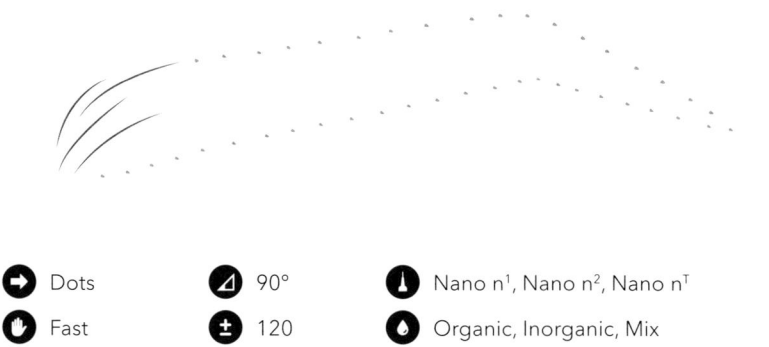

⮕ Dots ◢ 90° ◖ Nano n[1], Nano n[2], Nano n[T]

◔ Fast ± 120 ◗ Organic, Inorganic, Mix

Continue marking the outline using the dotted technique in order to preserve the sketch. We recommend tracing the outline dots very lightly, so that no traces remain visible after 30 days.

In countries where the law permits it, apply a numbing solution; this not only inhibits pain but also decongests the area, preventing bleeding which could dilute the color. Wait 1–3 minutes and wipe off if necessary. The sketched skin area will turn into a lighter color due to the vasoconstrictive properties of the solution, which makes the design even more visible.

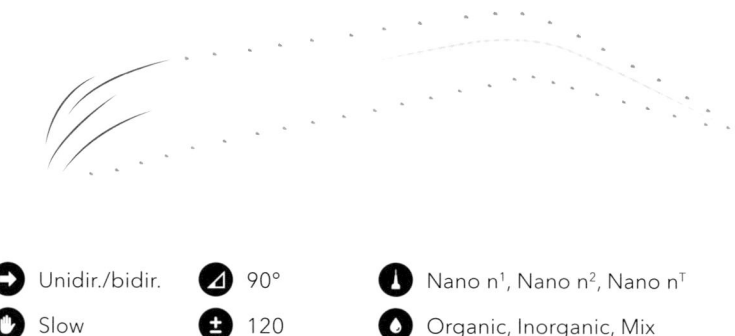

⮕ Unidir./bidir. ◢ 90° ◖ Nano n[1], Nano n[2], Nano n[T]

◔ Slow ± 120 ◗ Organic, Inorganic, Mix

At this point, add an additional line which begins from the end of the tail of the eyebrow, and ends at the center of the body, creating a sort of back bone. Trace this line with diluted pigment to differentiate it from the outline hairs.

18 ASCENDING HAIRS

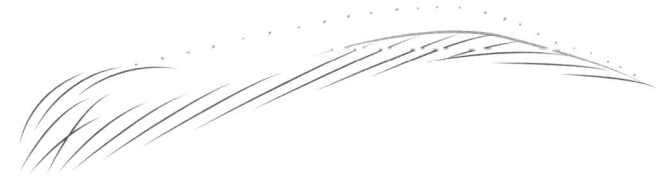

- ➡ Unidir./bidir.
- ✋ Slow
- ◿ 45°, 60°, 90°
- ± 120/140
- ⬇ Nano n¹, Nano n², Nano nᵀ, 1-Liner
- 💧 Organic, Inorganic, Mix

Given that the first hairs are always ascending, begin with the lower ascending hairs, following a domino effect and maintaining a minimum distance of half a millimeter between them.

REMEMBER
Hairstrokes with 1 point configurations

⬤	◿ 90°	⬤	◿ 45°	◿ 60°

Hairstrokes with 3-slope

⬤	◿ 60°

19 DESCENDING HAIRS

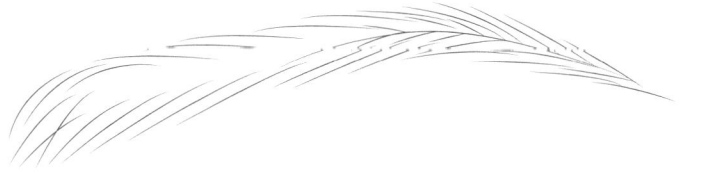

- ➡ Unidir./bidir.
- ✋ Slow
- ◿ 45°, 60°, 90°
- ± 120/140
- ⬇ Nano n¹, Nano n², Nano nᵀ, 1-Liner
- 💧 Organic, Inorganic, Mix

Continue with the upper descending hairs: these hairs will start descending down to the "back bone" and extend to the tail, with the opposite orientation of the previous hairs. It is important that the hairs do not cross over each other at the end, since this would pose the risk of the undesirable "Christmas Tree" effect.

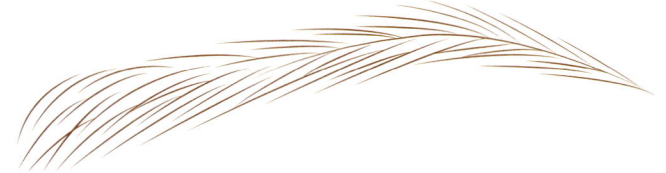

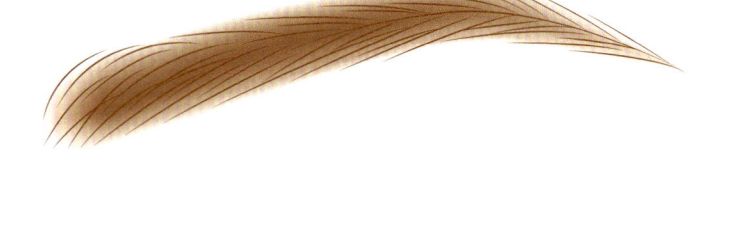

Unidir./bidir.   **45°, 60°, 90°**   Nano n[1], Nano n[2], Nano n[T], 1-Liner
Slow   **120/140**   Organic, Inorganic, Mix

Zigzag bidir.   **90°**   Nano n[1], Nano n[2], Nano n[T], 1-Liner
Fast   **100**   Organic, Inorganic, Mix

Procced to the center density hairs, which at first will follow the same orientation as the previous hairs, but will gradually take on a more horizontal angle, almost parallel to the floor, as they reach the center part of the body.

At this point, also shade in density if necessary. Once again, this shaded-in density should not cover up hairs, but serves to create added color to make the eyebrows more three-dimensional. The correct color intensities (10-8-6...) are mapped out in the drawing.

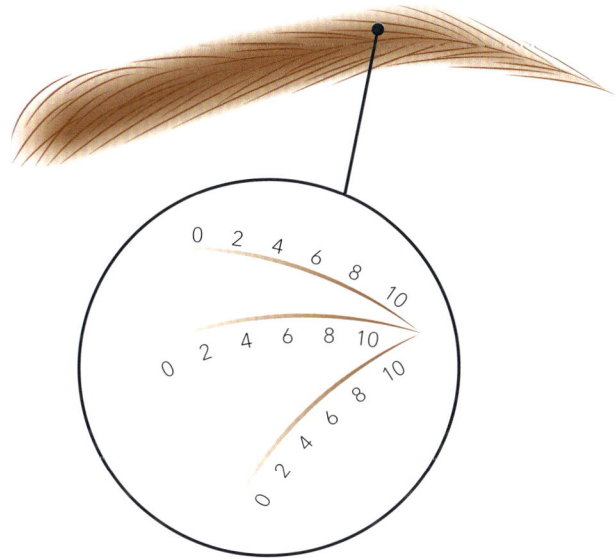

Starting from the center, the shading will perfectly follow the direction of the ascending, descending, and density hairs without ever reaching the outline area which should be the most transparent. The number 10 indicates the darker central color, while the number sequence 8-6-4... indicates that the color gradually lightens until it reaches 0, which is the very light shading around the external outline of the eyebrow.

"Don't seek the recipe for happiness;
invent one that tastes like you."
TONI BELFATTO

EYEBROWS

LIPS

EYES

13.1.3. COVERING TECHNIQUES

Defined techniques require more perfection: the eyebrows are more defined, but appear less natural. The effect is closer to that of daily makeup, when they are filled in with a pencil. This includes two techniques: SHADING and FILLING.

SHADING

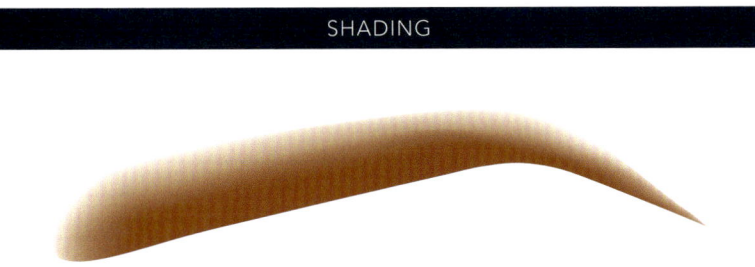

FILLING IN

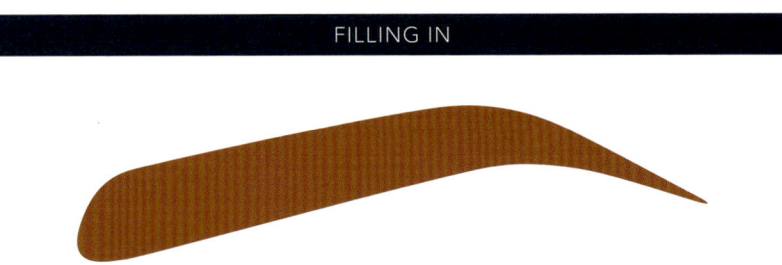

The lower part of the arch of the brow will generally be darkened to add more volume, then lightened towards the tail as the color gradually fades to reveal two areas: the first, slightly darker, and the upper one slightly lighter. In shaded eyebrows, the area should be filled in very lightly.

Meanwhile, the filling technique is the earliest, as well as the easiest. Once the contours are established, just proceed by simply coloring it in evenly. This technique shouldn't be thought of as the vulgar, full-color tattoo of many years ago when permanent makeup was little known, and performed by a few inexperienced tattoo artists. Although it is out of fashion and not requested often, you can sometimes achieve beautiful results when it is done with very light, subtle colors to guarantee saturation on difficult skin types, or for maximum definition on clients who are used to obvious makeup. It is also often used for camouflaging prior work, as an alternative to laser.

13.1.3.1. SHADING

1 INITIAL SITUATION

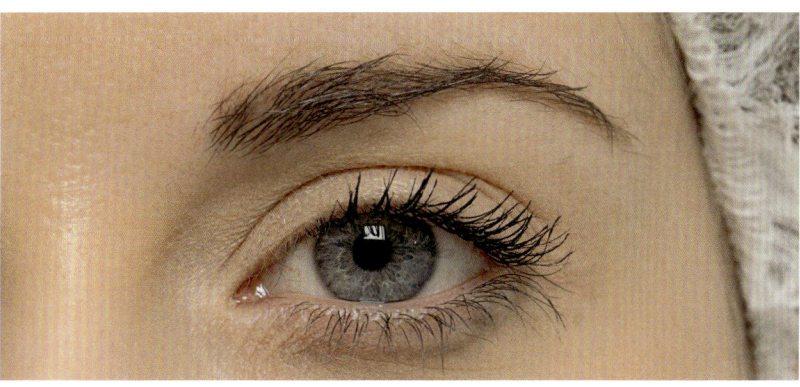

Before applying permanent makeup, the eyebrow ridge must be hygienically prepared.

2 CLEANING

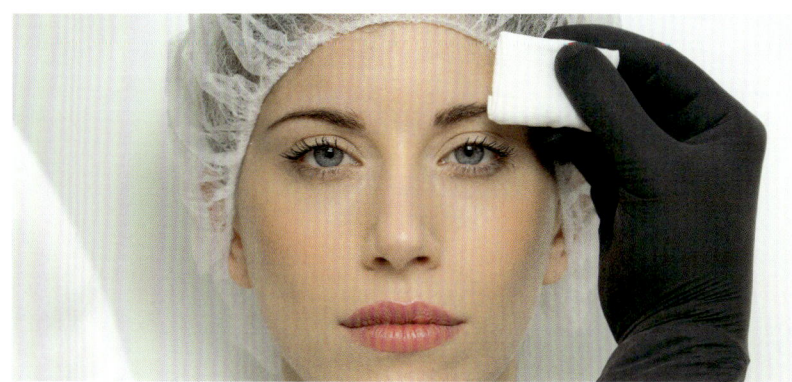

The first phase involves deep-cleaning the area to remove any previously applied makeup or cosmetic products, and to eliminate any potential non-pathogenic microorganisms. We recommend not re-using the dirty part of the wipe.

3 HAIR REMOVAL

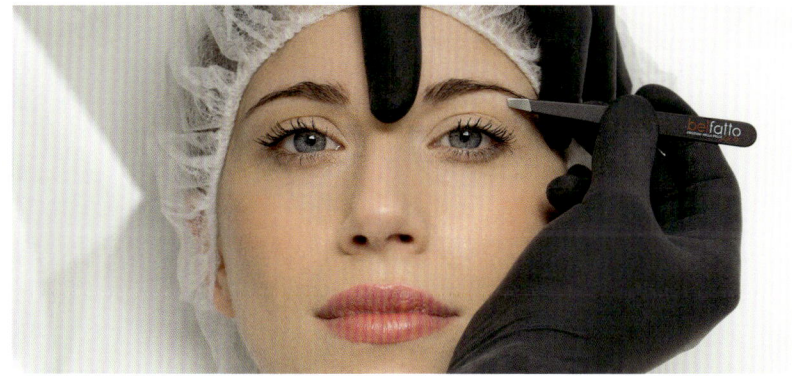

This step is done with tweezers instead of traumatic hair removal methods such as waxing or shaving, making sure to sterilize the tweezers in an autoclave to avoid cross-contamination between clients. First, we remove the hairs that clearly lie outside of our sketch; a second, more precise hair removal phase takes place after drawing in our new eyebrow, to perfect it.

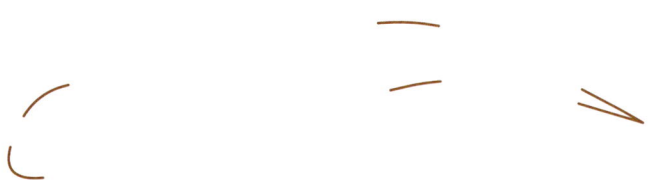

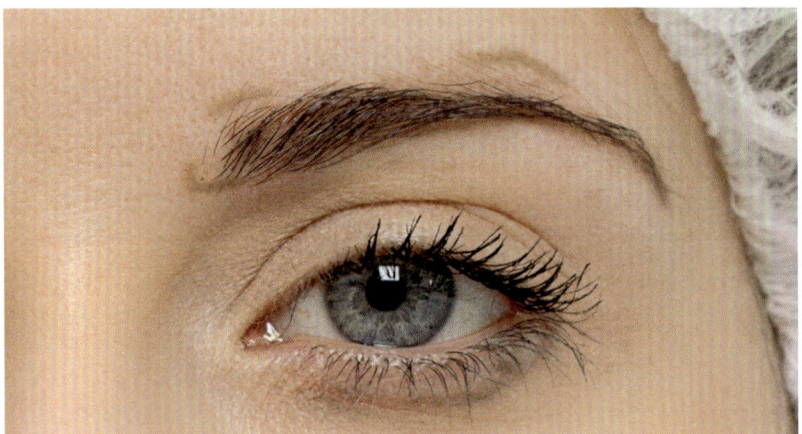

Before beginning any sketch, you should have a clear vision of what you want to achieve for the client, and never leave anything up to improvisation. There are five specific reference points that will help you achieve the desired results as accurately and quickly as possible. The first two points serve to lay out the base of the body and its thickness, while the other two indicate the height of the brow and the width of the vertex, and the last point determines the length and thickness of the tail.

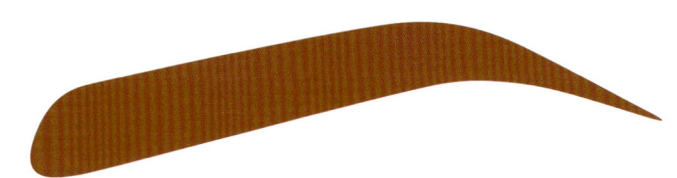

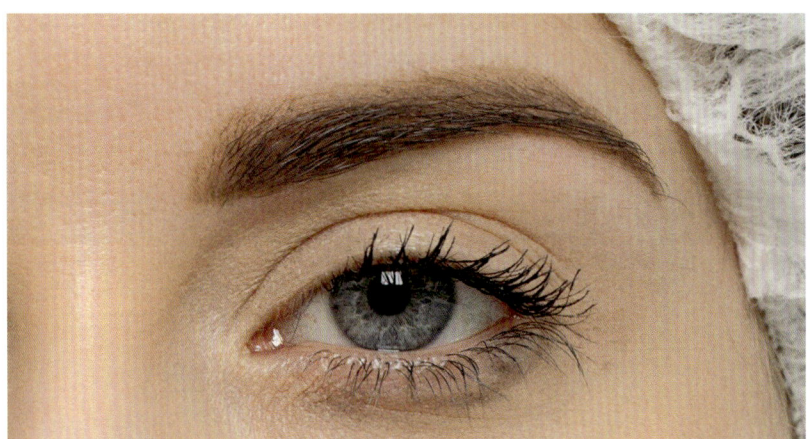

Once these five points are determined and drawn in, all you need to do is connect them and fill in the outline in order to see the chosen shape, and if necessary, make corrections and adjustments.

6 VERTICAL GUIDELINE

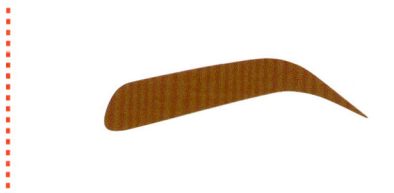

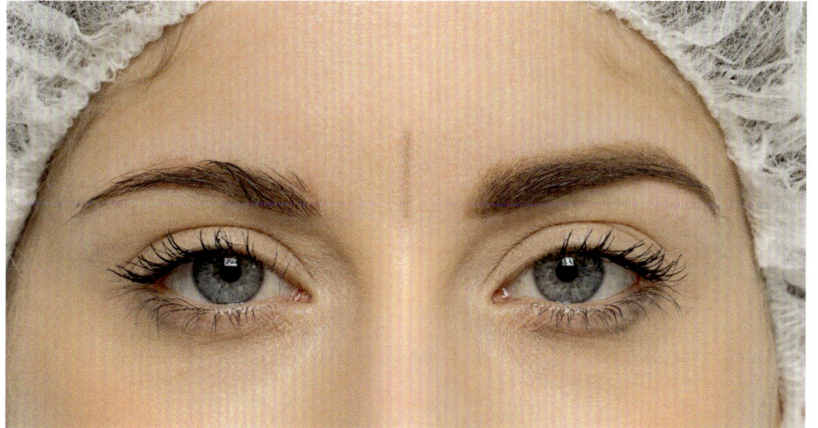

Using a sketching tool and the pigment chosen for the procedure, trace a vertical line at the center of the face, using the forehead, eyes, and nose as reference points. This guideline will be useful for verifying that the distance between the two eyebrows is correct and centered according to the part of the face in question.

⚠ ATTENTION

In some countries only sterile, single-use markers are allowed for this purpose.

7 FIRST HORIZONTAL GUIDELINE

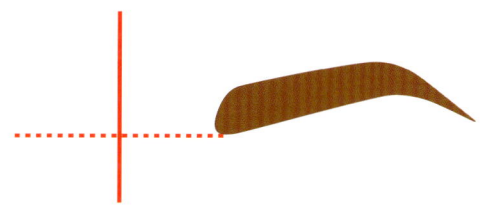

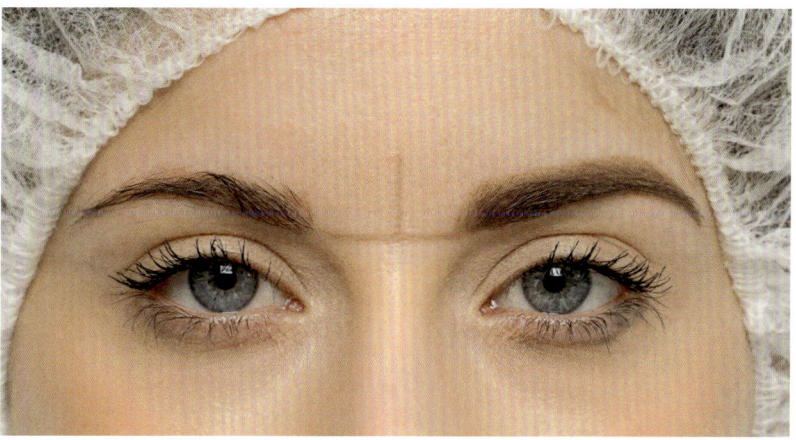

Next, we establish the first horizontal guideline, which is a line that runs parallel to the ground; it starts from the previously drawn eyebrow and leads to the point chosen for the beginning of the second eyebrow. The first horizontal guideline serves to ensure that the eyebrows are placed at the correct height compared to the eyes.

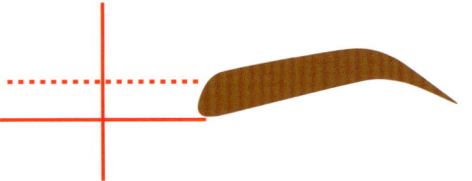

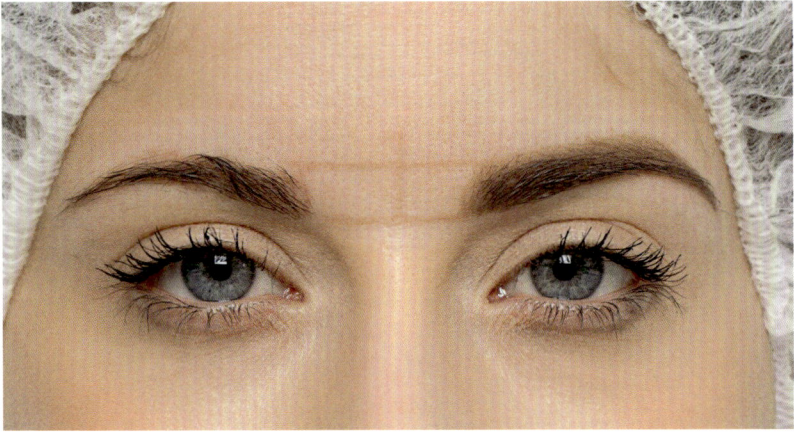

The second, upper horizontal reference point indicates the maximum height of the base of the body of the eyebrow and therefore the width of the base of the eyebrow.

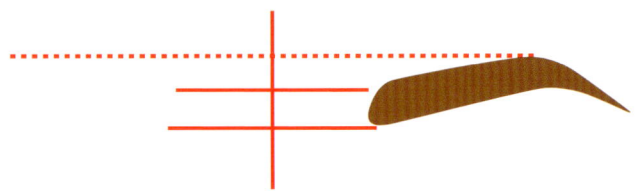

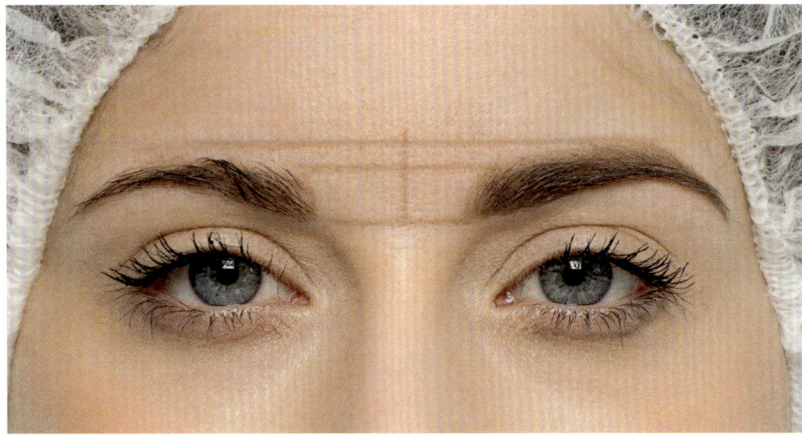

The third horizontal guideline concerns the vertex: a line that runs parallel to the floor and connects the brow arches and determines the highest point of the entire eyebrow. The vertex is one of the most important parts in characterizing a face's non-verbal expression, which is why the original intentions should be considered very carefully.

10 FIRST OBLIQUE GUIDELINE

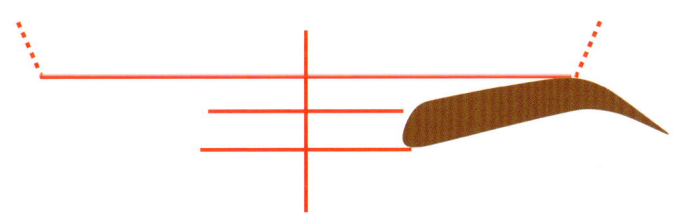

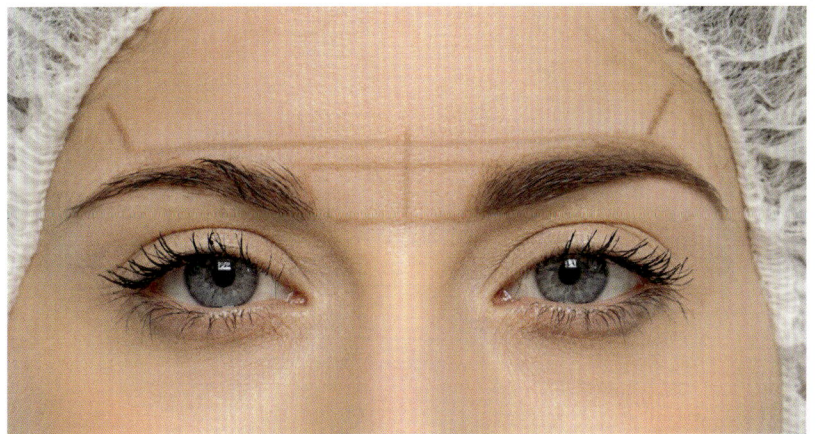

Now it is time to determine the innermost or outermost position of the vertex. not just its height. The best way to prevent the client from continuously moving their eyes is to firmly place a finger in front of their face, at a distance of about 40 cm, and ask them to stare at it to align the center of the pupil. Only then should you begin tracing an imaginary oblique line that starts from the wing of the nose, passes through the center of the pupil, and therefore indicates the correct placement of the vertex. Repeat the same process for the other eye.

11 SECOND OBLIQUE GUIDELINE

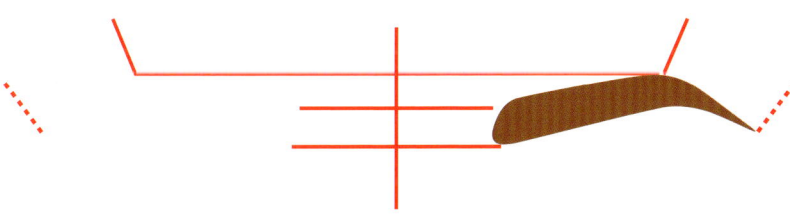

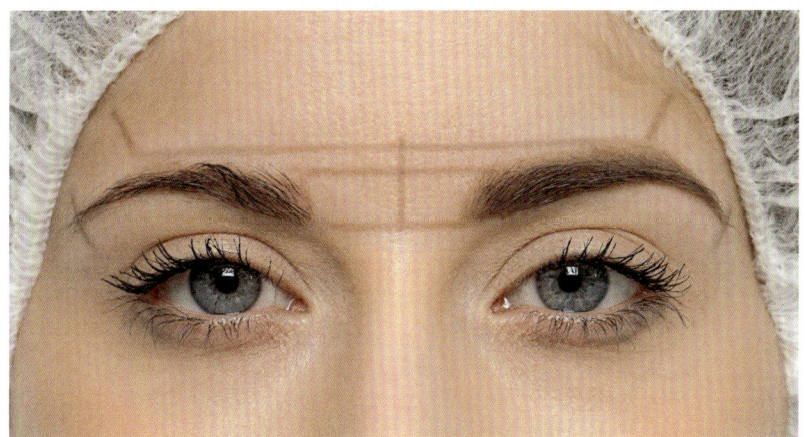

The second oblique guideline determines the length of the tail of the eyebrow. Starting from the wing of the nose once again, trace a second imaginary line, which this time passes through the outer corner of the eye, indicating the maximum length of the tail.

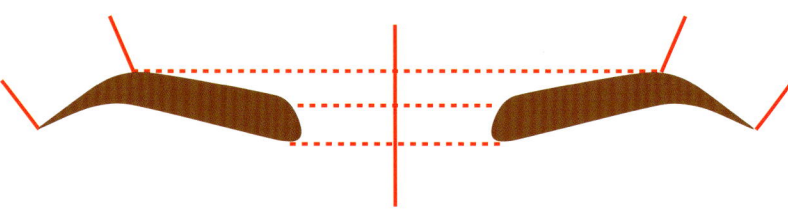

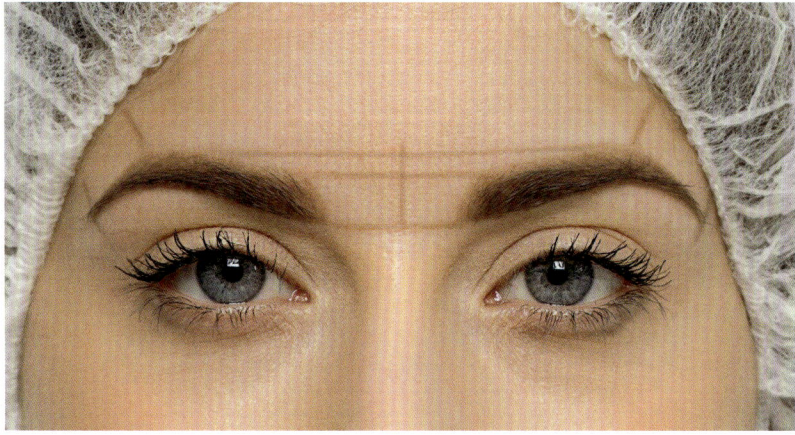

Once this is done, we'll have a grid within which we can quickly position the second eyebrow.

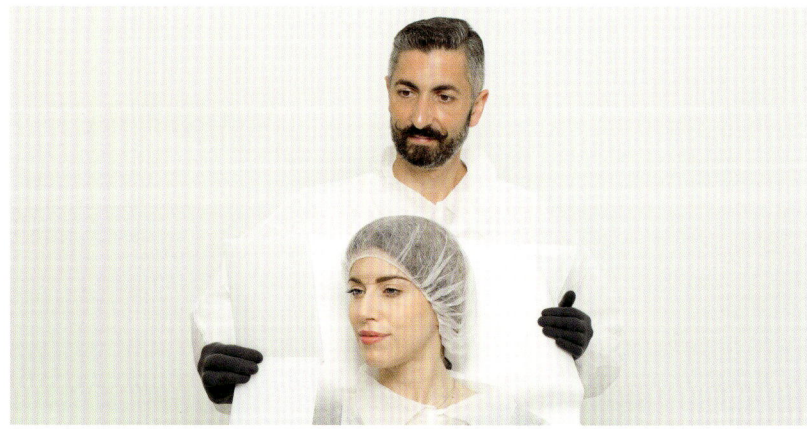

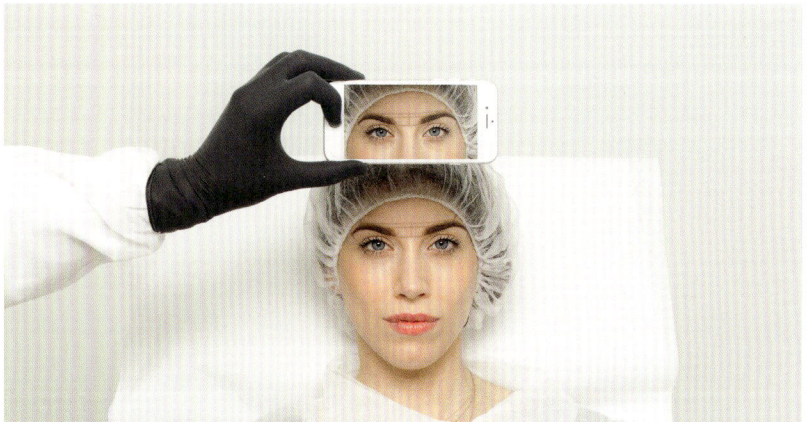

Using these reference points creates a symmetrical and accurate sketch, which should be checked, first through a direct, frontal observation of the client, then through an indirect observation made using two fundamental tools: the mirror and the camera (or a cell phone, if more convenient). This will guarantee the quality of the final results.

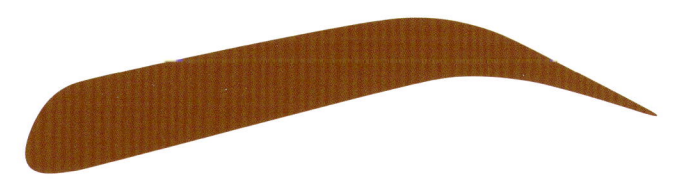

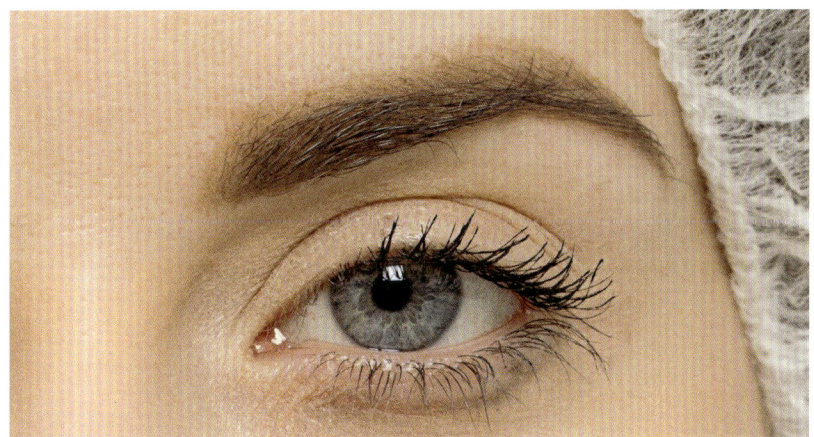

After having created a careful sketch, proceed by marking out the outline.

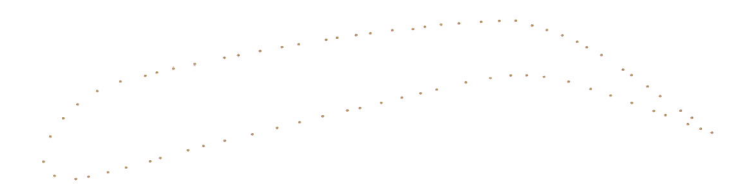

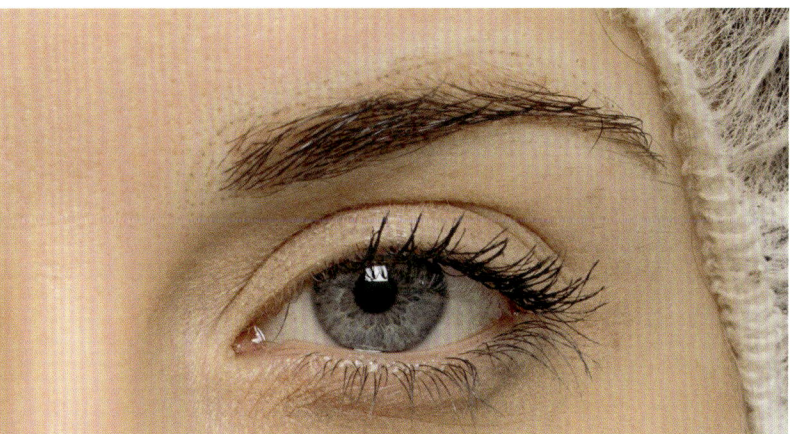

➡	Dots	◢	90°	🌡	3-Liner
✋	Fast	±	100	💧	Organic, Inorganic, Mix

We recommend tracing the outline dots very lightly, so that no traces remain visible after 30 days.

EYEBROWS

LIPS

EYES

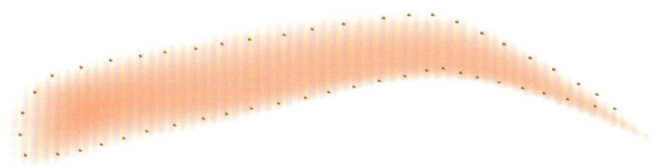

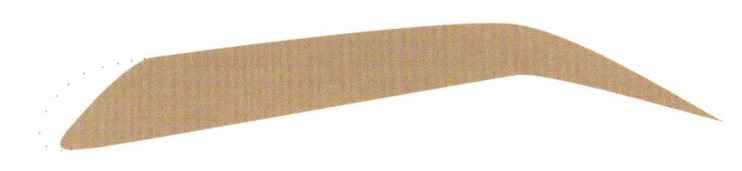

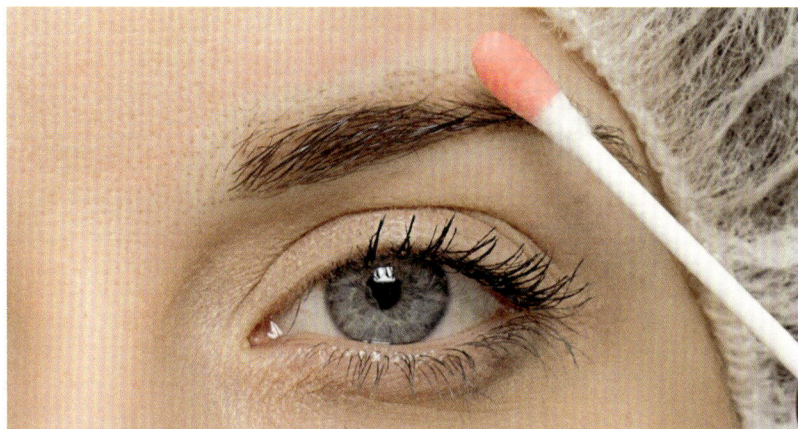

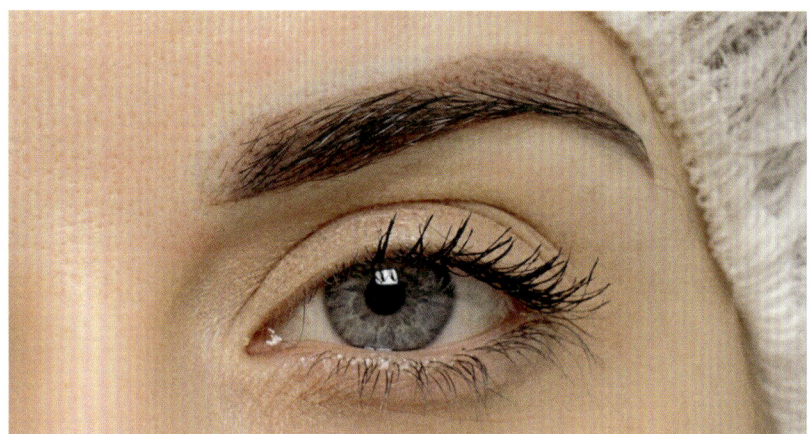

In countries where the law permits it, apply a numbing solution, not just to inhibit pain stimuli but also to decongest the area, preventing bleeding which could dilute the color.

Wait 1–3 minutes and wipe off if necessary. The sketched skin area will turn into a lighter color due to the vasoconstrictive properties of the solution, which makes the design even more visible.

➡ Unidir./bidir.   ◢ 90°   ⬇ 3-Liner

✋ Medium   ± 100–120   💧 Organic, Inorganic, Mix

Start shading with a medium brown color: instead of starting from the beginning of the eyebrow, begin around 2/3 mm after the start of the body, as shown in the image. The movements will be monodirectional, moving from the lower outline to the upper outline. Each line should rest on the next, without leaving "empty spaces". They should all be slightly angled, at approximately a 25° angle compared to the lower outline.

18 2ND LEVEL OF SHADING

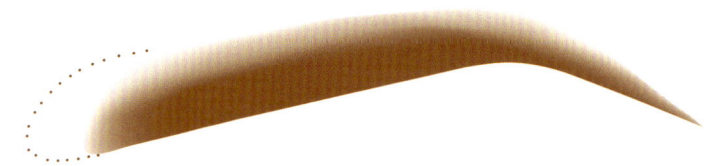

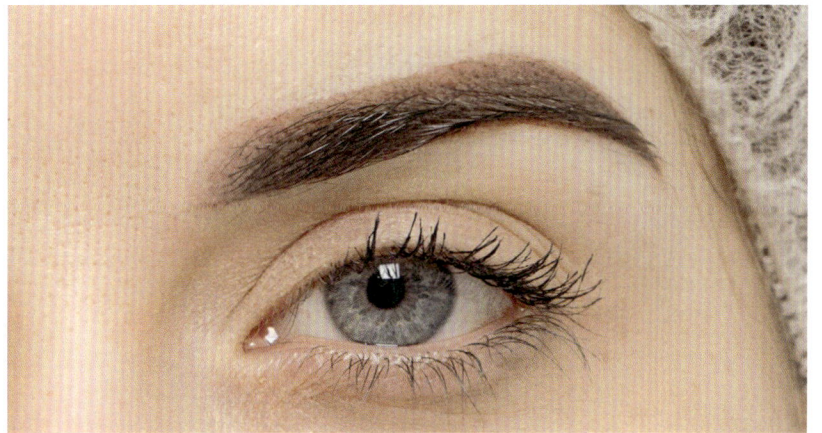

- ➡ Unidirectional
- ✋ Medium
- ◹ 90°
- ± 100–120
- 🌡 3-Liner
- 💧 Organic, Inorganic, Mix

With a different color and needle, perform a second pass with the same technique as above, choosing a darker brown color for this step. This step is only performed on the area that extends from the lower outline to the eyebrow's central axis.

19 SHADING THE BASE

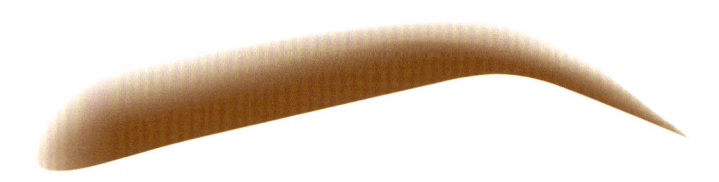

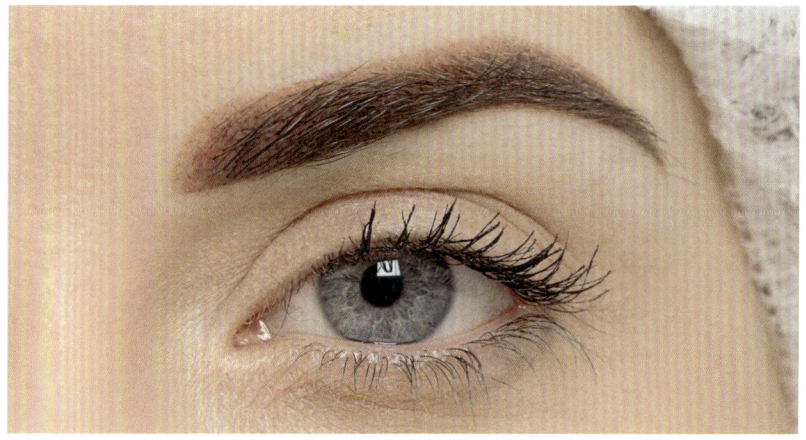

- ➡ Unidirectional
- ✋ Fast
- ◹ 90°
- ± 100–120
- 🌡 3-Liner
- 💧 Organic, Inorganic, Mix

With the same needle and using diluted medium brown pigment as we were using in the first level of shading, proceed to the initial body base area.

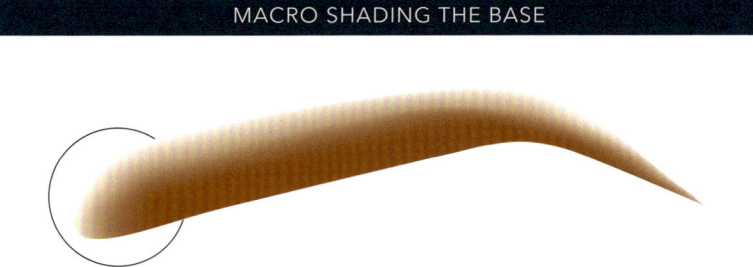

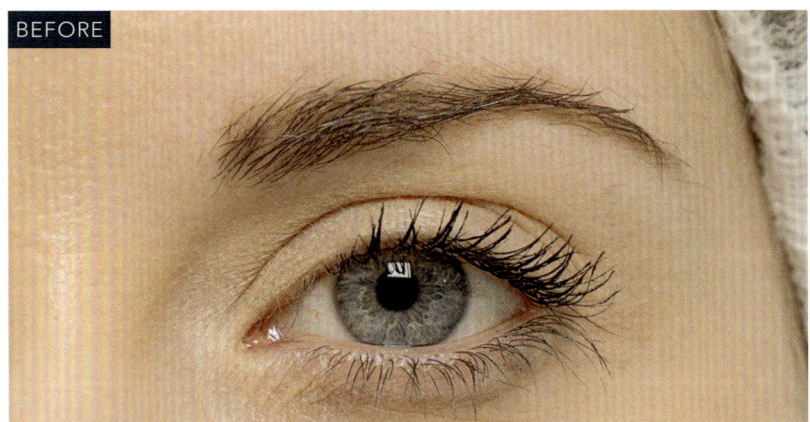

BEFORE

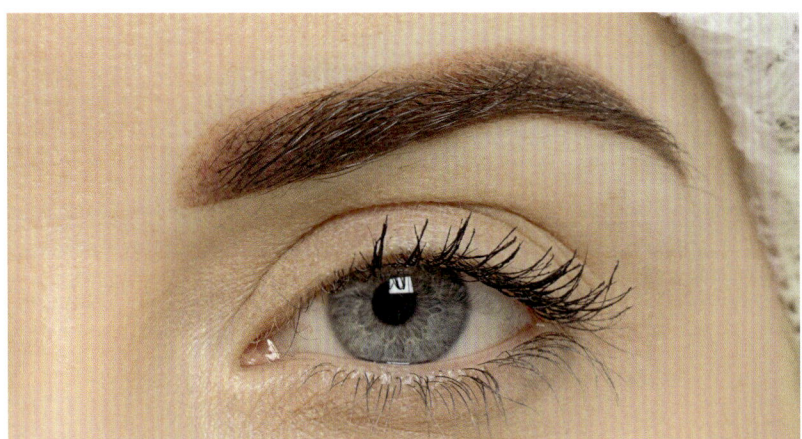

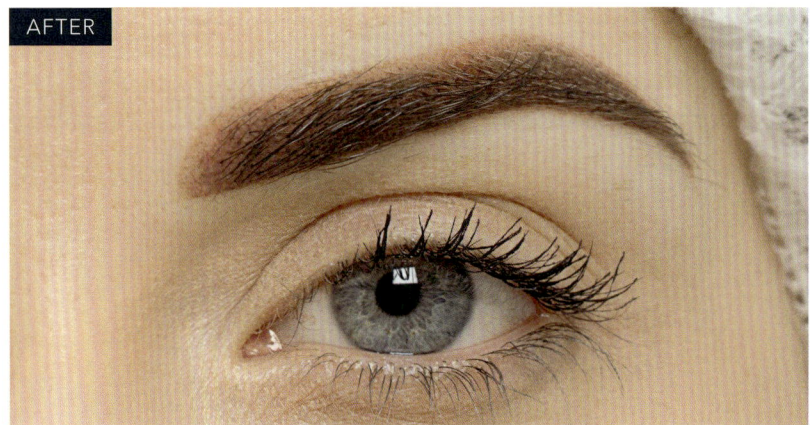

AFTER

The macro view of the base of the eyebrow shows a light gradient. This step is done with rapid unidirectional movements. For beginners, it is best to use the lighter pigment applied earlier in the first level of shading.

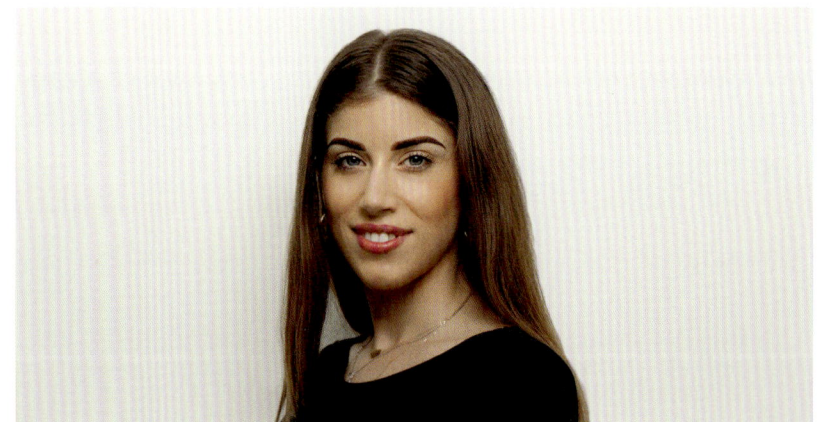

13.1.3.2. FILLING IN (Unusual technique, e.g. correction, cover-up)

1 INITIAL SITUATION

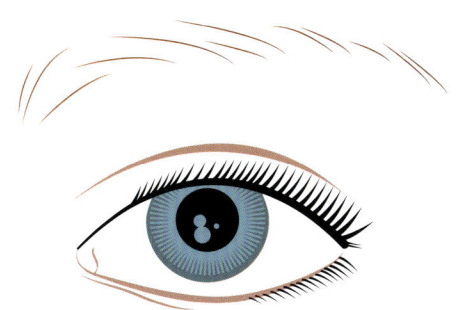

Before applying permanent makeup, the eyebrow ridge must be hygienically prepared.

2 CLEANING

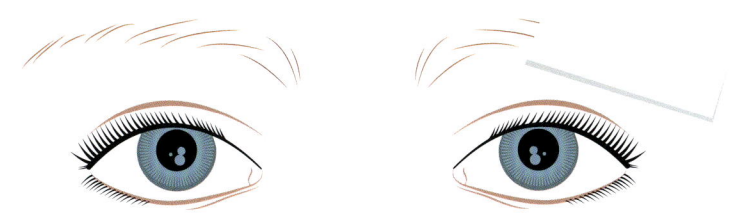

The first phase involves deep-cleaning the area to remove any previously applied makeup or cosmetic products, and to eliminate any potential non-pathogenic microorganisms. We recommend not re-using the dirty part of the wipe.

3 HAIR REMOVAL

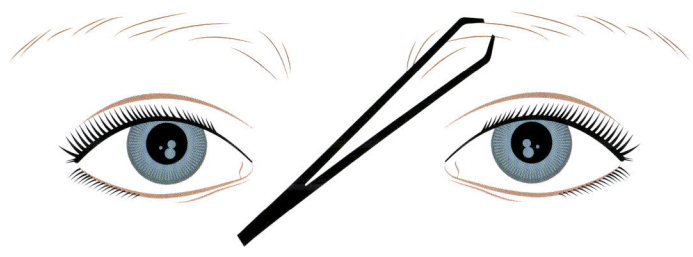

This step is done with tweezers instead of traumatic hair removal methods such as waxing or shaving, making sure to sterilize the tweezers in an autoclave to avoid cross-contamination between clients. First, we remove the hairs that clearly lie outside of our sketch; a second, more precise hair removal phase takes place after sketching in our new eyebrow, to perfect it.

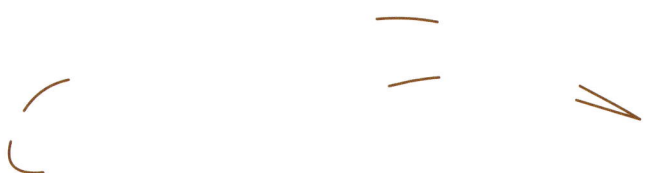

Before starting any sketch, we need a clear and precise vision of what we aim to achieve for our client. We don't want to improvise anything. There are five specific reference points that help us achieve the desired results in the most scrupulous and precise way possible. The first two points determine the base and thickness of the body, the other two indicate the height of the eyebrow and the thickness of the angle, and the last point indicates the thickness and length of the tail.

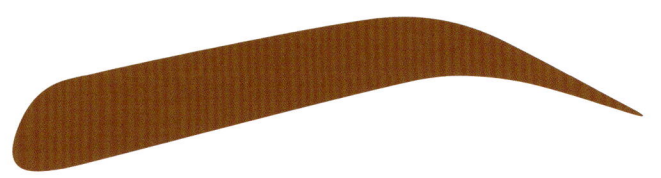

Once these five points are determined and drawn in, all you need to do is connect them and fill in the outline in order to see the chosen shape, and if necessary, make corrections and adjustments.

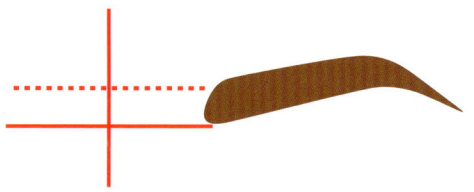

The second, upper horizontal reference point indicates the maximum height of the base of the body of the eyebrow and therefore the width of the base of the eyebrow.

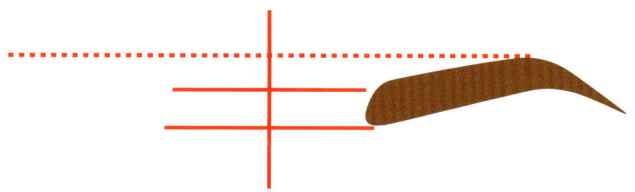

The third horizontal guideline concerns the vertex: a line that runs parallel to the floor and connects the brow arches and determines the highest point of the entire eyebrow. The vertex is one of the most important parts in characterizing a face's non-verbal expression, which is why the original intentions should be considered very carefully.

6 VERTICAL GUIDELINE

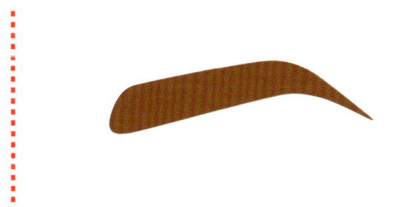

Using a sterile, single-use sketching tool and the pigment chosen for the procedure, trace a vertical line at the center of the face, using the forehead, eyes, and nose as reference points. This guideline will be useful for verifying that the distance between the two eyebrows is correct and centered according to the part of the face in question.

7 FIRST HORIZONTAL GUIDELINE

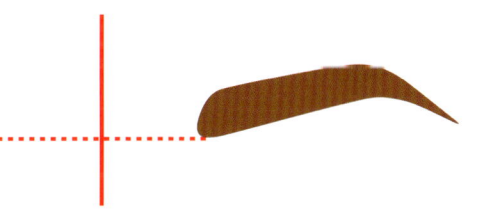

Next, we establish the first horizontal guideline, which is a line that runs parallel to the ground; it starts from the previously drawn eyebrow and leads to the point chosen for the beginning of the second eyebrow. The first horizontal guideline serves to ensure that the eyebrows are placed at the correct height compared to the eyes.

10 FIRST OBLIQUE GUIDELINE

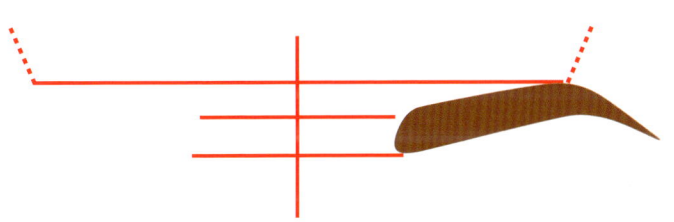

Now it is time to determine the innermost or outermost position of the vertex. not just its height. The best way to prevent the client from continuously moving their eyes is to firmly place a finger in front of their face, at a distance of about 40 cm, and ask them to stare at it to align the center of the pupil. Only then should you begin tracing an imaginary oblique line that starts from the wing of the nose, passes through the center of the pupil, and therefore indicates the correct placement of the vertex. Repeat the same process for the other eye.

11 SECOND OBLIQUE GUIDELINE

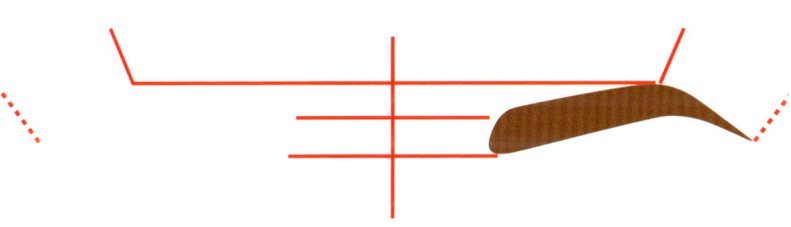

The second oblique guideline determines the length of the tail of the eyebrow. Starting from the wing of the nose once again, trace a second imaginary line, which this time passes through the outer corner of the eye, indicating the maximum length of the tail.

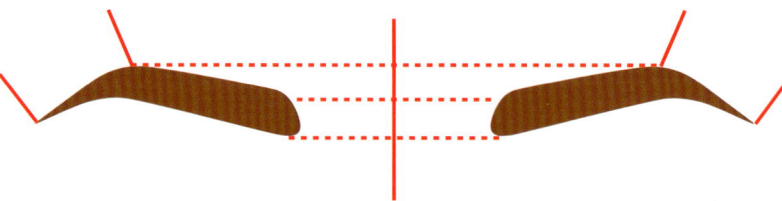

Once this is done, we'll have a grid within which we can quickly position the second eyebrow. The sketch obtained won't be perfect; since the face is asymmetrical, it should adapt to the expression and differences that exist between one side and the other, in order to look natural.

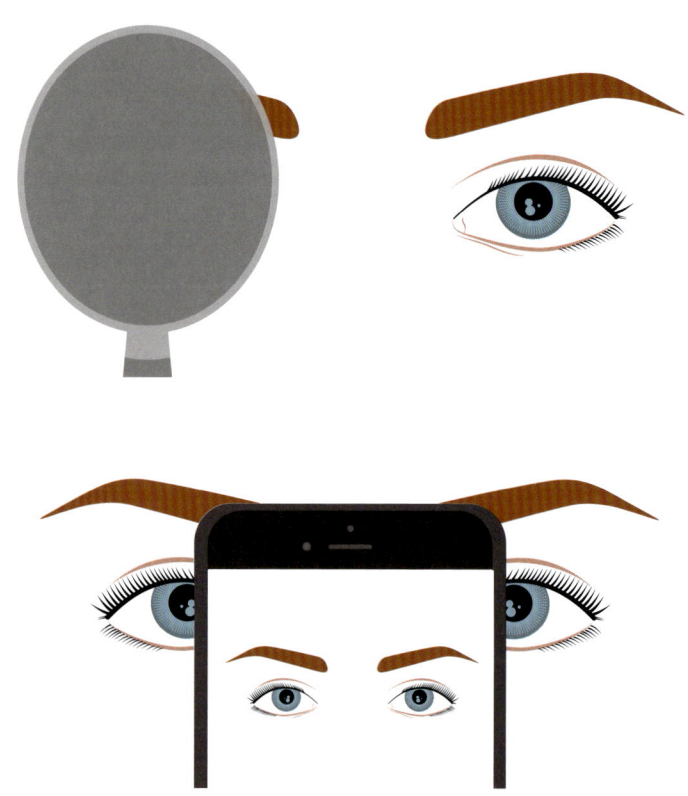

Using these reference points creates a symmetrical and accurate sketch, which should be checked, first through a direct, frontal observation of the client, then through an indirect observation made using two fundamental tools: the mirror and the camera. This will guarantee the quality of the final results.

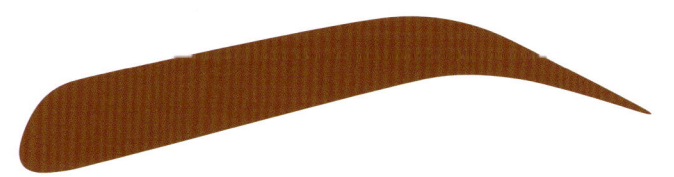

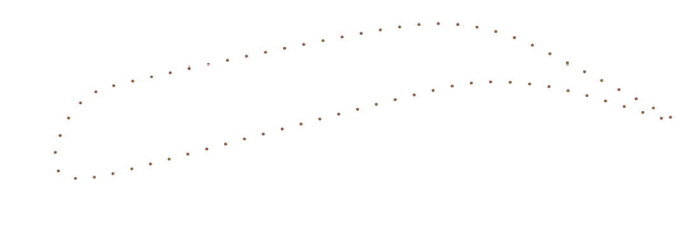

After having created an accurate sketch, it is time to pick up the handpiece and begin the procedure. First, mark out the outline: this ensures that you will not lose the shape and that final results will be correct, despite any swelling that may give the appearance of a mistake.

| ➡ Dots | ◢ 90° | 🖊 Nano n[1], Nano n[2], 1-Liner |
| 👆 Fast | ± 80/90 | 💧 Organic, Inorganic, Mix |

With a 1-point needle, gently mark out the outline: this provides a linear reference outline on the epidermis that defines and ensures the correct shape. Be careful not to go too deep, as this could leave an undesirable outline mark after the scarring phase. Use small, very transparent dots that disappear within a few days. This technique is mostly recommended for students who are just starting out; it may be less useful for professionals who can begin filling in the brow immediately, without needing to define the outline.

In countries where the law permits it, apply a numbing solution; this not only inhibits pain but also decongests the area, preventing bleeding which could dilute the color. Wait 1–3 minutes and wipe off if necessary. The sketched skin area will turn into a lighter color due to the vasoconstrictive properties of the solution, which makes the design even more visible.

EYEBROWS

LIPS

EYES

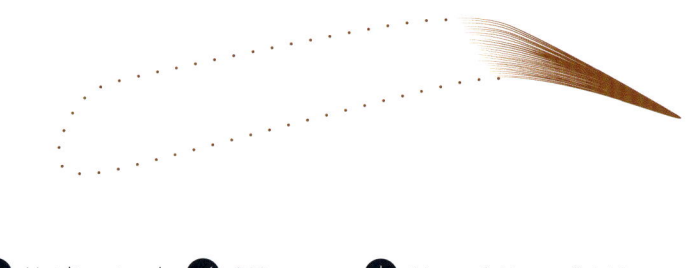

- ➡ Unidirectional
- 🕐 Fast
- ◪ 90°
- ± 100/110
- 🖊 Nano n^1, Nano n^2, 1-Liner
- 💧 Organic, Inorganic, Mix

Use the same needle to fill in the tail. Always use very thin needles to avoid going past the outline of the sketch. This would lead to results that are too thick and displeasing to clients who like absolute precision. Since the needle is very thin, it is crucial to follow guidelines regarding skin trauma: work very superficially, and use quick, but repeated passes to achieve perfect saturation of the area. Only after having perfectly filled in the tail should you change needles for the next phase.

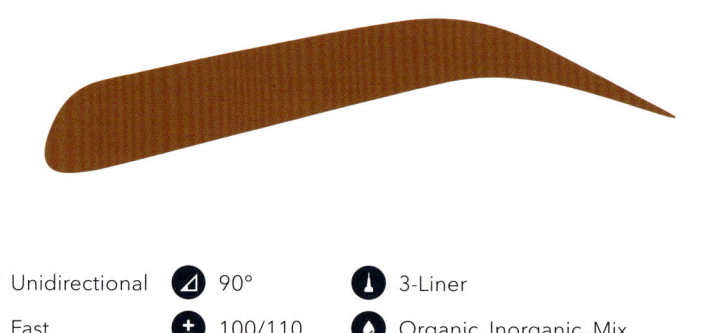

- ➡ Unidirectional
- 🕐 Fast
- ◪ 90°
- ± 100/110
- 🖊 3-Liner
- 💧 Organic, Inorganic, Mix

Start working from the tail of the eyebrow towards the beginning drawing dots in a unidirectional movement. Hand motion is fast and work at an angle of 90 degrees. Important! Work very superficially and control the saturation and intensity of the color with your passes. Not more than 3 passes for each area. The final result should look like dots. Start with the upper part of the eyebrow and continue in the medium and bottom part. In case you would like to make lower part darker, perform more passes on these areas.

13.1.4. MIXED TECHNIQUE

Mixed techniques are techniques in between natural and defined approaches. For the base of the eyebrow, the hair-by-hair technique is used; starting from halfway through the body, the hair-by-hair technique is gradually transformed into a kind of shading. While the lower body and the tail are more filled in, the upper part of the body is shaded in with hairs. This procedure is mostly chosen by clients who can't decide between a natural and defined look in permanent makeup: usually, after an initial session in which the natural, hair-by-hair technique is suggested, the second session may lead to a mixed technique if they desire a fuller, more obvious effect.

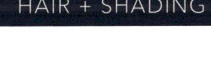

HAIR + SHADING

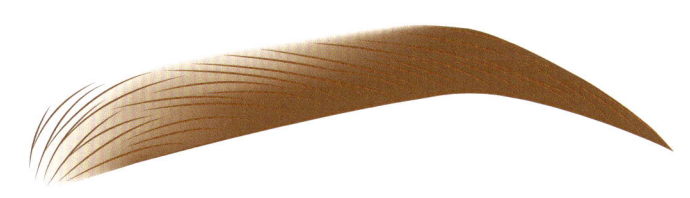

EYEBROWS

LIPS

EYES

13.1.4.1. HAIR + SHADING

1 INITIAL SITUATION

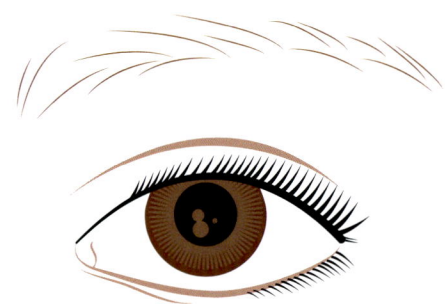

Before applying permanent makeup, the eyebrow ridge must be hygienically prepared.

2 CLEANING

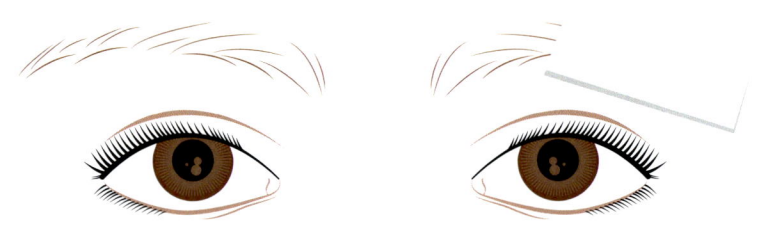

The first phase involves deep-cleaning the area to remove any previously applied makeup or cosmetic products, and to eliminate any potential non-pathogenic microorganisms. We recommend not re-using the dirty part of the wipe.

3 HAIR REMOVAL

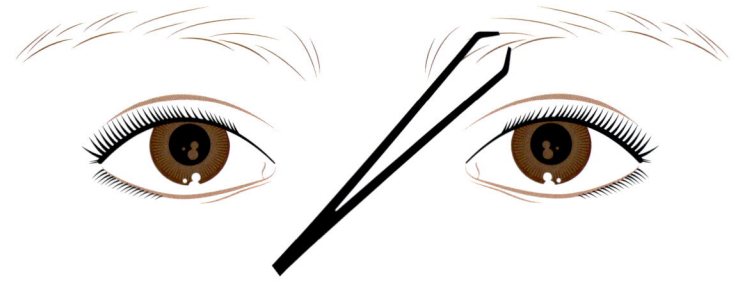

This step is done with tweezers instead of traumatic hair removal methods such as waxing or shaving, making sure to sterilize the tweezers in an autoclave to avoid cross-contamination between clients. First, we remove the hairs that clearly lie outside of our sketch; a second, more precise hair removal phase takes place after sketching in our new eyebrow, to perfect it.

4   THE 5 REFERENCE POINTS

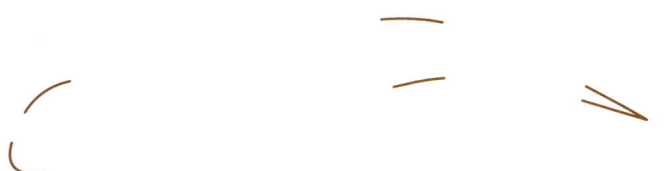

Before starting any sketch, we need a clear and precise vision of what we aim to achieve for our client. We don't want to improvise anything. There are five specific reference points that help us achieve the desired results in the most scrupulous and precise way possible. The first two points determine the base and thickness of the body, the other two indicate the height of the eyebrow and the thickness of the angle, and the last point indicates the thickness and length of the tail.

5   SKETCH

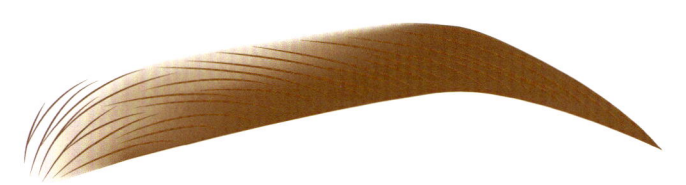

Once these five points are determined and drawn in, all you need to do is connect them and fill in the outline in order to see the chosen shape, and if necessary, make corrections and adjustments.

6   VERTICAL GUIDELINE

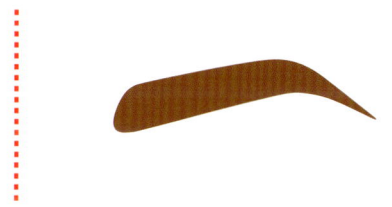

Using a sterile, single-use sketching tool and the pigment chosen for the procedure, trace a vertical line at the center of the face, using the forehead, eyes, and nose as reference points. This guideline will be useful for verifying that the distance between the two eyebrows is correct and centered according to the part of the face in question.

7   FIRST HORIZONTAL GUIDELINE

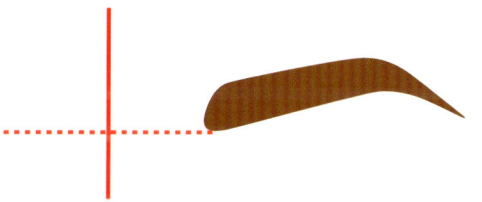

Next, we establish the first horizontal guideline, which is a line that runs parallel to the ground; it starts from the previously drawn eyebrow and leads to the point chosen for the beginning of the second eyebrow. The first horizontal guideline serves to ensure that the eyebrows are placed at the correct height compared to the eyes.

8   SECOND HORIZONTAL GUIDELINE

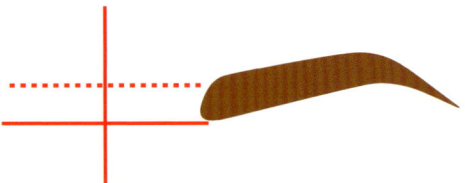

The second, upper horizontal reference point indicates the maximum height of the base of the body of the eyebrow and therefore the width of the base of the eyebrow.

9   THIRD HORIZONTAL GUIDELINE

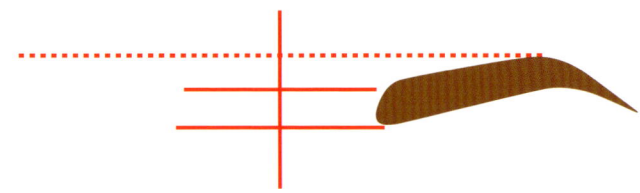

The third horizontal guideline concerns the vertex: a line that runs parallel to the floor and connects the brow arches and determines the highest point of the entire eyebrow. The vertex is one of the most important parts in characterizing a face's non-verbal expression, which is why the original intentions should be considered very carefully.

10   FIRST OBLIQUE GUIDELINE

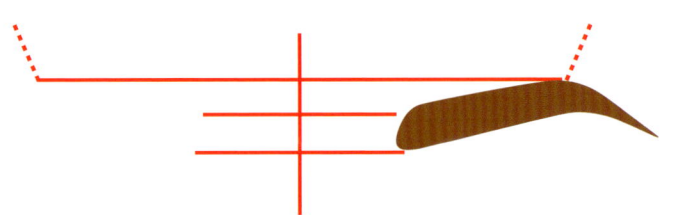

Now it is time to determine the innermost or outermost position of the vertex, not just its height. The best way to prevent the client from continuously moving their eyes is to firmly place a finger in front of their face, at a distance of about 40 cm, and ask them to stare at it to align the center of the pupil. Only then should you begin tracing an imaginary oblique line that starts from the wing of the nose, passes through the center of the pupil, and therefore indicates the correct placement of the vertex. Repeat the same process for the other eye.

11   SECOND OBLIQUE GUIDELINE

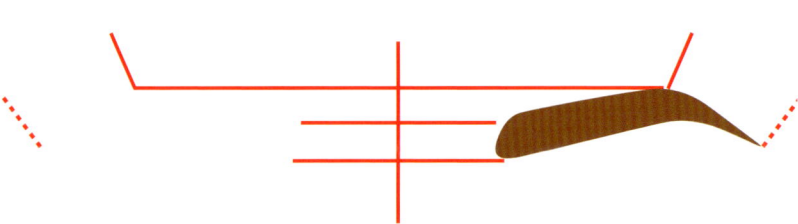

The second oblique guideline determines the length of the tail of the eyebrow. Starting from the wing of the nose once again, trace a second imaginary line, which this time passes through the outer corner of the eye, indicating the maximum length of the tail.

12 SKETCHING THE SECOND EYEBROW

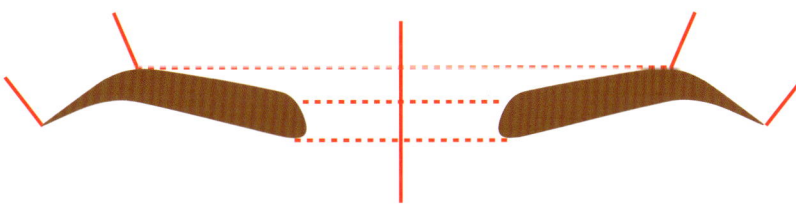

Once this is done, we'll have a grid within which we can quickly position the second eyebrow.

13 MIRROR AND TEST PHOTO

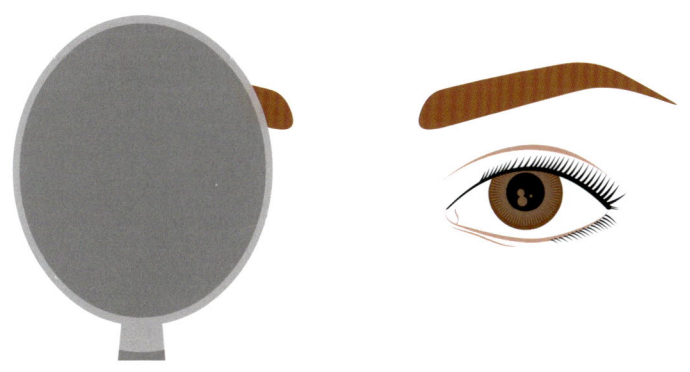

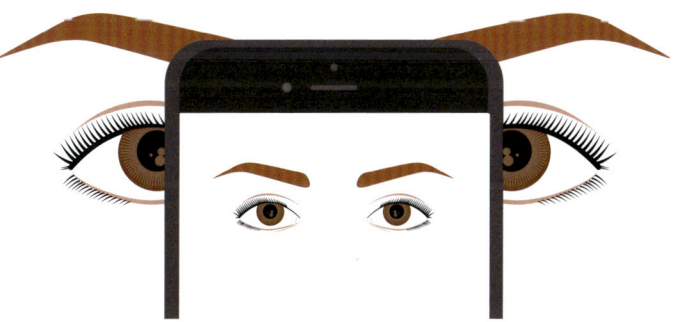

Using these reference points creates a symmetrical and accurate sketch, which should be checked, first through a direct, frontal observation of the client, then through an indirect observation made using two fundamental tools: the mirror and the camera (or a cell phone, if more convenient). This will guarantee the quality of the final results.

14 DRAWING THE HAIR + SHADING

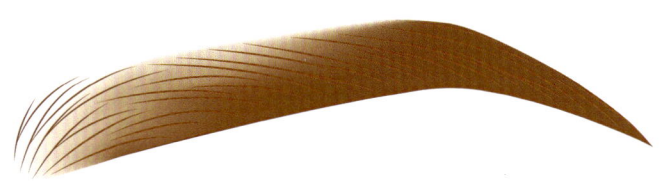

The sketch is always the starting point. When drawing in the shape, the goal is to create what will be the final result, attempting to create a sort of shadow in the lower part and leaving more transparency at the beginning and at the top.

15 MARKING THE OUTLINE

➡ Unidir./bidir.   ◨ 90°   🌡 Nano n^1, Nano n^2, Nano n^T, 1-Liner
✋ Slow   ± 100   💧 Organic, Inorganic, Mix

Draw the first hairs within the outline. Continue marking the outline using the dotted technique in order to preserve the sketch. We recommend tracing the outline dots very lightly, so that no traces remain visible after 30 days.

16 NUMBING SOLUTION

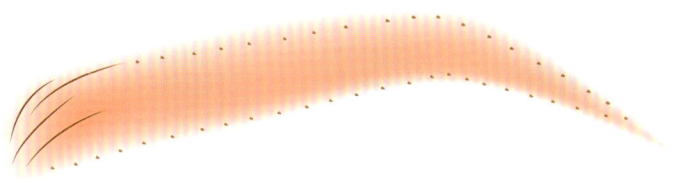

In countries where the law permits it, apply a numbing solution; this not only inhibits pain but also decongests the area, preventing bleeding which could dilute the color. Wait 1–3 minutes and wipe off if necessary. The sketched skin area will turn into a lighter color due to the vasoconstrictive properties of the solution, which makes the design even more visible.

17 ASCENDING HAIRS

➡ Unidir./bidir.   ◨ 90°   🌡 Nano n^1, Nano n^2, Nano n^T, 1-Liner
✋ Slow   ± 120/140   💧 Organic, Inorganic, Mix

Proceed to draw three additional ascending hairs, right next to the first ones.

18 DESCENDING HAIRS

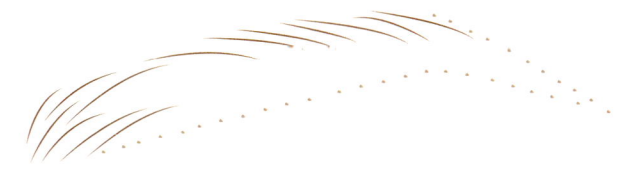

➡ Unidir./bidir.   ◢ 45°, 60°, 90°   ⬥ Nano n[1], Nano n[2], Nano n[T], 1-Liner

✋ Slow   ± 120/140   💧 Organic, Inorganic, Mix

Proceed to draw some descending hairs in the upper part of the body until they reach the vertex, thus creating a structure to be filled in with shading. We recommend creating each hair starting from the central part and moving towards the upper part, to avoid any excess pigment deposits. A slow, monodirectional motion is best for beginners, while more advanced professionals may use a faster, bidirectional movement.

REMEMBER
Hairstrokes with 1 point configurations

| ⬤ | ◢ 90° | | ⬤ | ◢ 45° | ◢ 60° |

Hairstrokes with 3-slope

| ⬤ | ◢ 60° |

19 1ST LEVEL OF SHADING

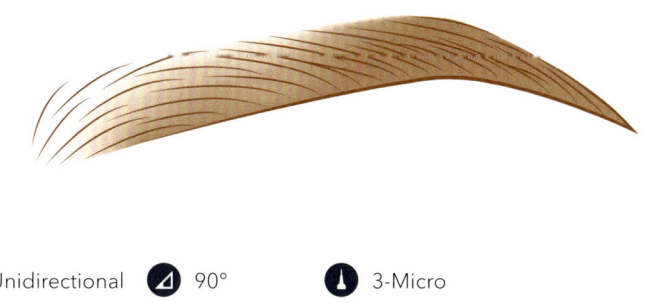

➡ Unidirectional   ◢ 90°   ⬥ 3-Micro

✋ Fast   ± 100   💧 Organic, Inorganic, Mix

Proceed to create a more defined shading effect. Work with unidirectional movements. For a natural looking effect, make sure that the tail and upper external part of the eyebrow are darker and more compact, while leaving the upper central part and beginning part more translucent. You can control the density of the color by drawing more passes on the darker areas.

EYEBROWS

LIPS

EYES

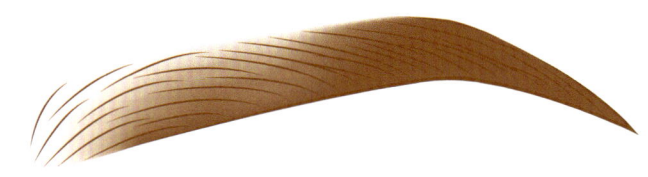

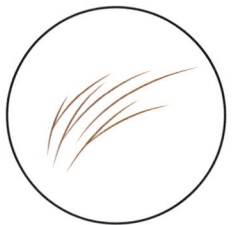

➡ Unidirectional ◢ 90° ⬍ 3-Micro
✋ Fast ± 100 💧 Organic, Inorganic, Mix

➡ Unidir./bidir. ◢ 45°, 60°, 90° ⬍ Nano n^1, Nano n^2, Nano n^T, 1-Liner
✋ Slow ± 120/140 💧 Organic, Inorganic, Mix

Proceed to create a more defined shading effect. Work with unidirectional movements. For a natural-looking effect, make sure that the tail and upper external part of the eyebrow are darker and more compact, while leaving the upper central part and beginning part more translucent. You can control the density of the color by drawing more passes on the darker areas.

The base of the body, which will have remained lighter and sparser compared to the rest of the eyebrow, is enhanced with Y-shaped hairs, meaning the initial hairs will be split into a Y shape. This phase is crucial for ensuring a very natural effect for the eyebrow. It would be unnatural, on the other hand, to place hairs of the same lengths from bottom to top, which would create a "gate" effect.

22 Y HAIRS

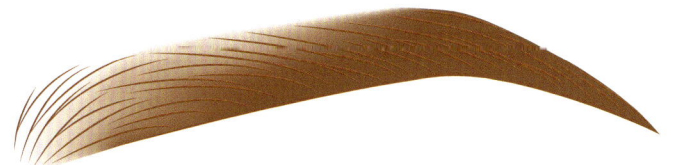

Y hairs are done at the end of the procedure creating an effect that is between the natural and defined look. In this way, permanent makeup satisfies clients who are undecided between the two possible effects, and often this technique is chosen during the second, retouching session, when the hair-by-hair technique is not deemed to fill in the brows as much as is desired.

EYEBROWS

LIPS

"If you think that your training is expensive today think about how much your ignorance will cost tomorrow."

TONI BELFATTO

EYES

13.2.

LIPS
STEP BY STEP

There are three different application techniques used to achieve these results:

LIP LINER TATTOO

The lip line can be emphasized with a pencil that is darker than the mucous membranes themselves. This technique is chosen for lips whose shape is more or less perfect and no asymmetries need to be corrected.

SHADING TECHNIQUE

This technique includes lining the lips and then filling in the color inwards, to hide the difference between the lip line and the natural color of the mucous membranes. The lips look more polished and their outline is well-defined. This technique is also often used to correct asymmetries.

FILLING-IN TECHNIQUE

This technique is also called the lipstick or gloss effect, and involves filling in the entire mucous membrane, leaving intentionally lighter areas at the center to create a more voluminous effect. This technique is preferred by people with very light lip colors who want a dramatic change in color.

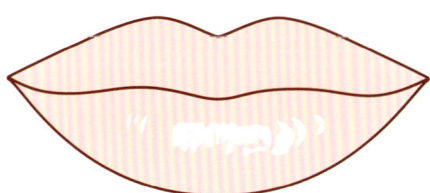

LINER

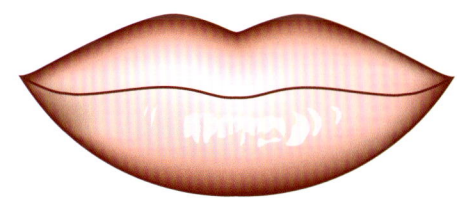

SHADING

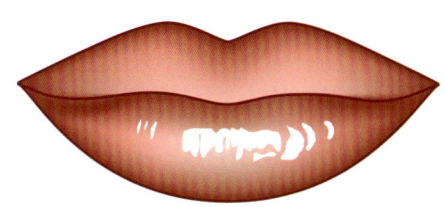

FILLING IN

EYEBROWS

LIPS

EYES

13.2.1. MARKING THE OUTLINE

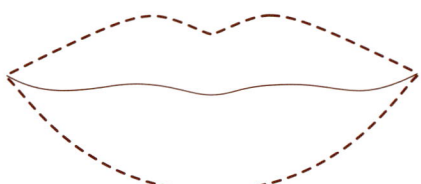

The correct procedure for marking out the outline on the skin, given that the professional is seated to the right of the client, is to start from the outer left-hand corner of the lower lip line at a 45° to 60° degree angle to the professional's stomach, using a rapid bi-directional movement. Pigment is transferred very lightly into the epidermis, just to mark out the sketch. Repeat the same process on the upper lip line.

When applying pigment to the outline, it is extremely important not to pause on the vertices: this leads to the risk of depositing color there and creating an unnatural Cupid's bow.

When working on the outer corner, to the right of the client, the movement of the handpiece will be inverted: it will no longer move towards the professional's stomach, but away from it. The professional's grip on the handpiece also switches from the classic grip to the "reverse" grip.

Numbing substance can then be applied again to the area without cleansing beforehand, so that through precipitation, the color will be absorbed more easily by the epidermis and the line

will be made clearer. After 10 more minutes have passed, cleanse the area.

Once the outline has been marked out on the skin, it is time to choose the application technique that best suits the client's wishes: an outline, light shading, or filling in the entire lip.

To draw the lip line, it is best for the professional to sit on the client's right side, resting the outside of their hand directly on the client's jaw. To avoid wiping away the sketch, start from the lower lip line. Start from the outer corner of the mouth (which corresponds with the client's left side), then trace a line using a very light bidirectional movement.

Bidirectional movement of the needle looks exactly like the motion of a pendulum as it swings: The needle should also follow the same path in the skin in a perfectly perpendicular manner (90° to the skin) without creating uncertain oscillations that would create totally imprecise lines.

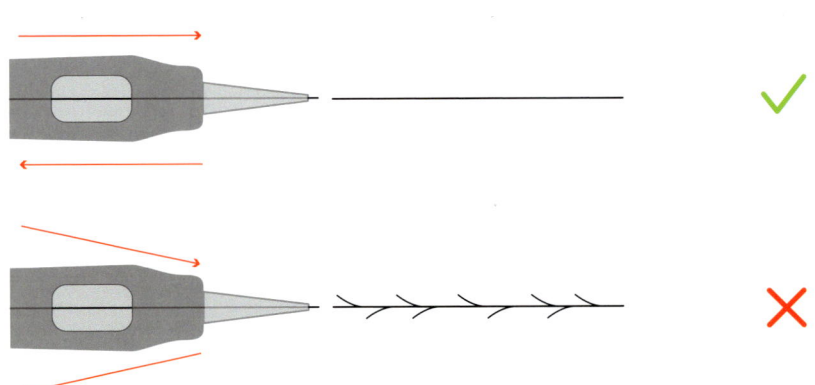

The hand's sensitivity is crucial in this exercise. Being able to perceive even the smallest vibrations as the needle comes in contact in the skin will help us understand if the movement we are performing is right or wrong. Experience and consistency will allow the professional's hands to become an extension of their head, eyes, and aesthetic taste.

"It is time to stop believing in miracles: every goal in our life is achieved by fighting to reach it."

TONI BELFATTO

13.2.2. CONTOUR – LIP LINER

1 INITIAL SITUATION

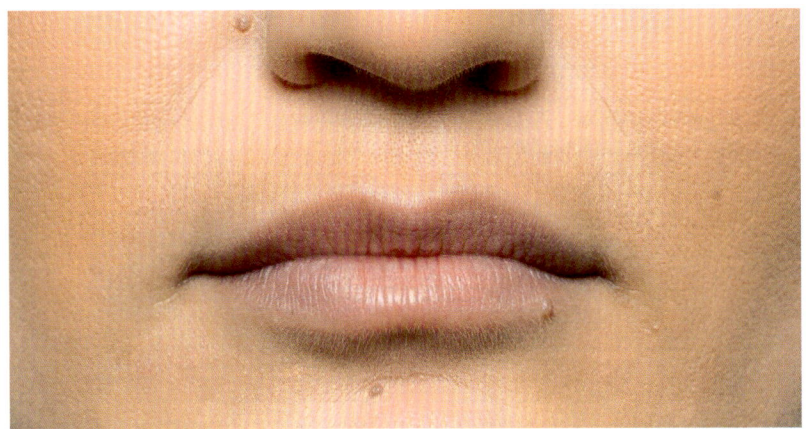

2 CLEANING

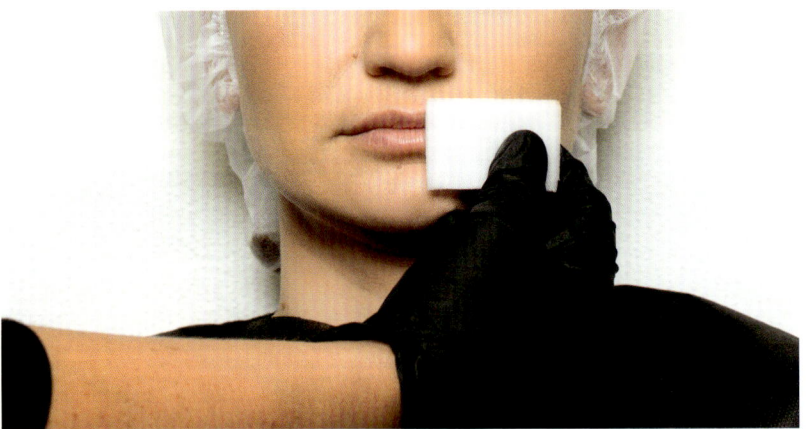

Before starting the lip procedure, it is important to take into account all relevant hygienic aspects for the lip area. Remember that lip tissue has a completely different morphology and sensibility than the eyebrow area and it is more prone to inflammation, infections, and other reactions. Therefore, it is of crucial importance to follow the highest safety and hygienic standards.

Treatment steps and pictures by Olga Kravchenko.

In the first stage, the professional will proceed to remove any makeup or cosmetic products and clean off the lip area with antibacterial tissue to eliminate any potential non-pathogenic microorganisms. We recommend not re-using the dirty part of the wipe. If the client is wearing lipstick, the professional will use several antibacterial tissues until the makeup has been completely removed.

3   PHILTRAL COLUMNS

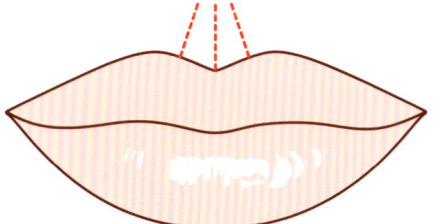

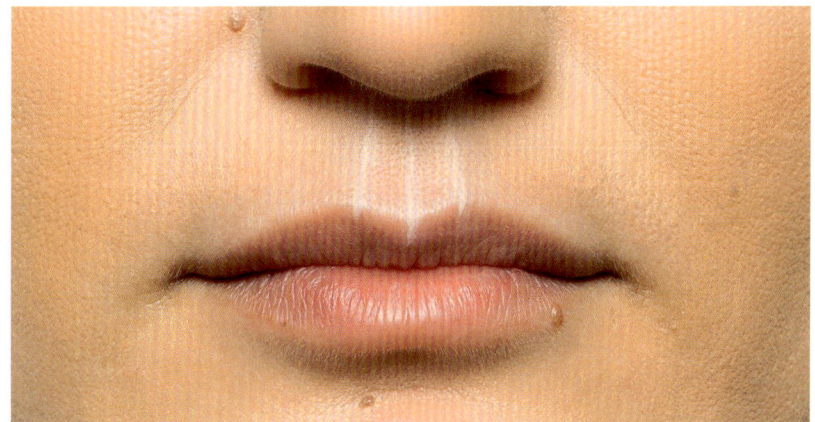

Mark the philtrum and Cupid's bow with a white marker in order to easily define lip symmetry and draw three lines as in the picture.

⚠ **ATTENTION**

In some countries only sterile, single-use markers are allowed for this purpose.

4   CUPID'S BOW

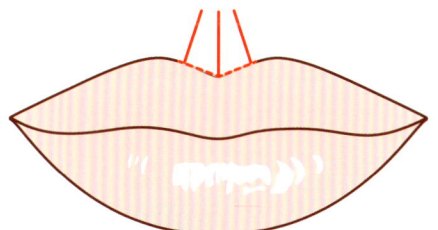

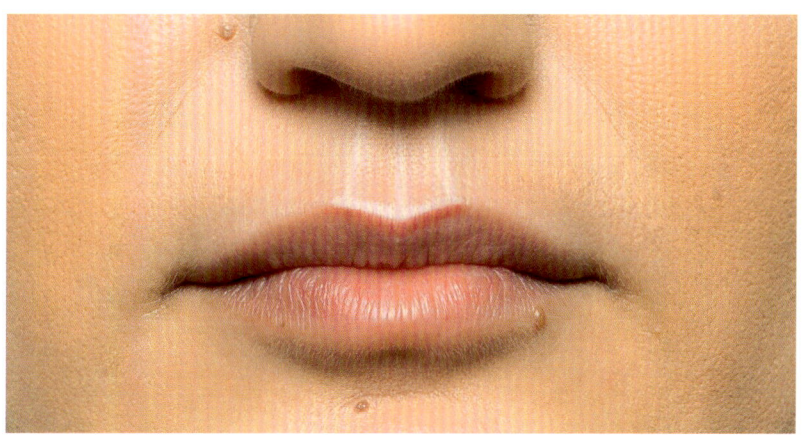

Outline the Cupid's bow and vermilion borders of the upper lip trying not go beyond the red border of the lips. This rule is of crucial importance in order to get a natural result after healing. Use two markers in different tones for the sketch: we will use a white or skin-tone marker for the external outline and a red or pink color marker for sketching the lip contour on the mucous membrane.

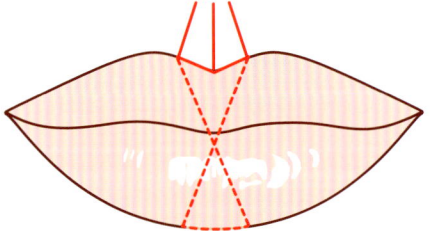

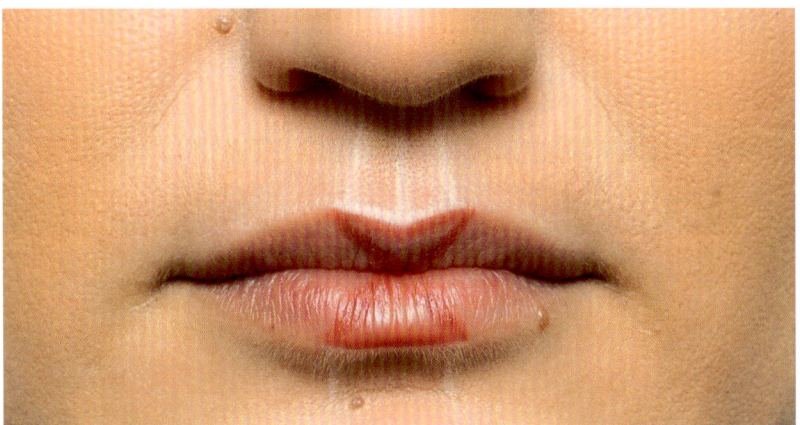

Proceed to draw the lower lip contour starting from the central area and making sure not to make it too round looking. Use the rule of creating a symmetric inversed triangle to the upper central part of the lip to create a balanced, natural design.

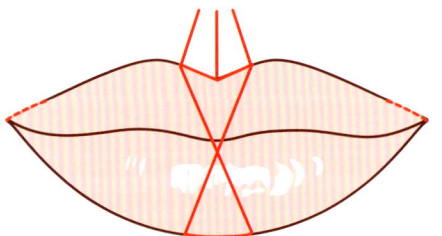

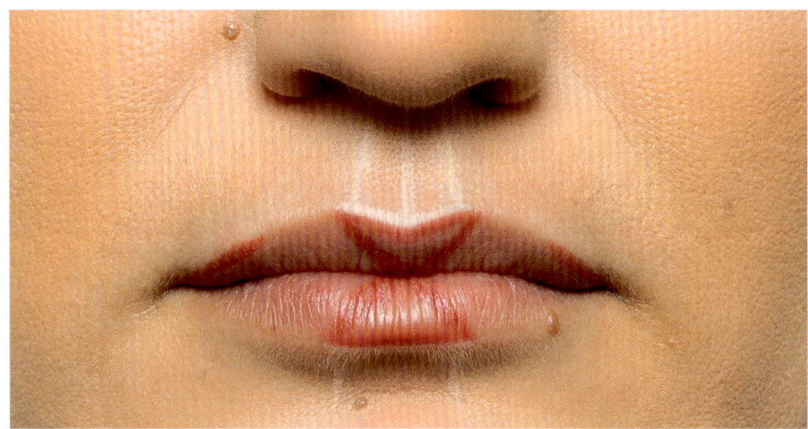

Continue drawing the external sketch outline of the upper lip by tracing two external corner lines around the upper lip and make them symmetric to each other.

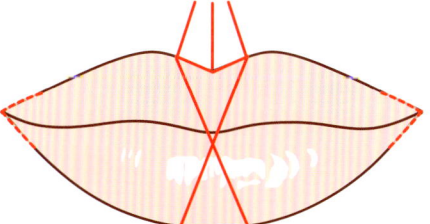

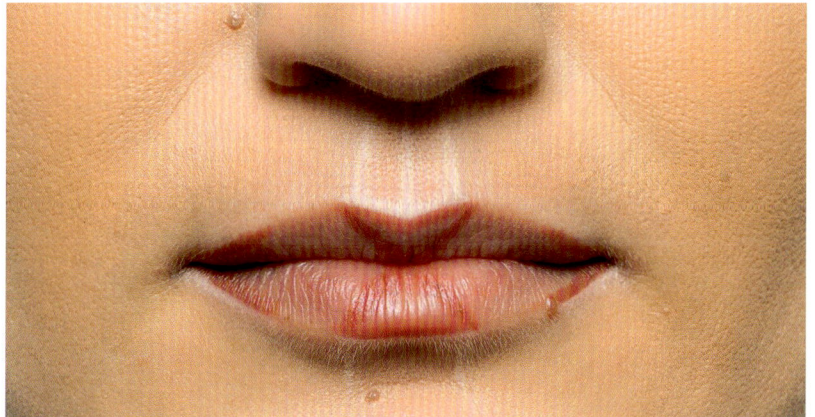

Continue drawing the external sketch outline of the bottom lip by tracing two external corner lines around the bottom lip and make them symmetric to each other. Also draw the external contour lines with the white or beige marker.

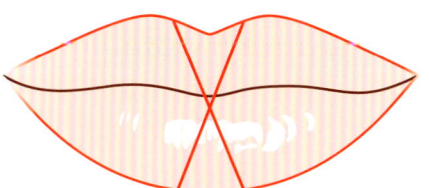

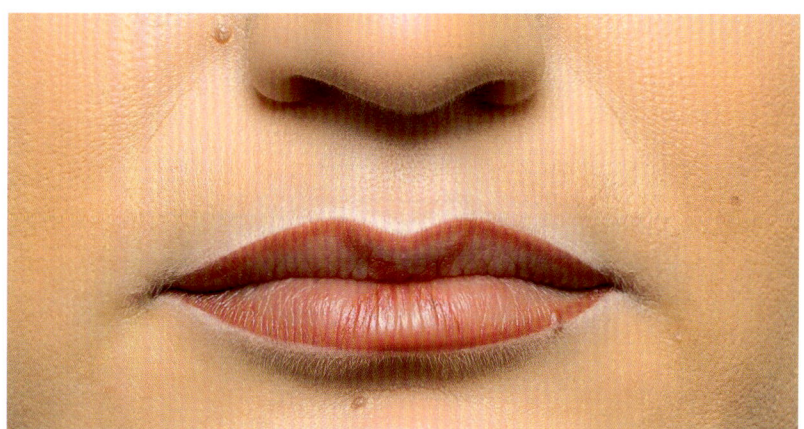

Connect all the contour lines in the sketch with the pink or red pencil. Also draw the external contour lines with the white or beige marker.

IMPORTANT NOTICE:

In case we want to correct asymmetry or to give more volume, it is allowed to draw the contour slightly outside of the client's mucous membrane, but never exceeding 1–1.5 mm.

EYEBROWS

LIPS

EYES

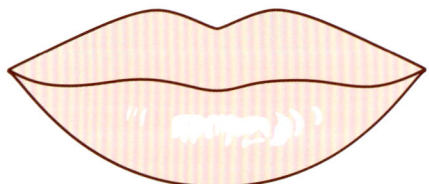

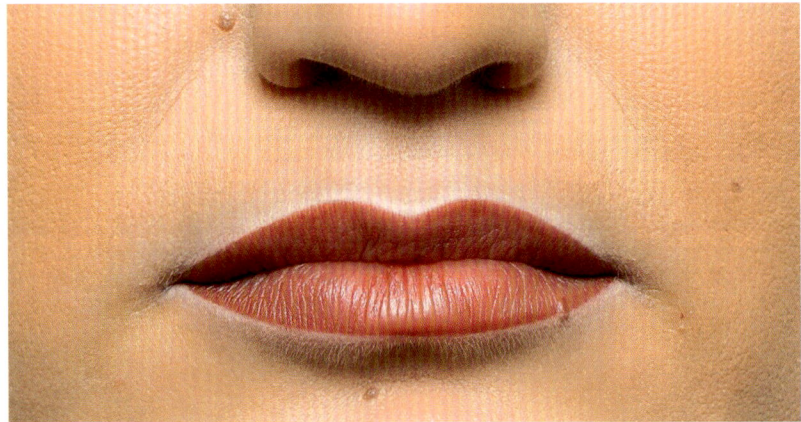

Fill in the inside part of the the lip area with red or pink color in a soft and homogeneous way. Make a visual check of symmetry of the design, paying attention to the dynamic aspect as well. It is recommended that the client talk or smile as a double check, as the symmetry and natural look of the lip design must also be guaranteed in motion.

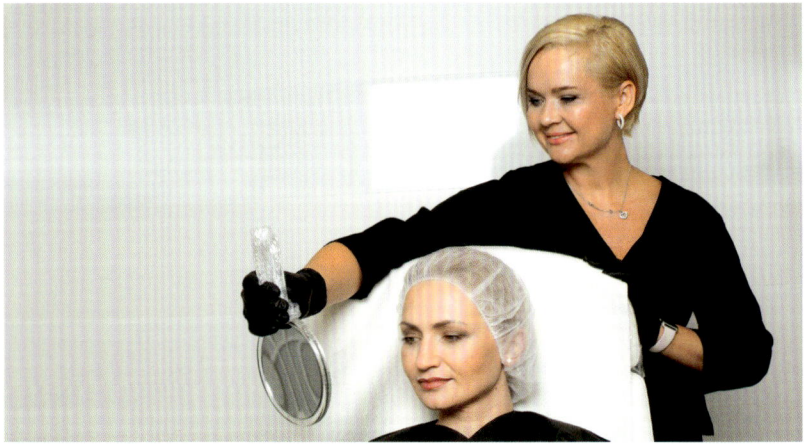

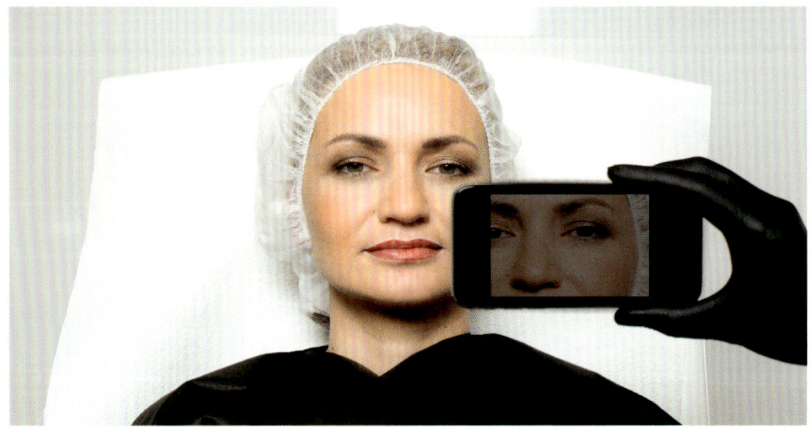

When the sketch is ready, it is time to show final design to the client and ask for approval. Two methods are recommended for a visualization of the sketch by our clients. The first and more classic method it is looking in a mirror from frontal and side angles. The second method consists in taking several pictures from different perspectives and showing them to the client. Don't underestimate this approval step, and take enough time when showing the sketch to your clients, pointing out the improvements in terms of definition, balance, and symmetry. It will increase customer satisfaction once the procedure has been performed.

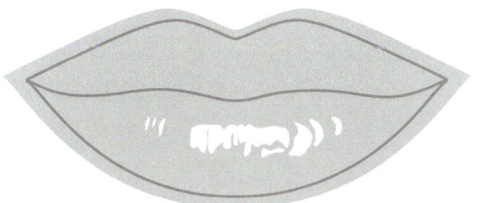

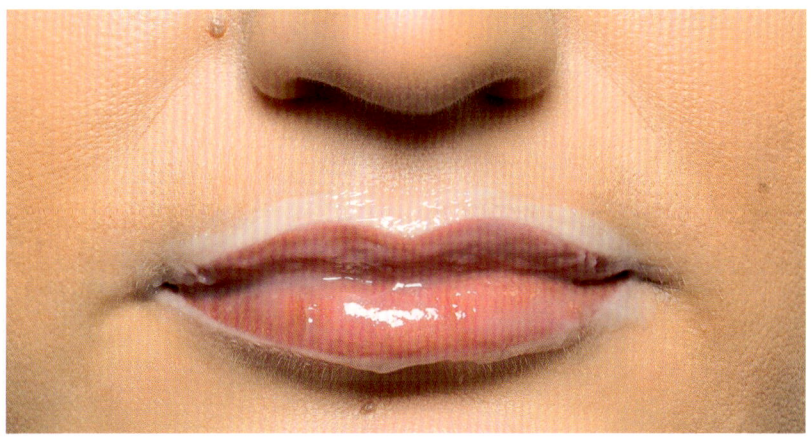

Carefully apply a numbing solution with sterilized cotton tips on the whole surface of the sketch and wait around 15-20 minutes before starting the procedure. It is important to follow the regulations in your own country and use only products authorized for permanent makeup professionals.

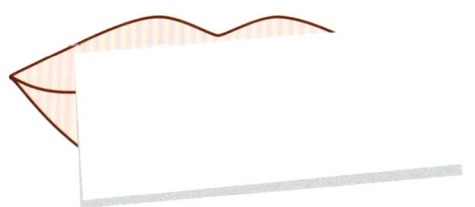

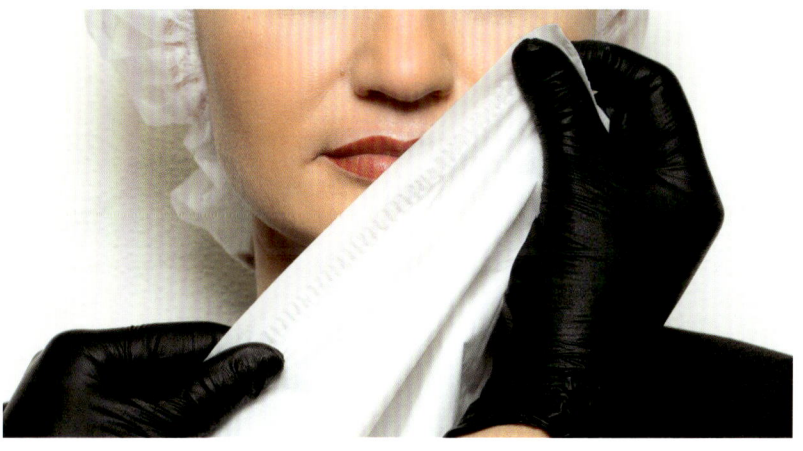

After 15-20 minutes, gently remove excess numbing solution with a tissue, taking care not to wipe off the lip contour design.

EYEBROWS

LIPS

EYES

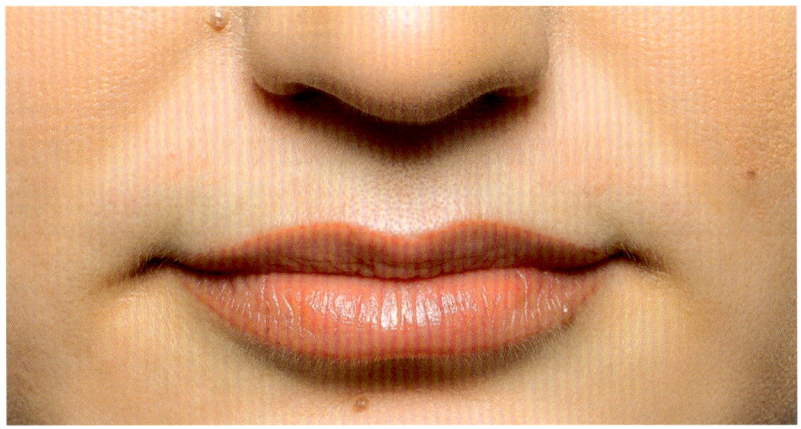

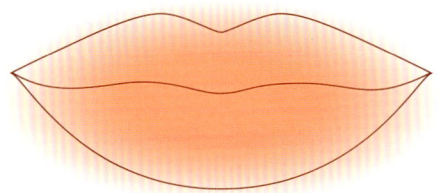

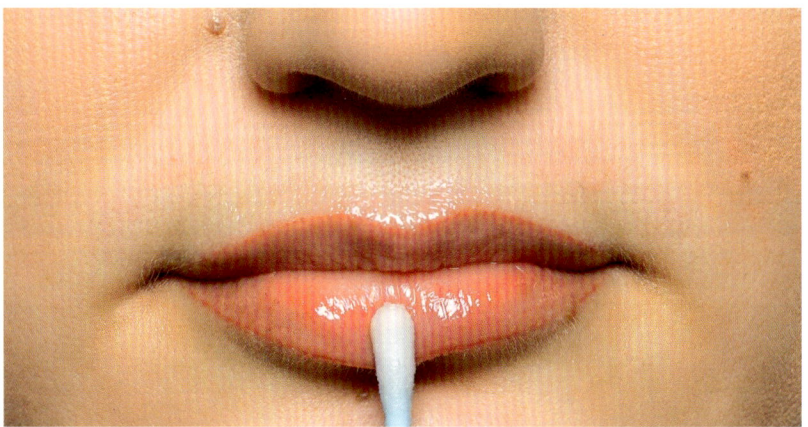

➡ Bidirectional   ◢ 60°   🌡 1-Liner, 3-Micro

🔄 Fast   ± 100/120   💧 Organic, Inorganic, Mix

Proceed to fix the sketch with our micropigmentation device and selected pigment starting from the left corner of the upper lip. Use 1-Liner or 3-Micro. Try to find the adequate needle depth and pressure with the first passes. Observe how thoroughly pigment is implanted in the skin and increase the pressure slightly if it is not saturated enough. Follow the directions as explained in the picture. Be careful that the contour line is clearly visible and you do not have to redraw the sketch. Open the skin gently with soft needle passes on the internal part of the lips after fixing the contour.

Carefully apply a numbing solution suitable for open skin with sterilized cotton tips on the whole surface of the sketch and wait around 2-3 minutes before continuing the procedure. It is important to follow the regulations in your own country and use only products authorized for permanent makeup professionals. In some countries, use of this solution by aestheticians is absolutely forbidden by law.

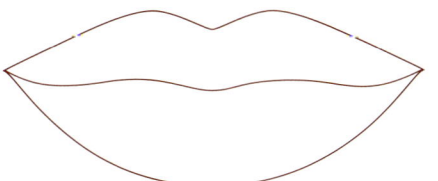

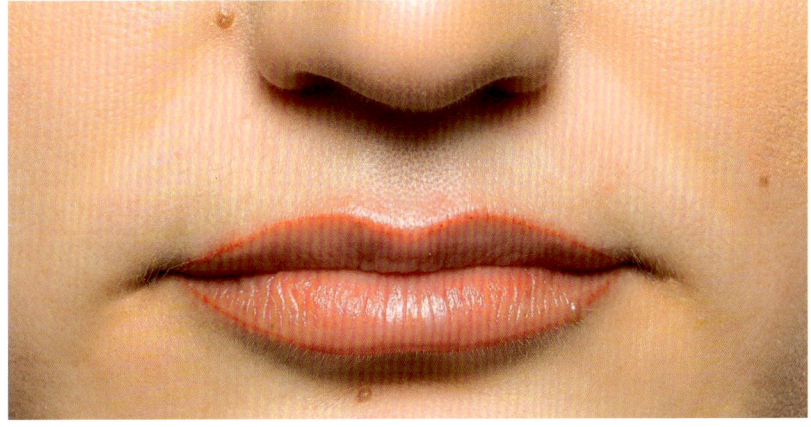

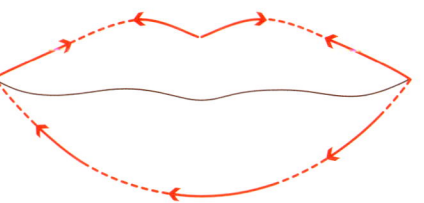

➡ Bidirectional   ◪ 90°   🌡 1-Liner, 3-Micro

✋ Medium/Slow   ± 100/120   💧 Organic, Inorganic, Mix

Follow the directions as explained in the picture. Move slowly with back-and-forth hand movements from the external corners of upper lip to the Cupid's bow. On the Cupid's bow area it is important to start from the center and move towards the sides. Proceed to start the contour micropigmentation on the bottom lip, fixing the contour from the left to right corner of the lip in the directions shown on the picture. Hold the needle perpendicularly but without applying too much pressure in a 90° degree angle.

➡ Bidirectional   ◪ 60°   🌡 1-Liner, 3-Micro

✋ Medium/Slow   ± 100/120   💧 Organic, Inorganic, Mix

Proceed with the first passes on the contour in order to define the outer lines and make them visible. The working technique is bidirectional, with slow or medium hand motion, the pen at a 60° angle, and slow frequency, no higher than 120 pps.

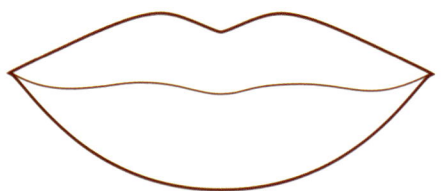

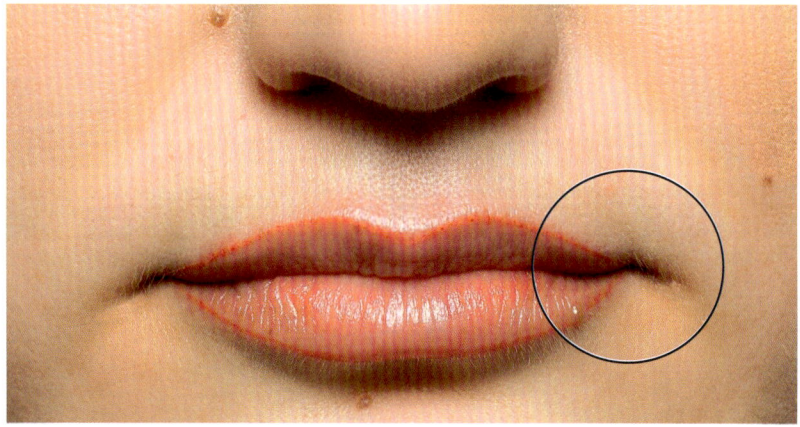

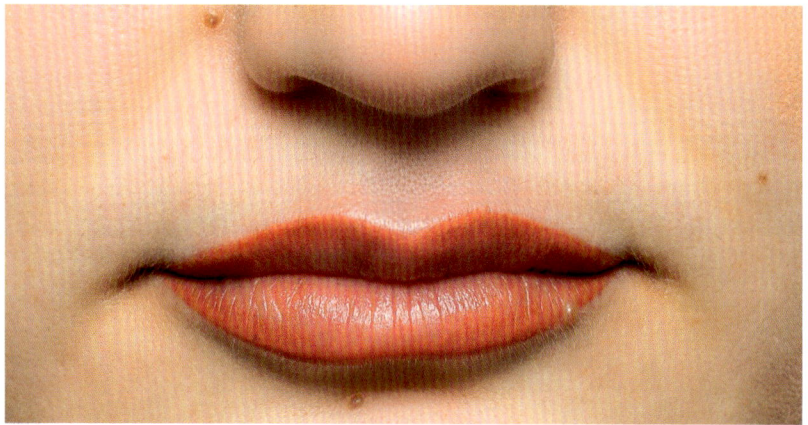

➡ Bidirectional   ◢ 60°   ⬍ 1-Liner, 3-Micro

✋ Medium/Slow   ± 100/120   ◈ Organic, Inorganic, Mix

➡ Bidirectional   ◢ 60°   ⬍ 1-Liner, 3-Micro

✋ Medium/Slow   ± 100/120   ◈ Organic, Inorganic, Mix

A very important rule is not connecting the contour lines on the external corners of the lips. The color implantation on the external corners must be smooth, in the same way as in the natural lip.

Do the second pass of lips contour micropigmentation, paying special attention to the uniformity and saturation of the pigment. Please follow the directions as explained in 16.

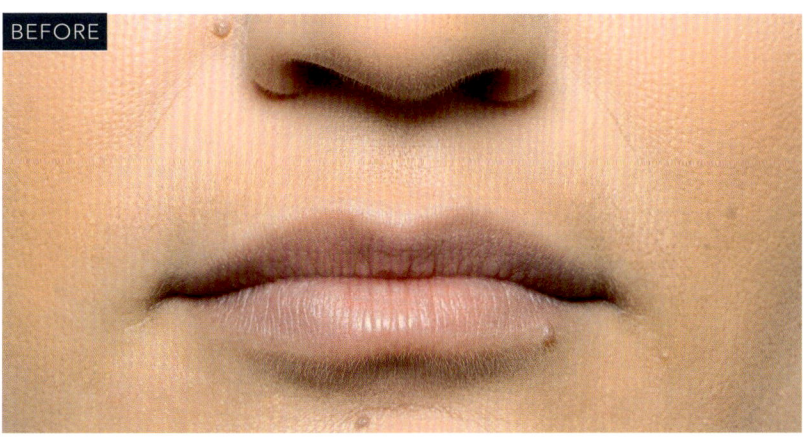

BEFORE

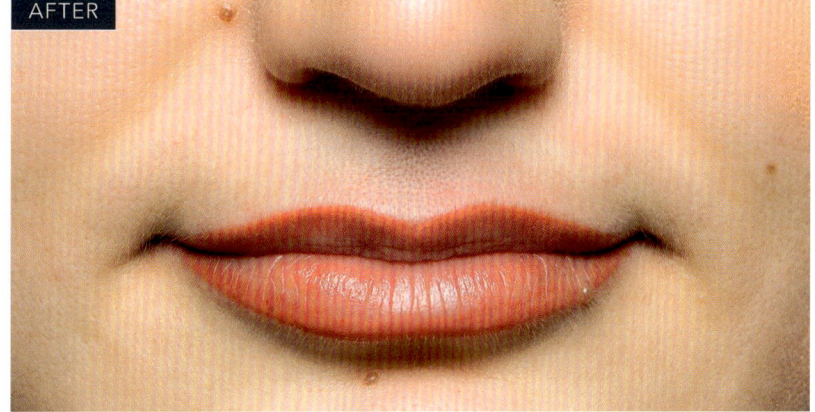

AFTER

After 40 days, the pigment will undergo a change in color in which the final result lightens and becomes much more natural.

13.2.3. SHADING

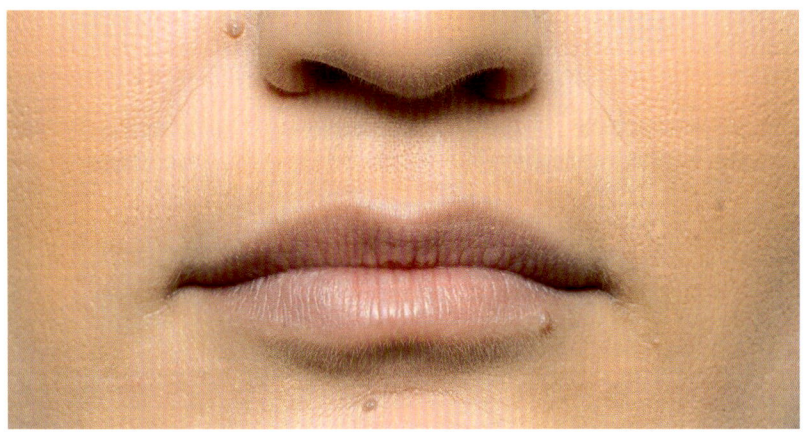

Before starting the lip procedure, it is important to take into account all relevant hygienic aspects for the lip area. Remember that lip tissue has a completely different morphology and sensibility than the eyebrow area and it is more prone to inflammation, infections, and other reactions. Therefore, it is of crucial importance to follow the highest safety and hygienic standards.

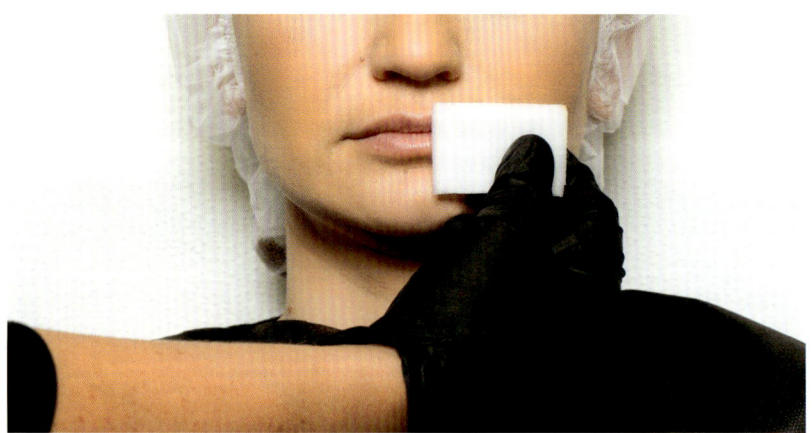

In the first stage, the professional will proceed to remove any makeup or cosmetic products and clean off the lip area with antibacterial tissue to eliminate any potential non-pathogenic microorganisms. We recommend not re-using the dirty part of the wipe. If the client is wearing lipstick, the technician will use several antibacterial tissues until the makeup has been completely removed.

3 PHILTRAL COLUMNS

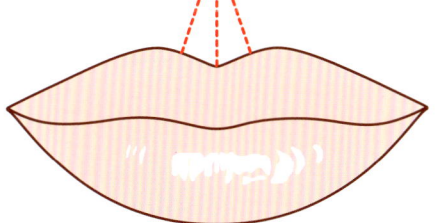

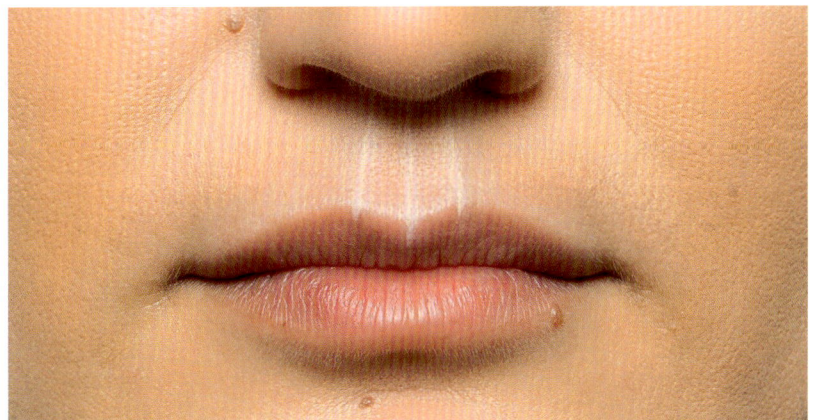

Mark the philtrum and Cupid's bow with a white marker in order to easily define lip symmetry and draw three lines as in the picture.

⚠ ATTENTION
In some countries only sterile, single-use markers are allowed for this purpose.

4 CUPID'S BOW

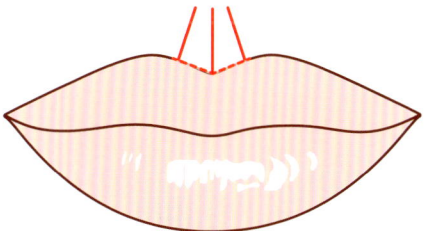

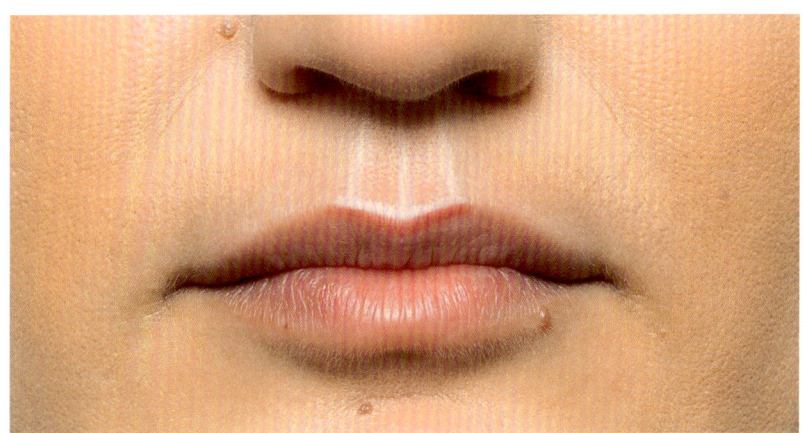

Outline the Cupid's bow and vermilion borders of the upper lip trying not go beyond the red border of the lips. This rule is of crucial importance in order to get a natural result after healing. Use two markers in different tones for the sketch: we will use a white or skin-tone marker for the external outline and a red or pink color marker for sketching the lip contour on the mucous membrane.

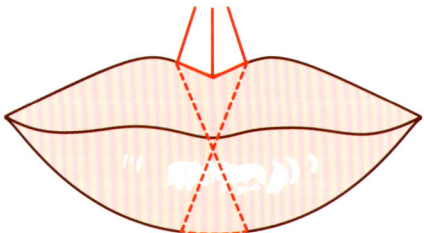

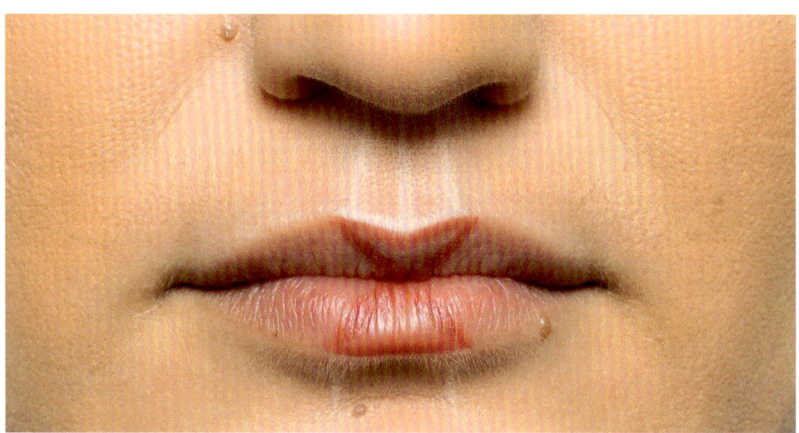

Proceed to draw the lower lip contour starting from the central area and making sure not to make it too round looking. Use the rule of creating a symmetric inversed triangle to the upper central part of the lip to create a balanced, natural design.

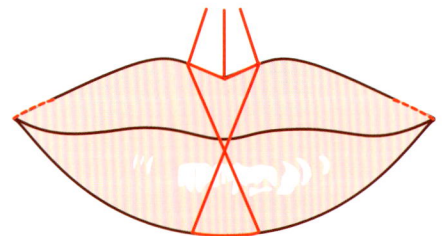

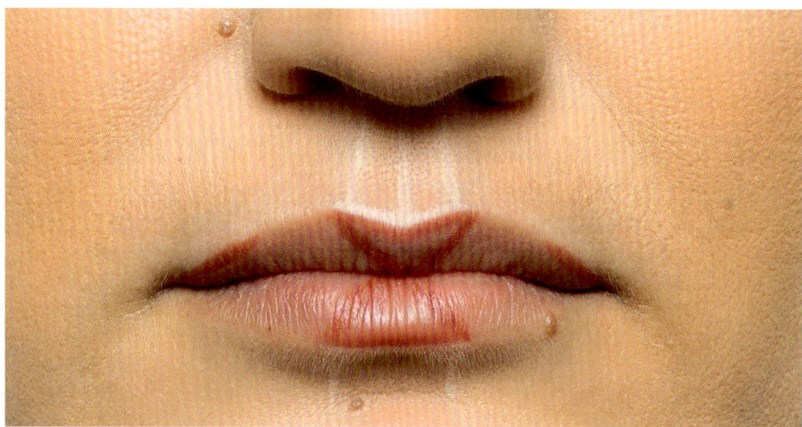

Continue drawing the external sketch outline of the upper lip by tracing two external corner lines around the upper lip and make them symmetric to each other.

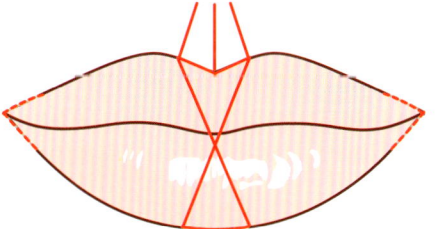

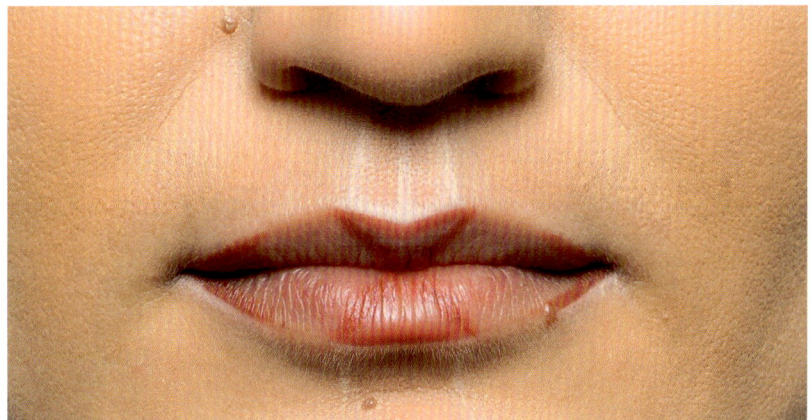

Continue drawing the external sketch outline of the bottom lip by tracing two external corner lines around the bottom lip and make them symmetric to each other. Also draw the external contour lines with the white or beige marker.

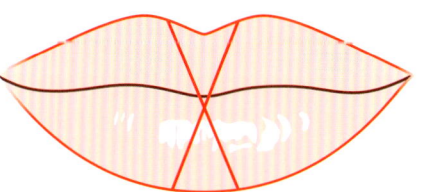

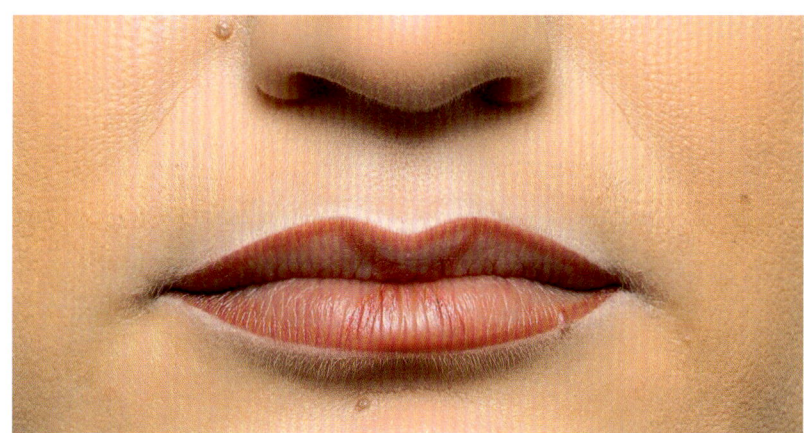

Connect all the contour lines in the sketch with the pink or red pencil. Also draw the external contour lines with the white or beige marker.

IMPORTANT NOTICE:

In case we want to correct asymmetry or to give more volume, it is allowed to draw the contour slightly outside of the client's mucous membrane, but never exceeding 1–1.5 mm.

EYEBROWS

LIPS

EYES

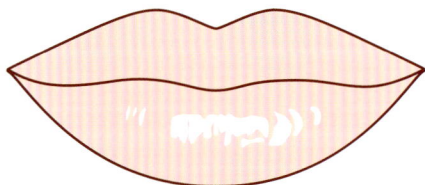

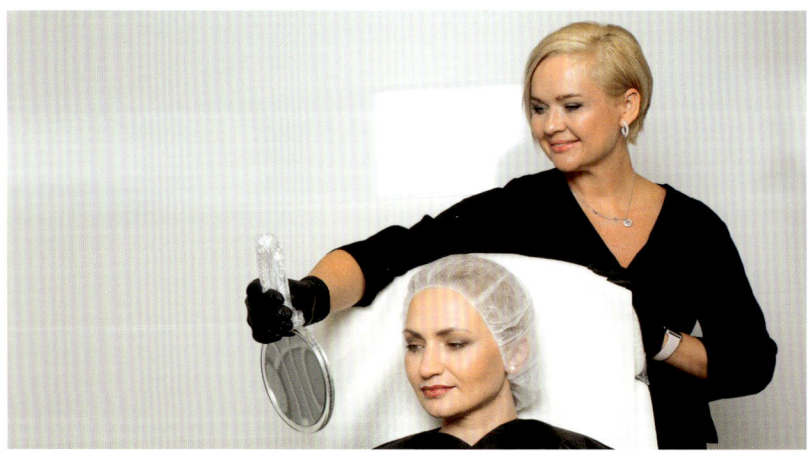

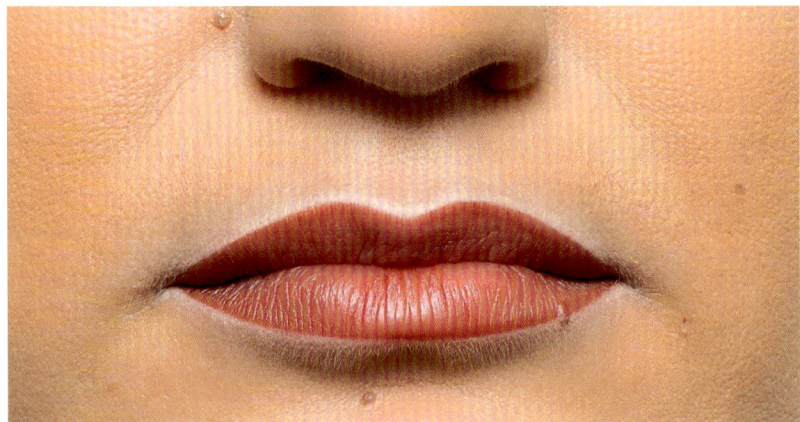

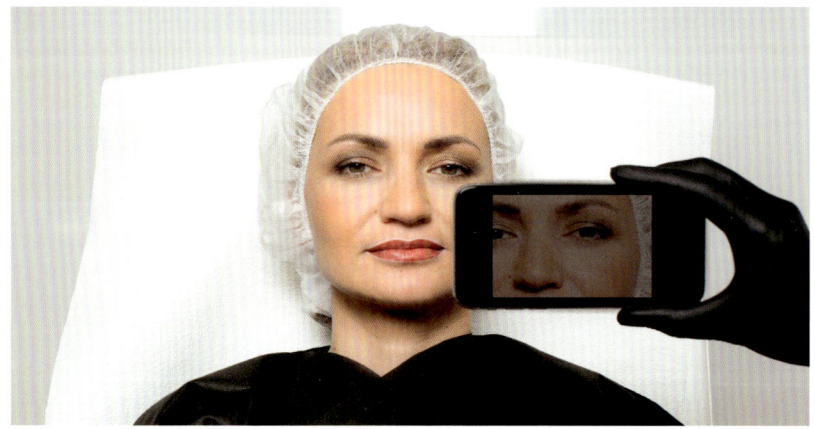

Fill in the inside part of the the lip area with red or pink color in a soft and homogeneous way. Make a visual check of symmetry of the design, paying attention to the dynamic aspect as well. It is recommended that the client talk or smile as a double check, as the symmetry and natural look of the lip design must also be guaranteed in motion.

When the sketch is ready, it is time to show final design to the client and ask for approval. Two methods are recommended for a visualization of the sketch by our clients. The first and more classic method it is looking in a mirror from frontal and side angles. The second method consists of taking several pictures from different perspectives and showing them to the client. Don't underestimate this approval step, and take enough time when showing the sketch to your clients, pointing out the improvements in terms of definition, balance, and symmetry. It will increase customer satisfaction once the procedure has been performed.

11 APPLYING 1ST NUMBING SOLUTION

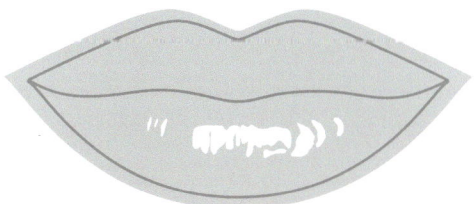

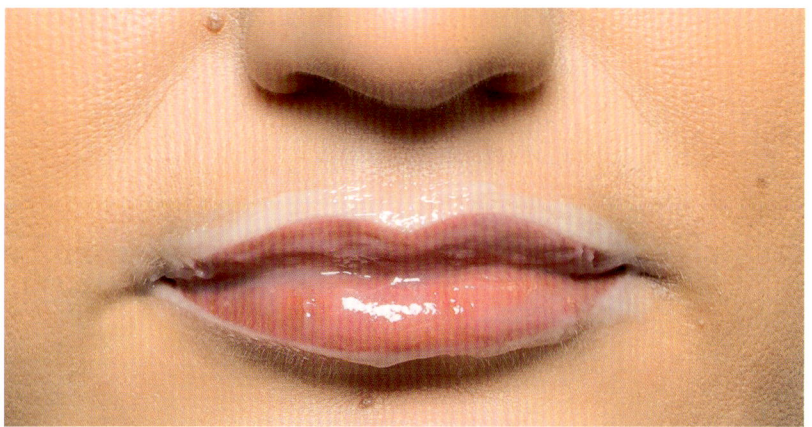

Carefully apply a numbing solution with sterilized cotton tips on the whole surface of the sketch and wait around 15-20 minutes before starting the procedure. It is important to follow the regulations in your own country and use only products authorized for permanent makeup professionals.

12 REMOVING THE NUMBING SOLUTION

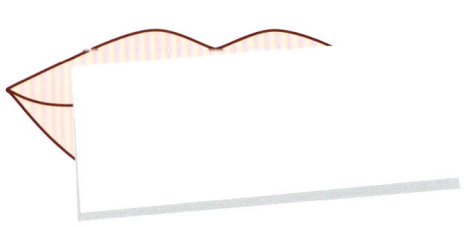

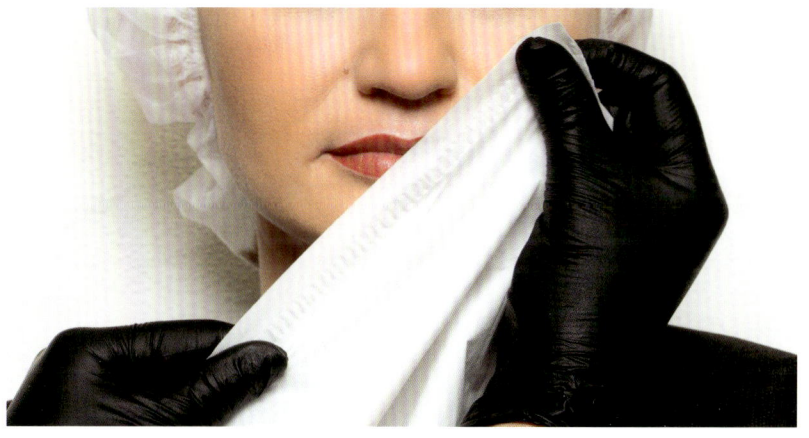

After 15-20 minutes, gently remove excess numbing solution with a tissue, taking care not to wipe off the lip contour design.

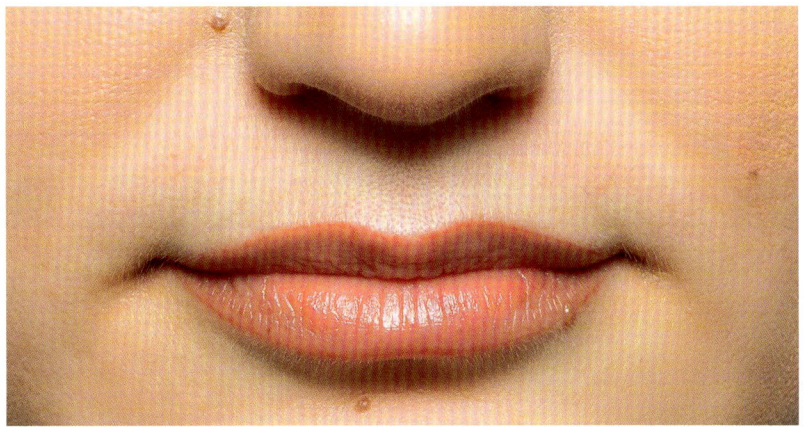

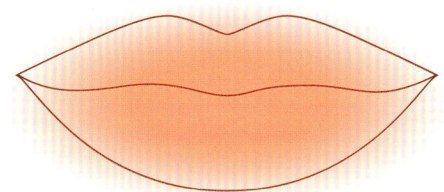

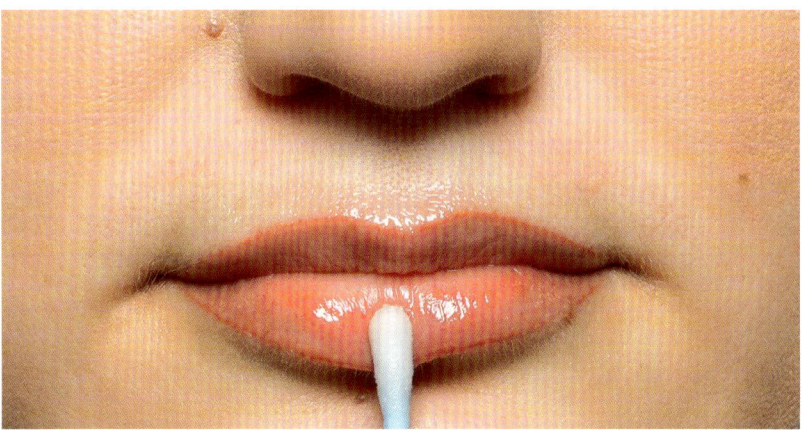

➡ Bidirectional   ◢ 60°   🖊 1-Liner, 3-Micro

✋ Fast   ± 100/120   💧 Organic, Inorganic, Mix

Proceed to fix the sketch with the amiea micropigmentation device and selected pigment starting from the left corner of the upper lip. Use 3-Micro. Try to find the adequate needle depth and pressure with the first passes. Observe how thoroughly pigment is implanted in the skin and increase the pressure slightly if it is not saturated enough. Follow the directions as explained in the picture. Make sure that the contour line is clearly visible and you do not have to redraw the sketch. Open the skin gently with soft needle passes on the internal part of the lips after fixing the contour.

Carefully apply a numbing solution suitable for open skin with sterilized cotton tips on the whole surface of the sketch and wait around 2–3 minutes before continuing the procedure. It is important to follow the regulations in your own country and use only products authorized for permanent makeup professionals. In some countries, use of this solution by aestheticians is absolutely forbidden by law.

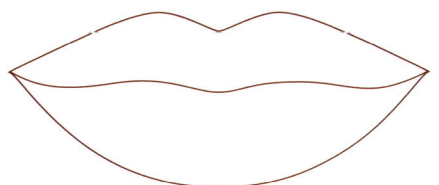

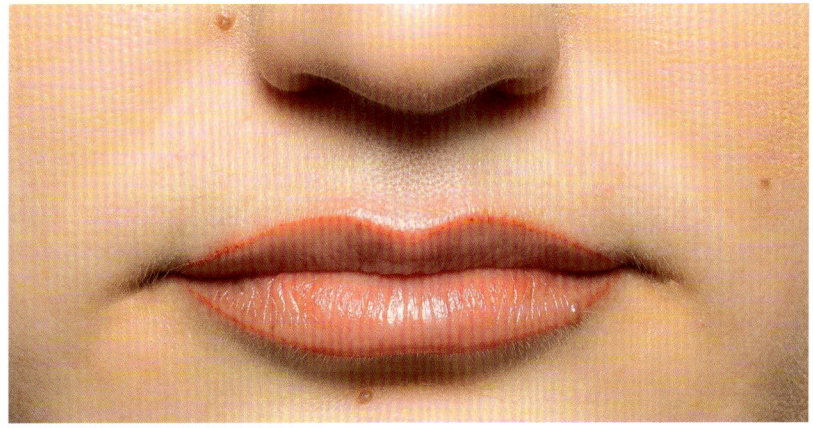

➡ Bidirectional   ◢ 60°   ⬍ 3-Micro

✋ Medium/Slow   ± 100/120   ◍ Organic, Inorganic, Mix

Proceed with the first passes on the contour in order to define the outer lines and make them visible. The working technique is bidirectional, with slow or medium hand motion, the pen at a 60° angle, and slow frequency, no higher than 120 pps.

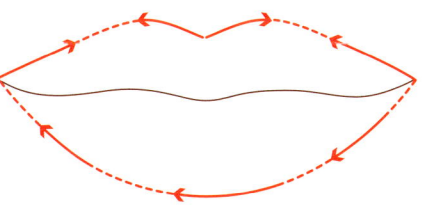

➡ Bidirectional   ◢ 90°   ⬍ 3-Micro

✋ Medium/Slow   ± 100/120   ◍ Organic, Inorganic, Mix

Follow the directions as explained in the picture. Move slowly with back-and-forth hand movements from the external corners of upper lip to the Cupid's bow. On the Cupid's bow area it is important to start from the center and move towards the sides. Proceed to start the contour micropigmentation on the bottom lip, fixing the contour from the left to right corner of the lip in the directions shown on the picture. Hold the needle perpendicularly but without applying too much pressure in a 90° degree angle.

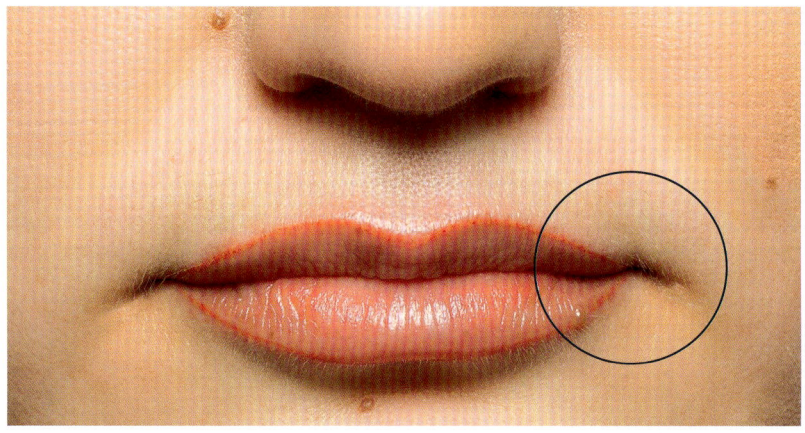

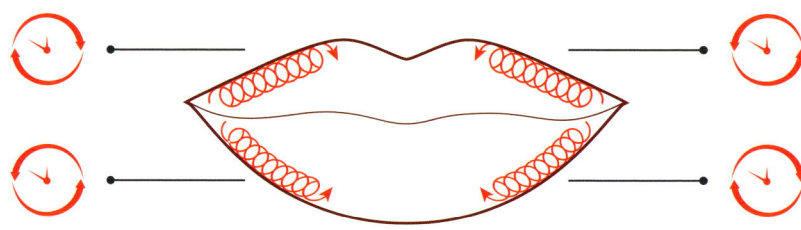

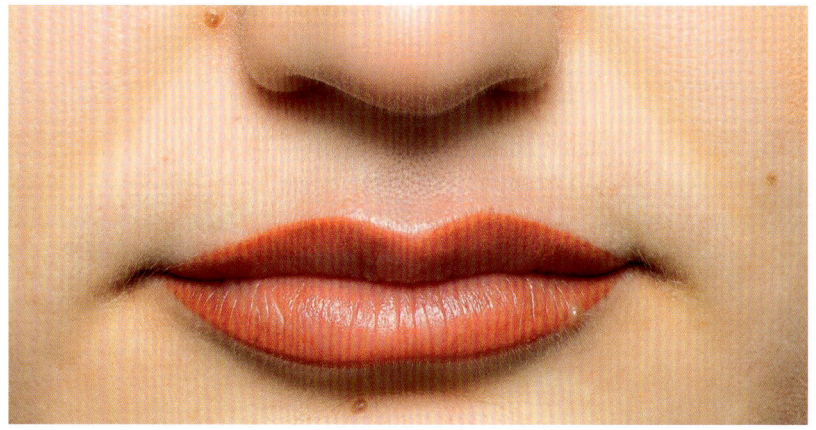

➡ Bidirectional   ◭ 60°   🖊 1-Liner, 3-Micro

✋ Medium/Slow   ± 100/120   💧 Organic, Inorganic, Mix

A very important rule is not connecting the contour lines on the external corners of the lips. The color implantation on the external corners must be smooth, in the same way as in the natural lip.

➡ Spiral movement   ◭ 60°   🖊 1-Liner, 3-Micro

✋ Medium/Slow   ± 100/120   💧 Organic, Inorganic, Mix

Proceed to start contour shading. Work with a 3-point micro needle at a 60° inclination with oval-spiral-like movements (ellipses) and medium hand motion. Start on the left edge of the upper lip moving towards to the center. Spiral-oval movements must not exceed the lip contour in any way. Pay attention to the stretching; it should be strong enough, especially in the center of the upper lip.

Movements must be confident and needle penetration rather shallow. The most important thing in the performance of spirals is to avoid uneven injection of the needle – "digging" effect. It is advisable not to do the spirals more than 2 times on the same area.

As a second step, we proceed with the lower lip contour shading. The same technique will apply, starting from the left edge and moving towards center, but ellipses should performed in a clockwise direction.

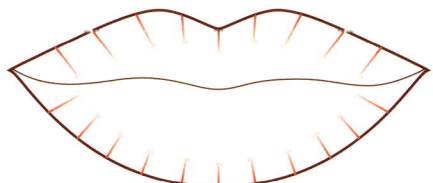

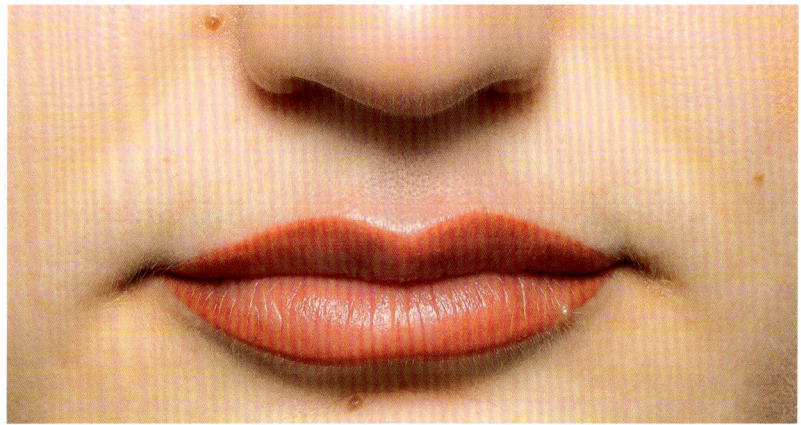

➡ Bidirectional	◢ 60°, 90°	🔧 3-Micro, 3-Slope, 5-Slope
✋ Fast	± 100/120	💧 Organic, Inorganic

We proceed to give a more homogeneous and compact look to the shading by drawing several straight lines starting from the contour and moving towards the central part of the mucous membrane. We use a 3-micro needle at an inclination of 60° and a medium hand motion.

Important! The distance between the lines is about 1 mm; do not trace too many lines. Our goal is to create a more compact look after tracing the spirals.

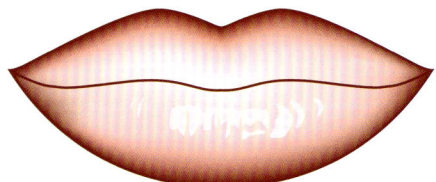

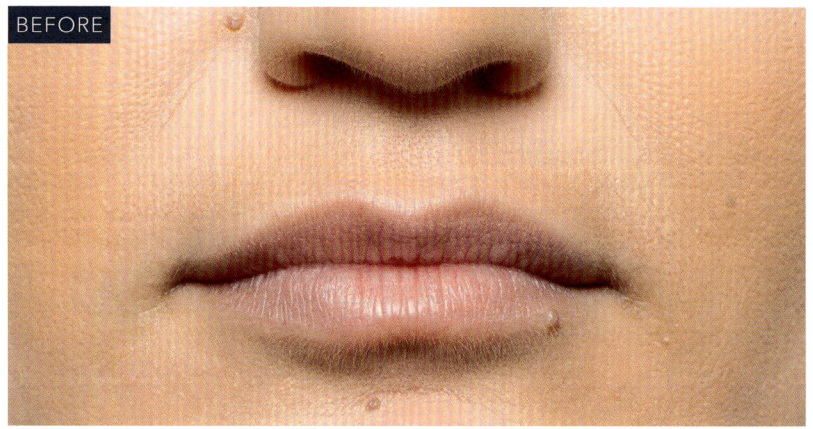
BEFORE

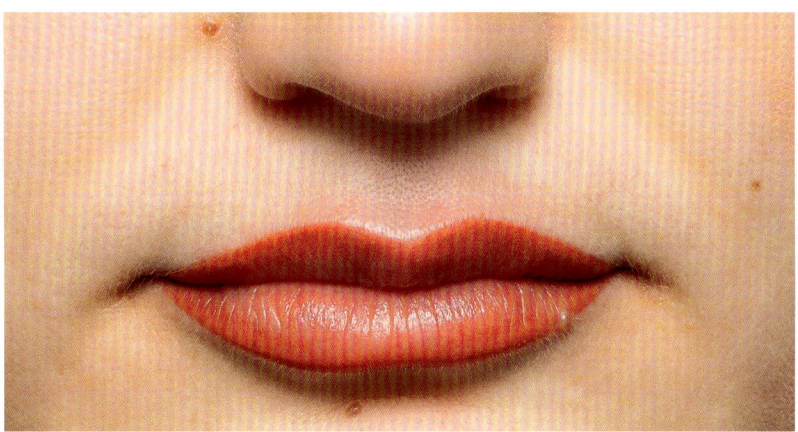

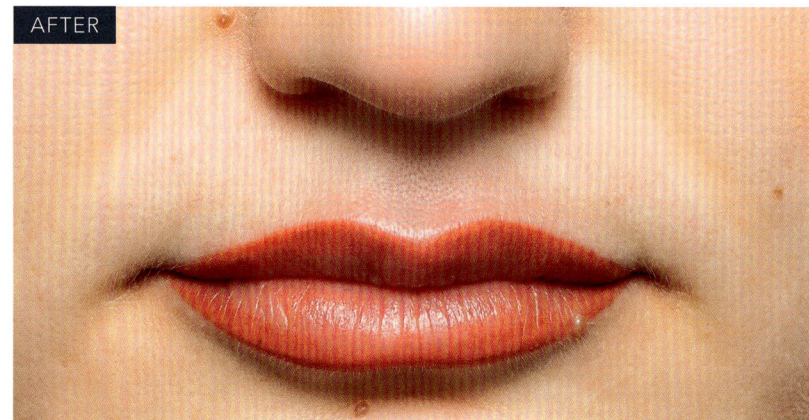
AFTER

Make a visual control of the final pigment implantation. It is important to avoid any unshaded sections between contour and shading, the connection should be smooth and natural looking.

The result immediately after treatment shows an intensive color. After 40 days, the pigment will undergo a change in color in which the final result lightens and becomes much more natural.

13.2.4. SHADING

1 INITIAL SITUATION

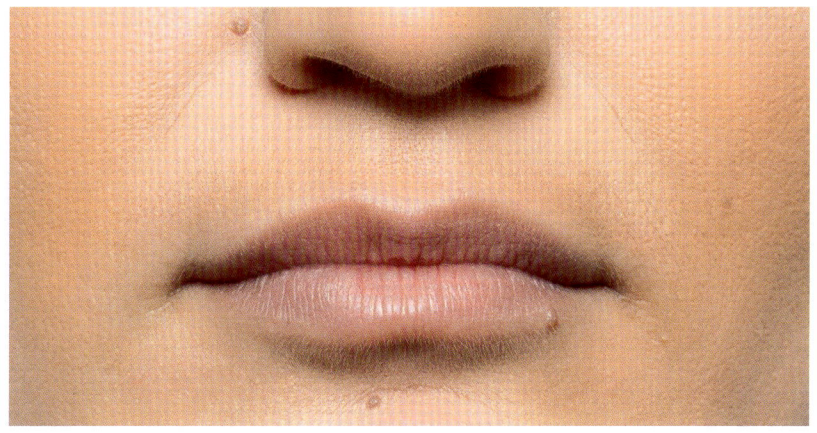

Before starting the lip procedure, it is important to take into account all relevant hygienic aspects for the lip area. Remember that lip tissue has a completely different morphology and sensibility than the eyebrow area and it is more prone to inflammation, infections, and other reactions. Therefore, it is of crucial importance to follow the highest safety and hygienic standards.

2 CLEANING

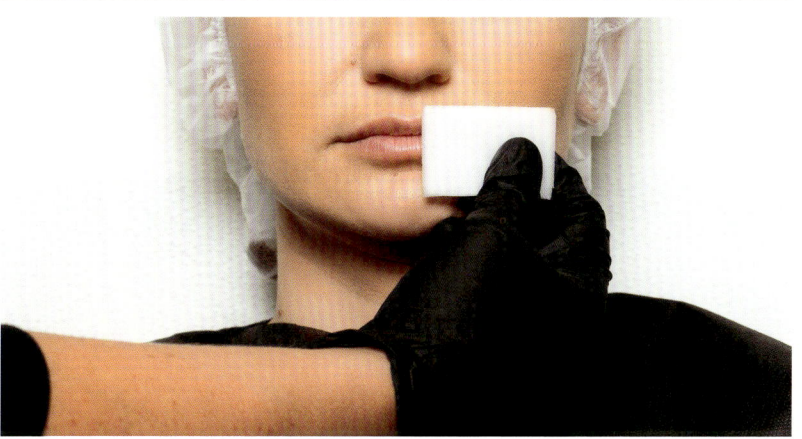

In the first stage, the professional will proceed to remove any makeup or cosmetic products and clean off the lip area with antibacterial tissue to eliminate any potential non-pathogenic microorganisms. We recommend not re-using the dirty part of the wipe. If the client is wearing lipstick, the technician will use several antibacterial tissues until the makeup has been completely removed.

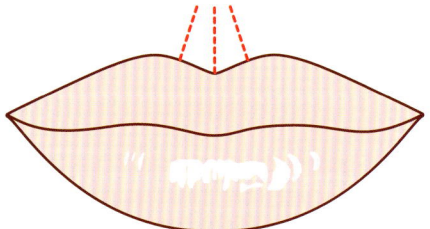

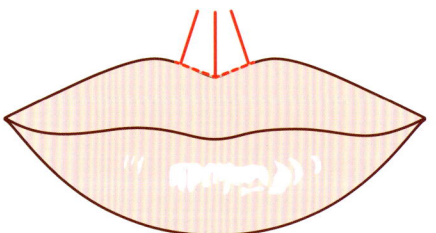

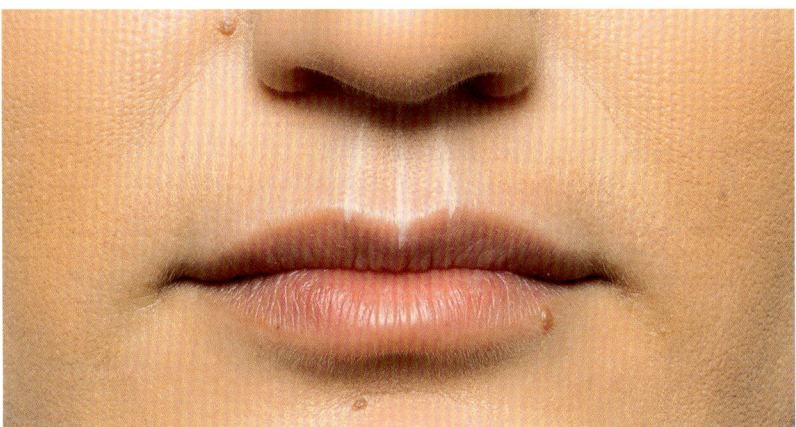

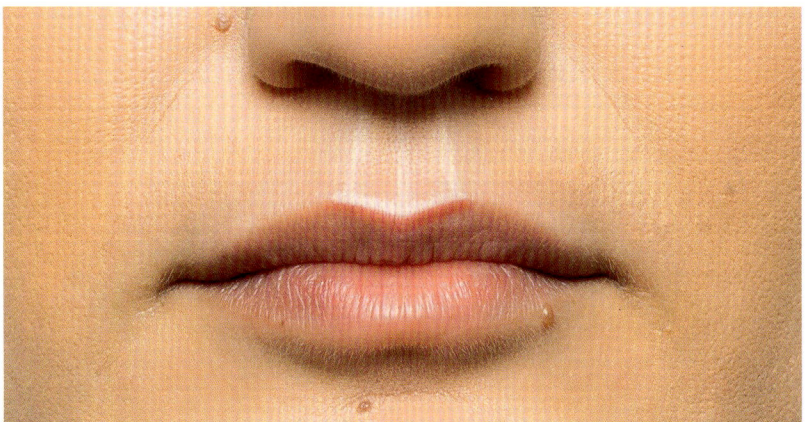

Mark the philtrum and Cupid's bow with a white marker in order to easily define lip symmetry and draw three lines as in the picture.

⚠ ATTENTION

In some countries only sterile, single-use markers are allowed for this purpose.

Outline the Cupid's bow and vermilion borders of the upper lip trying not go beyond the red border of the lips. This rule is of crucial importance in order to get a natural result after healing. Use two sharpened markers in different tones for the sketch: we will use a white or skin-tone marker for the external outline and a red or pink color marker for sketching the lip contour on the mucous membrane.

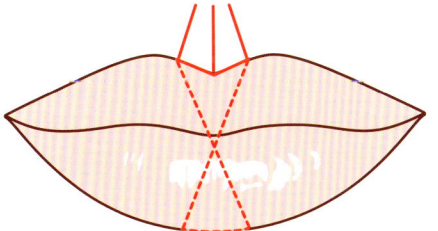

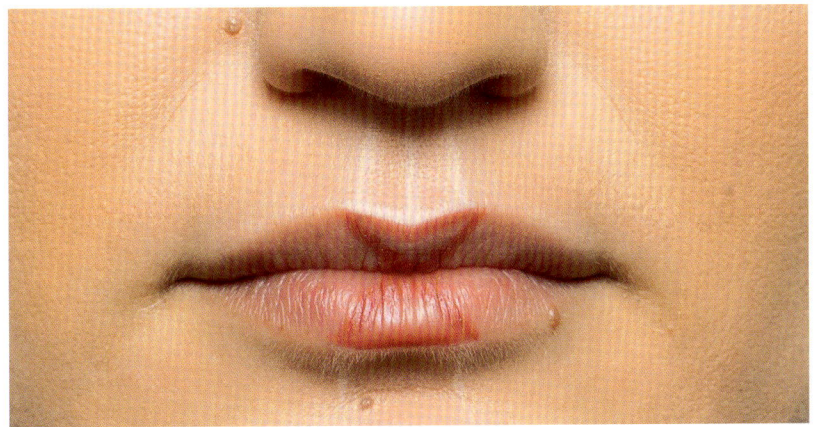

Proceed to draw the lower lip contour starting from the central area and making sure not to make it too round looking. Use the rule of creating a symmetric inversed triangle to the upper central part of the lip to create a balanced, natural design.

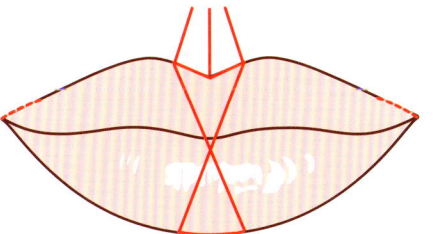

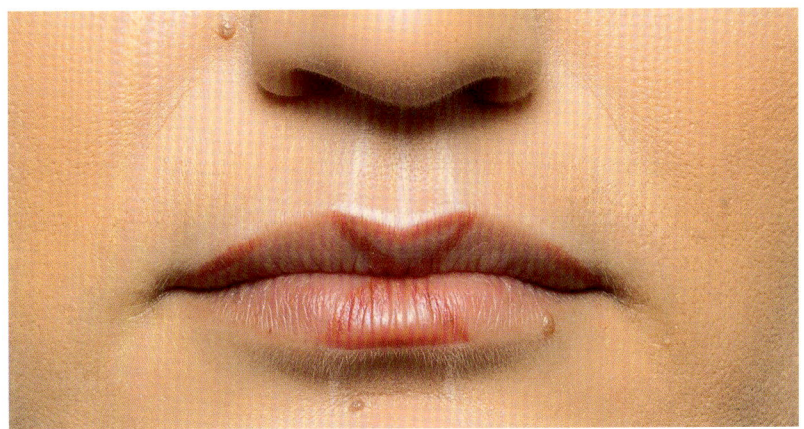

Continue drawing the external sketch outline of the upper lip by tracing two external corner lines around the upper lip and make them symmetric to each other.

EYEBROWS

LIPS

EYES

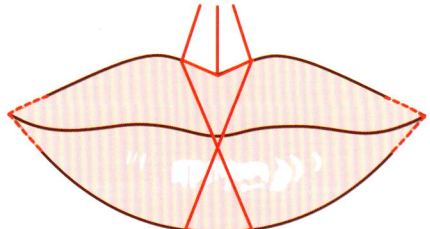

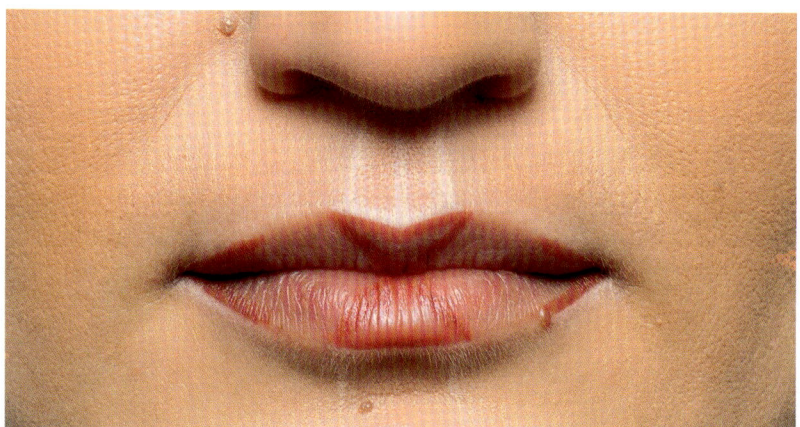

Continue drawing the external sketch outline of the bottom lip by tracing two external corner lines around the bottom lip and make them symmetric to each other. Also draw the external contour lines with the white or beige marker.

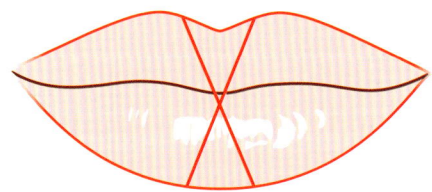

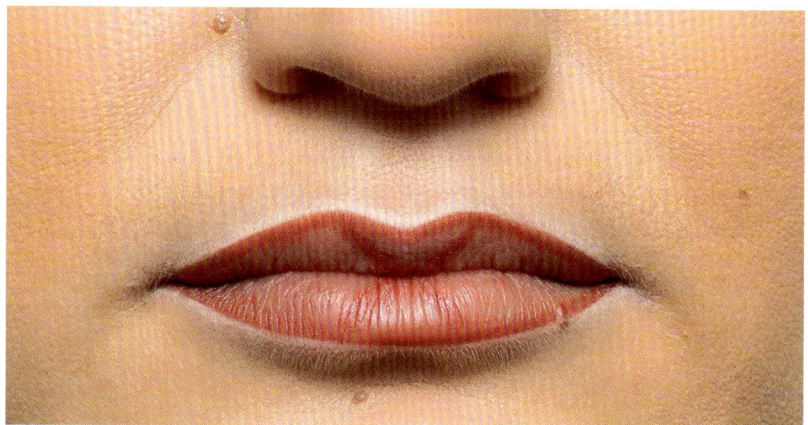

Connect all the contour lines in the sketch with the pink or red pencil. Also draw the external contour lines with the white or beige marker.

IMPORTANT NOTICE:

In case we want to correct asymmetry or to give more volume, it is allowed to draw the contour slightly outside of the client's mucous membrane, but never exceeding 1–1.5 mm.

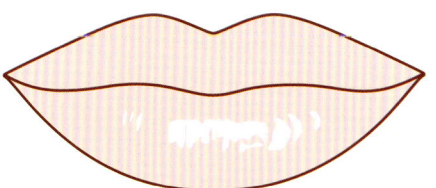

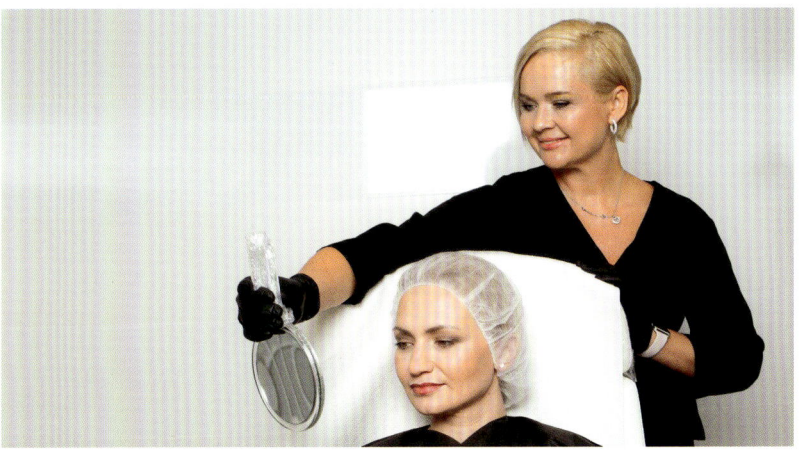

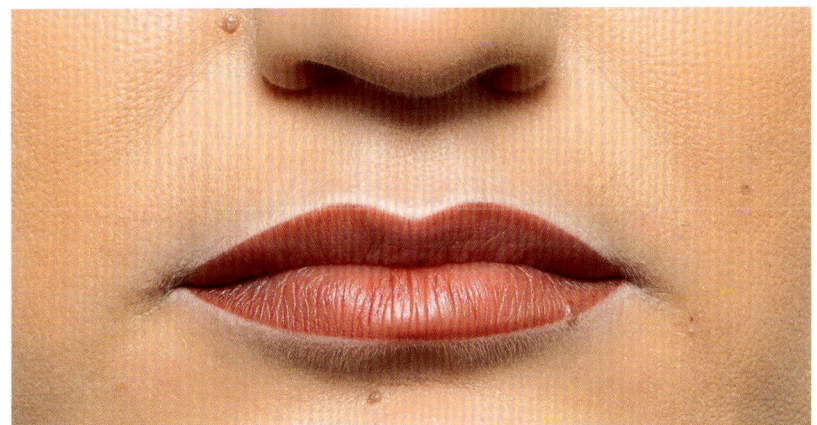

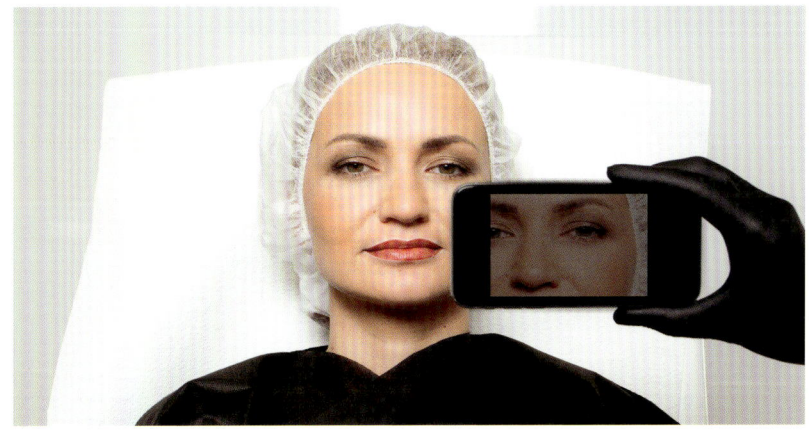

Fill in the inside part of the the lip area with red or pink color in a soft and homogeneous way. Make a visual check of the symmetry of the design, paying attention to the dynamic aspect as well. It is recommended that the client talk or smile as a double check, as symmetry and the natural look of the lip design must also be guaranteed in motion.

When the sketch is ready, it is time to show final design to the client and ask for approval. Two methods are recommended for a visualization of the sketch by our clients. The first and more classic method it is looking in a mirror from frontal and side angles. The second method consists of taking several pictures from different perspectives and showing them to the client. Don't underestimate this approval step, and take enough time when showing the sketch to your clients, pointing out the improvements in terms of definition, balance, and symmetry. It will increase customer satisfaction once the procedure has been performed.

EYEBROWS

LIPS

EYES

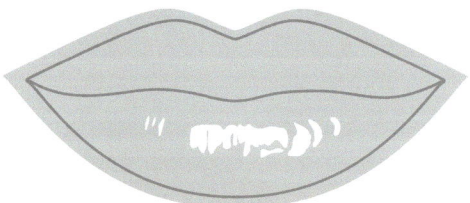

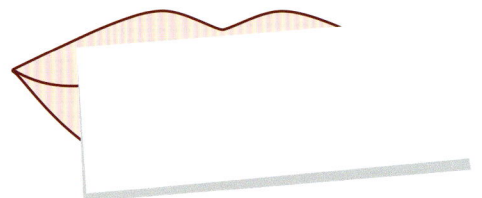

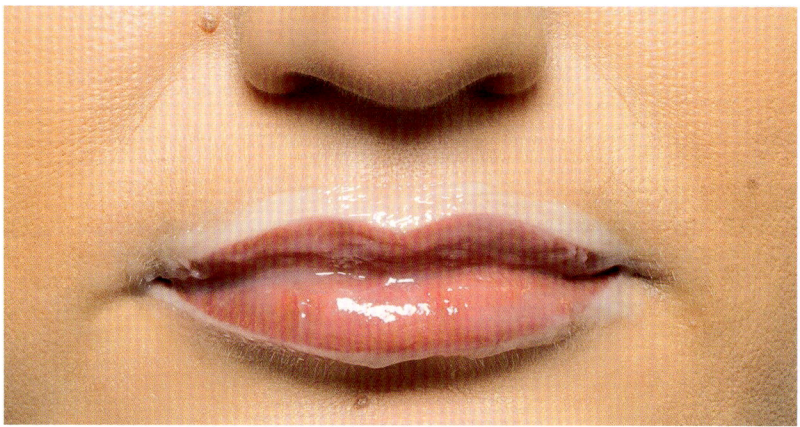

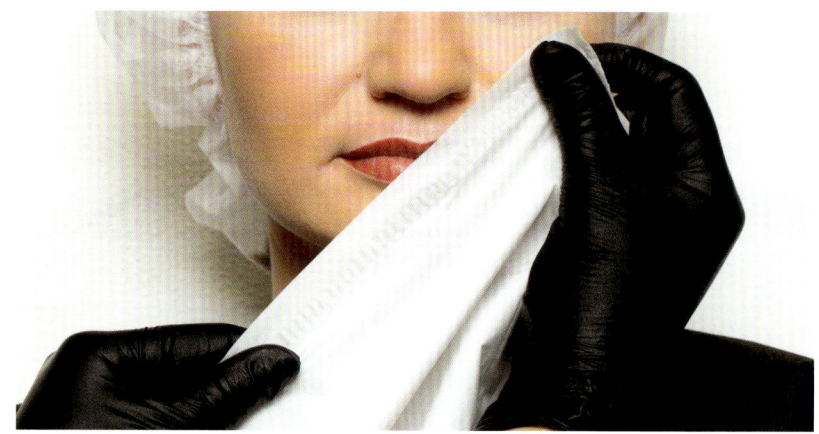

Carefully apply a numbing solution with sterilized cotton tips on the whole surface of the sketch and wait around 15–20 minutes before starting the procedure. It is important to follow the regulations in your own country and use only products authorized for permanent makeup professionals.

After 15–20 minutes, gently remove excess numbing solution with a tissue, taking care not to wipe off the lip contour design.

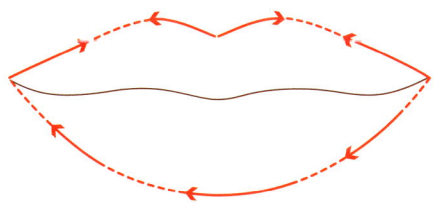

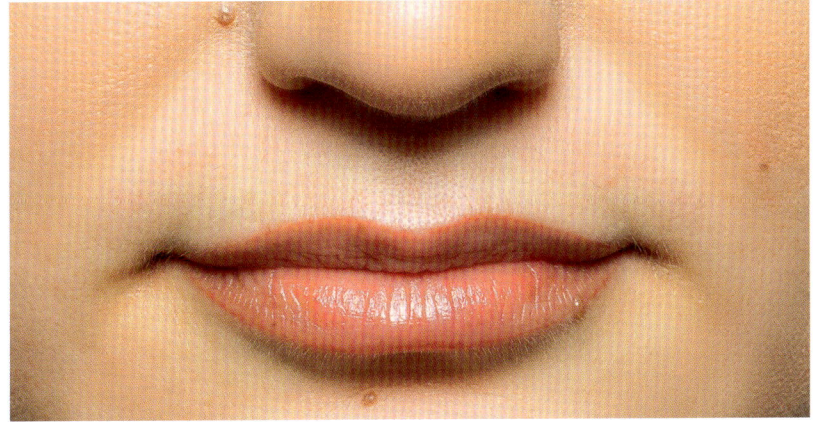

⮕ Bidirectional   ◳ 60°   🌡 1-Liner, 3-Micro

✋ Fast   ± 100/120   💧 Organic, Inorganic, Mix

Proceed to fix the sketch with our micropigmentation device and selected pigment starting from the left corner of the upper lip. Use 3-Micro. Try to find the adequate needle depth and pressure with the first passes. Observe how thoroughly pigment is implanted in the skin and increase the pressure slightly if it is not saturated enough. Follow the directions as explained in the picture. Make sure that the contour line is clearly visible and you do not have to redraw the sketch. Open the skin gently with soft needle passes on the internal part of the lips after fixing the contour.

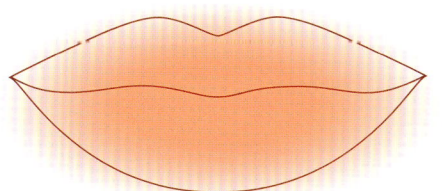

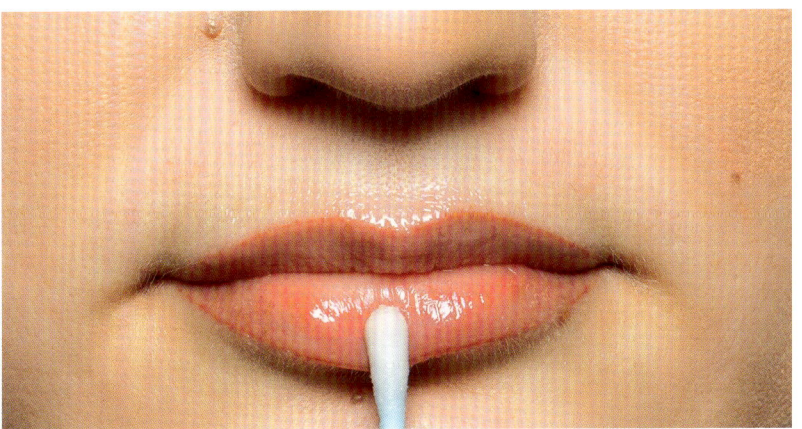

Carefully apply a numbing solution suitable for open skin with sterilized cotton tips on the whole surface of the sketch and wait around 2–3 minutes before continuing the procedure. It is important to follow the regulations in your own country and use only products authorized for permanent makeup professionals. In some countries, use of this solution by aestheticians is absolutely forbidden by law.

EYEBROWS

LIPS

EYES

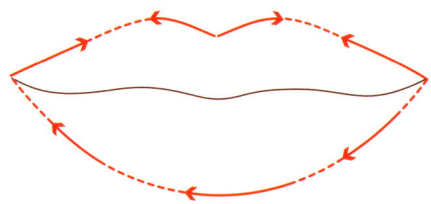

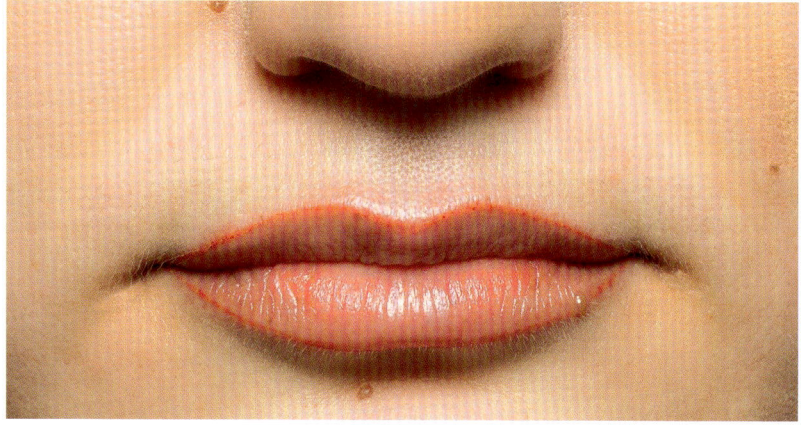

➡ Bidirectional	◢ 60°	🌡 3-Micro
✋ Medium/Slow	± 100/120	💧 Organic, Inorganic, Mix

Proceed with the first passes on the contour in order to define the outer lines and make them visible. The working technique is bidirectional, with slow or medium hand motion, the pen at a 60° angle, and slow frequency, no higher than 120 pps.

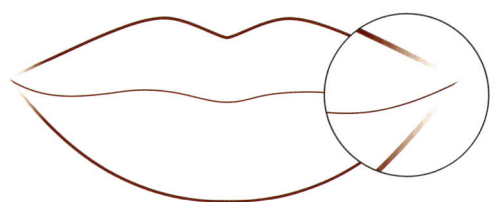

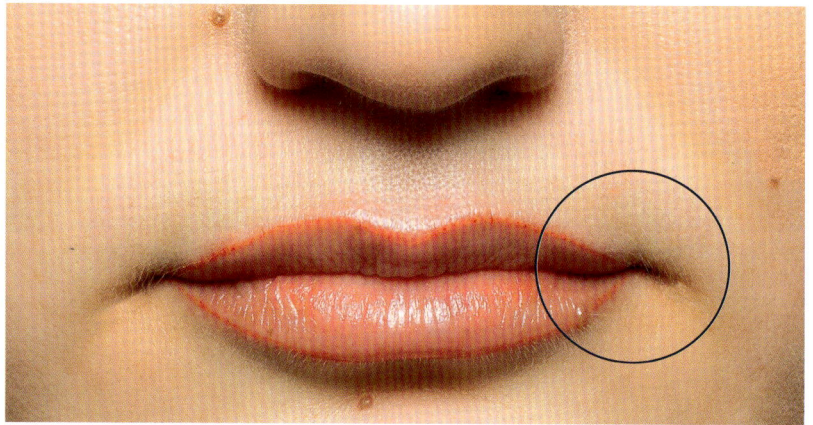

➡ Bidirectional	◢ 60°	🌡 3-Micro
✋ Medium/Slow	± 100/120	💧 Organic, Inorganic, Mix

A very important rule is not connecting the contour lines on the external corners of the lips. The color implantation on the external corners must be smooth, in the same way as in a natural lip.

17 SHADING THE OUTLINE

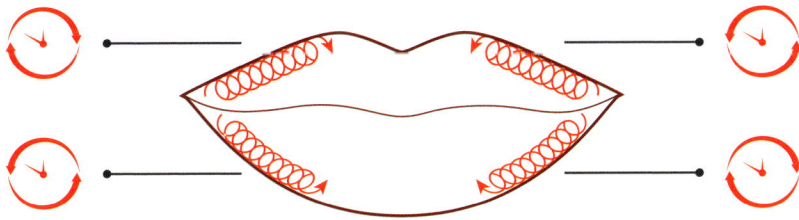

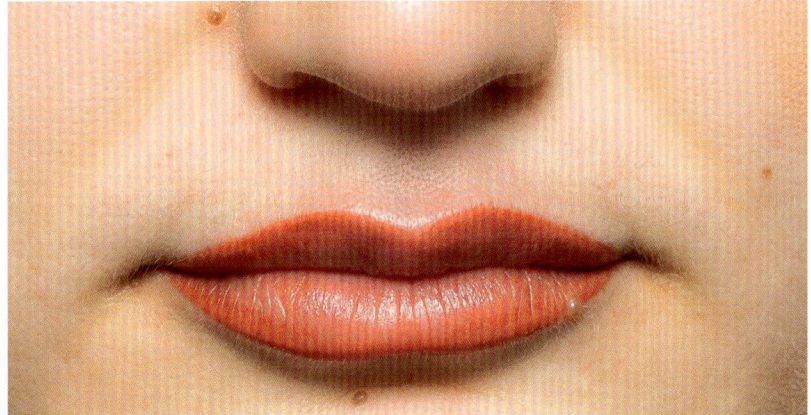

➡ Spiral movement   ◢ 60°   🌡 3-Micro

✋ Medium   ± 100/120   💧 Organic, Inorganic, Mix

Proceed to start contour shading. Work with a 3-point micro nee-dle at a 60° inclination with oval-spiral-like movements (ellipses) and medium hand motion. Start on the left edge of the upper lip moving towards to the center. Spiral-oval movements must not exceed the lip contour in any way. Pay attention to the stretching; it should be strong enough, especially in the center of the upper lip.

Movements must be confident and needle penetration rather shallow. The most important thing in the performance of spirals is to avoid uneven injection of the needle – "digging" effect. It is advisable not to do the spirals more than 2 times on the same area.

As a second step, we proceed with the lower lip contour shading. The same technique will apply, starting from the left edge and moving towards center, but ellipses should performed in a clockwise direction.

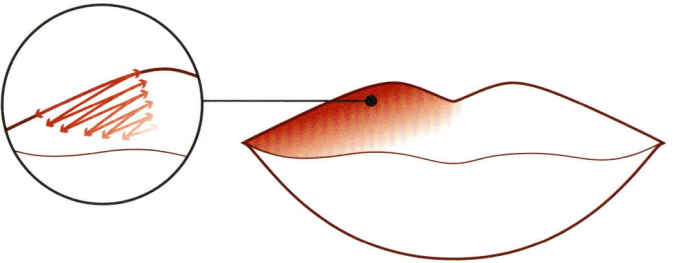

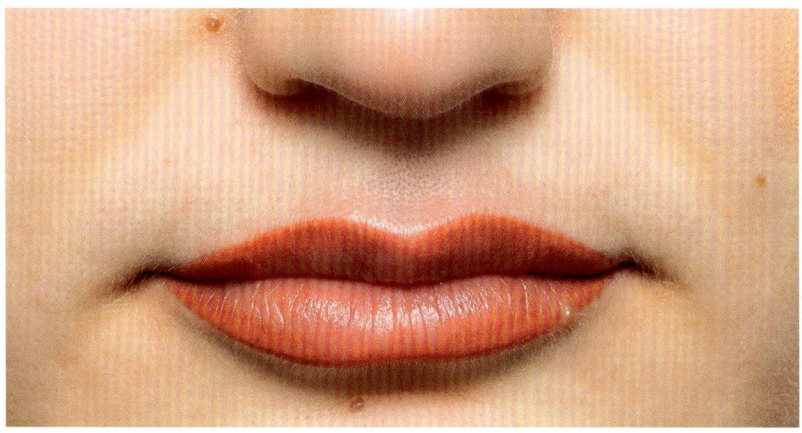

enough. After each step we add a secondary numbing solution (follow regulations of the country in which you are working).

2–3 passes are sufficient on each skin area. Recommendation for a natural result: it is important for the final frontal view of the lip to have different color saturations. Shading on the upper lip area below the contour should look lighter than the contour and interior central part of the upper mucous membrane. The central part of the bottom lip should look even lighter and more translucent in order to achieve the perfect result.

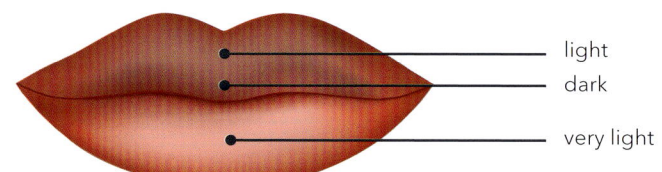

light
dark
very light

➡ Bidirectional ◐ 60°, 90° 🌡 3-Micro, 3-Slope, 5-Slope

✋ Fast ± 100/120 💧 Organic, Inorganic

We begin to fully fill the lips after completing the spirals. Start working from the contour and move towards center of the mucous membrane. We perform zigzag movements as indicated in the picture. This stage can be performed in two different ways: with 3-micro at a working angle of 60°. It is also possible to use the 3-slope and 5-slope needles, but with a working angle of 90°. Important! Hand movement must be even, slightly accelerating towards the center of the lips, and skin stretching should be strong

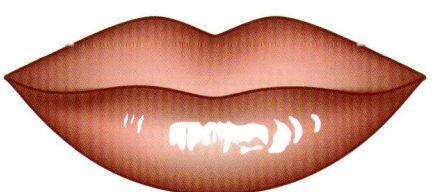

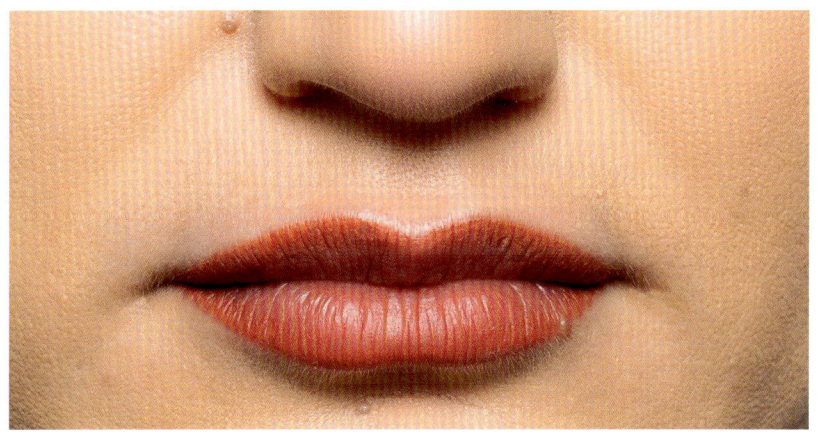

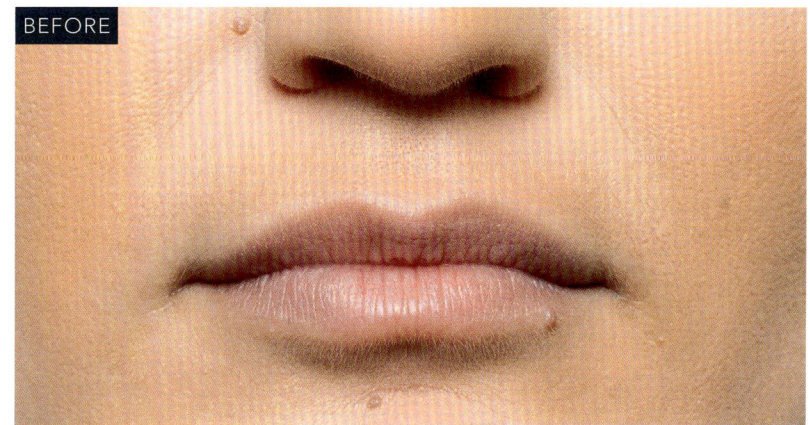

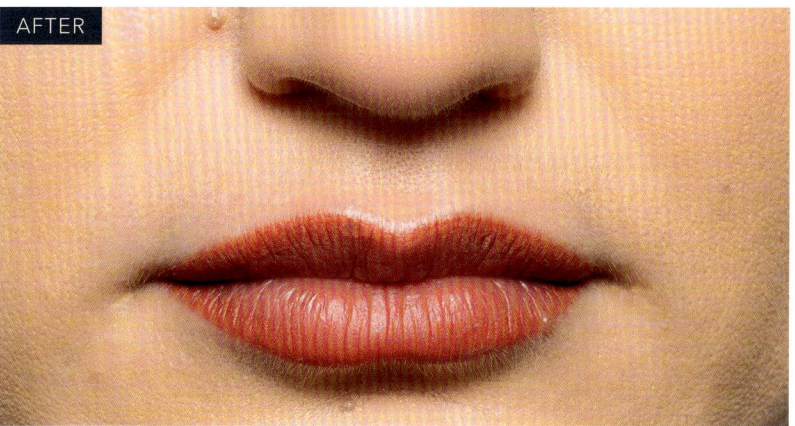

The result immediately after treatment shows an intensive color. After 40 days the pigment will undergo a change in color in which the final result lightens and becomes much more natural.

EYEBROWS

LIPS

EYES

13.3.

EYES
STEP BY STEP

EYEBROWS

LIPS

EYES

LINER

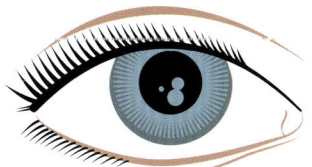

SHADING

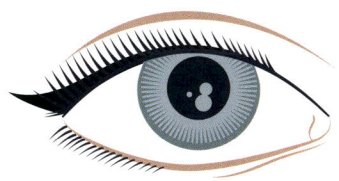

FILLING IN

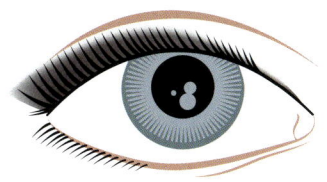

There are different application techniques in permanent makeup, which aim to give the eye a more or less emphasized, made-up, natural, or deep effect.

Applying pigment between the lashes creates the most subtle effect and is often used among men with alopecia, or for clients who want to enhance their eyes without the look of visible makeup.

Graphic eyeliner application, on the other hand, has more obvious purposes: it is done in order to change the anatomical appearance of the eye area, to replace daily makeup, or simply to create a more attractive gaze.

Shading is a technique specifically aimed at people who don't want a completely natural look, as with inter-eyelash pigment, but don't want an effect that is too defined and obvious.

The shadow technique creates a light shadow on the skin of the upper lash line resembling the effect created by eyeshadow. It is definitely a beautiful and high-impact technique, but it is not common since it is very difficult for the professional to get it right and it can be too constricting should the client ever want a fresh-faced look.

Following the step-by-step instructions is more important than ever for this essential technique in order to get the desired effect.

13.3.1. LASH ENHANCEMENT

1   INITIAL SITUATION

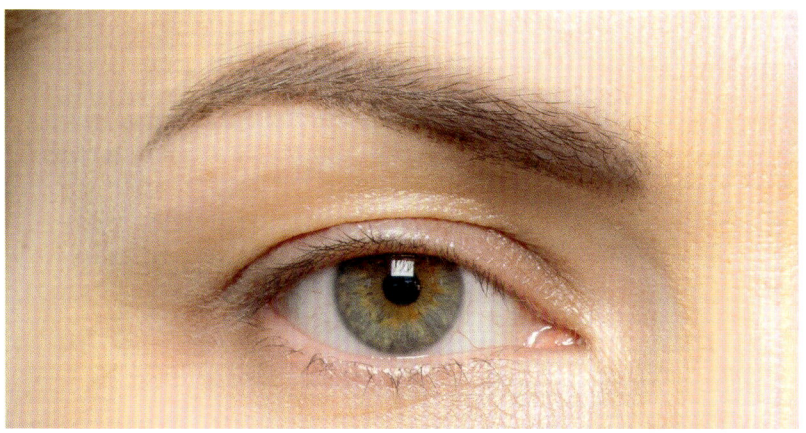

Before starting the eyelash enhancement procedure, it is advisable to ask your client how they draw their eyeliner in their daily makeup in order to discover the preferred color and thickness. At the same time, we analyze the shape and position of the eyes in our client´s face, so we will be able to correct the shape and make the eyes' expression more balanced.

Treatment steps and pictures by Elena Nikora.

2   CLEANING

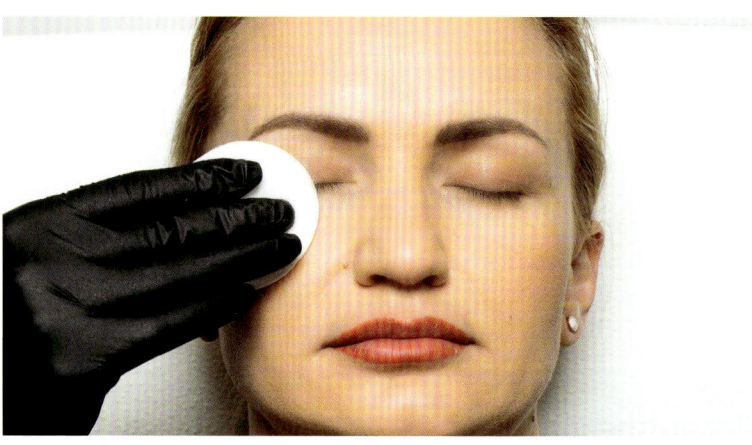

Before starting the procedure, it is important to take into account all relevant hygienic aspects for the eye area. Remember that tissue between the lashes has a different morphology and sensibility than the eyebrow area, and it is more prone to inflammation, infections and other reactions. Therefore, it is of crucial importance to follow the highest safety and hygienic standards. We proceed to gently clean the upper lid area with antiseptic liquid until makeup and other cosmetic products have been completely removed.

3 SKETCHING

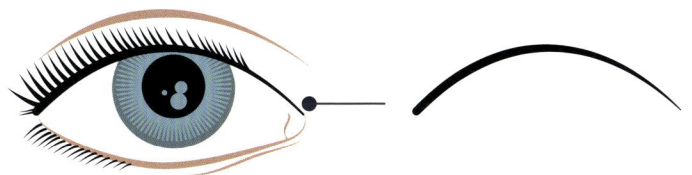

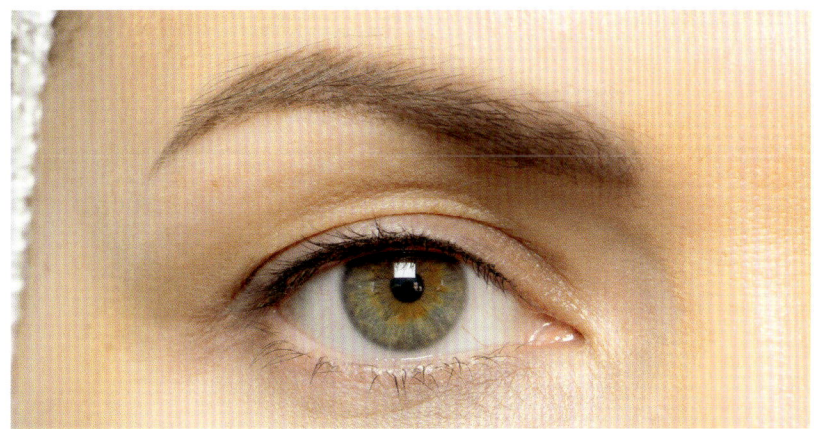

Proceed by sketching the design on the client. Use one sharp cosmetic pencil in the desired color following the common visagistic rules for eye area.

4 MIRROR AND TEST PHOTO

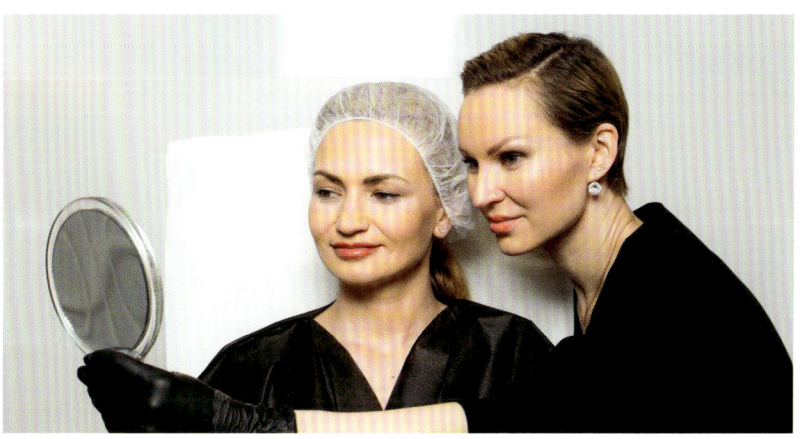

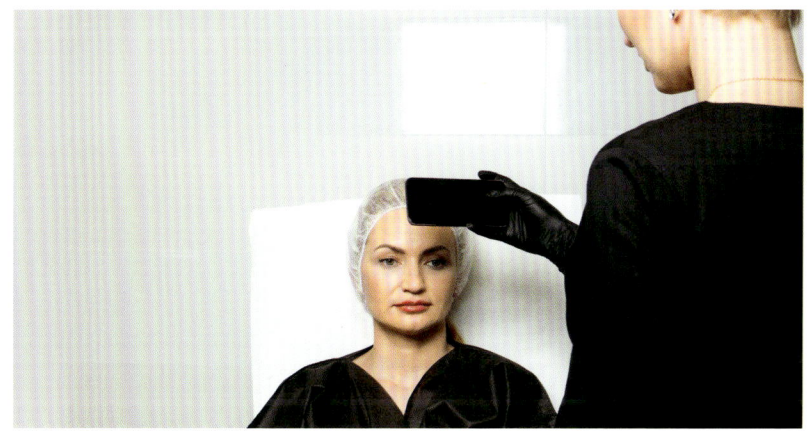

Once the sketch is ready, it is time to show the final design to the client and ask for approval. Two methods are recommended to help the client visualize the sketch. The first and more classic method is to view the sketch in a mirror from frontal and side angles. The second method consists of taking several pictures from different perspectives and showing them to the client. Take enough time to show the sketch to your clients, pointing out the improvements in terms of definition, balance, and symmetry. It will increase customer satisfaction once the procedure has been performed.

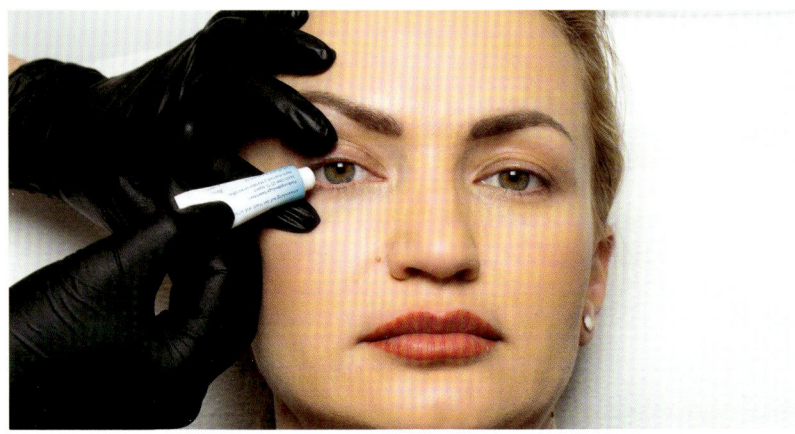

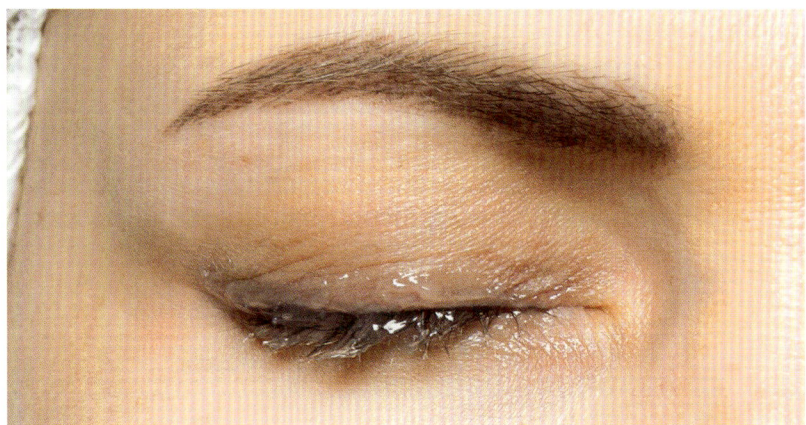

To avoid eye irritation from contact with pigments or other products, we will apply an ophthalmological cream which will create a sort of transparent, protective layer that will temporarily obstruct vision and disappear within a few minutes.

In countries that allow the use of topical numbing ointment, proceed by applying it to the external eye area, making sure not to let it come in contact with the eye itself. Let the solution sit for around 15 minutes then remove it with the special wipes and plenty of water.

7   1ST PASS OF MICROPIGMENTATION

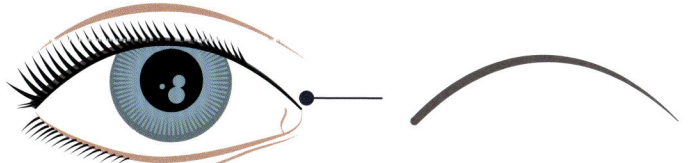

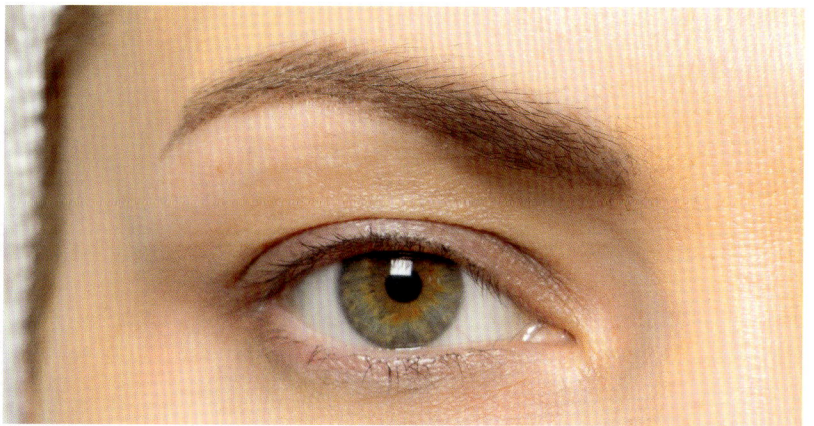

➡ Bidirectional   ◢ 60°, 90°   ✎ 3-Micro

✋ Medium/Slow   ± 100   💧 Organic, Inorganic, Mix

We start the first micropigmentation pass moving from the external corner of the eye towards the internal corner with short, bidirectional zigzag movements that go back and forth. Then proceed to draw a line in the area between the lashes following same zigzag movement.

We recommend using the 3 point micro cartridge and a working angle of 60° or 90°. Advanced students could use also a 3-Power or 1-Liner for this step.

8   2ND PASS OF MICROPIGMENTATION

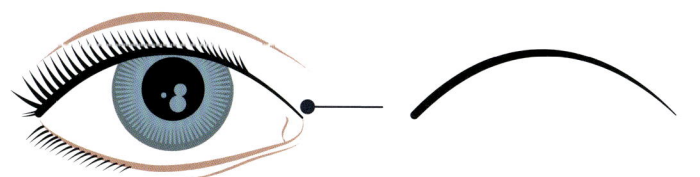

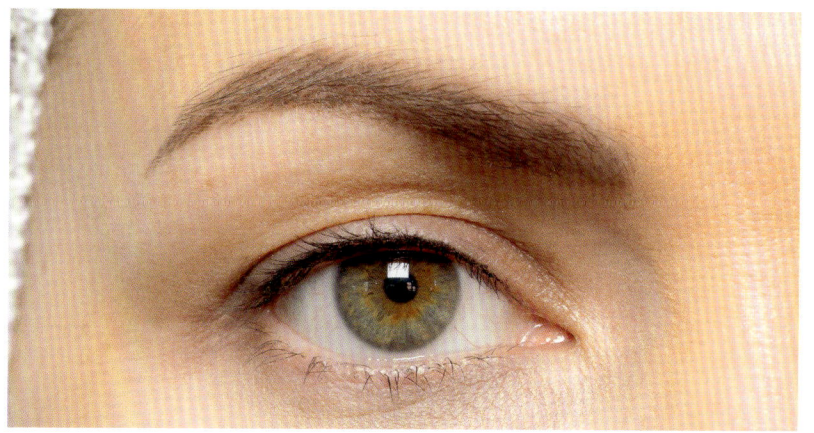

➡ Bidirectional   ◢ 60°, 90°   ✎ 3-Micro

✋ Medium/Slow   ± 100   💧 Organic, Inorganic, Mix

If necessary, proceed to perform a second or even a third pass on the area following same technique and movements until we achieve a very intensive and saturated fine line. However, please do not perform more than three passes on the same area.

Please remember! We are working on a very sensitive area, close to the eyeball. It is of crucial importance to stretch the skin properly.

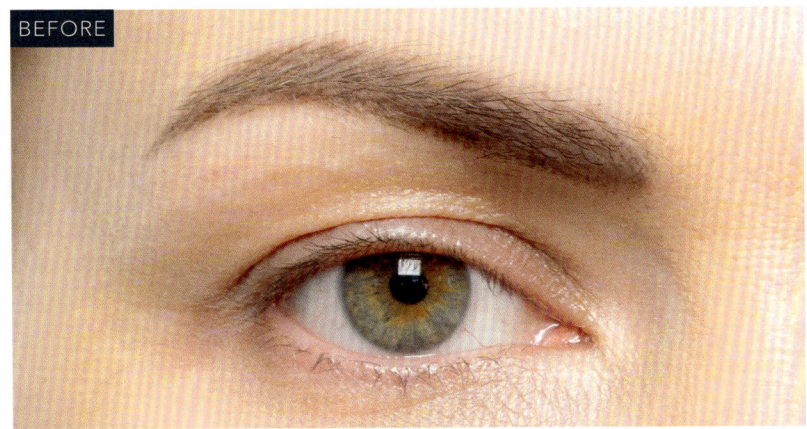

BEFORE

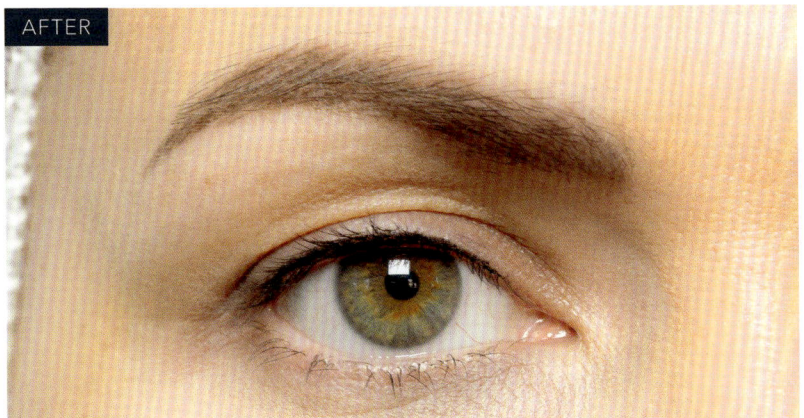

AFTER

Since procedures in the eye area deal with two different kinds of tissue, the skin and the conjunctiva, there is a risk of greater irritation compared to procedures for the eyebrows.

As usual, the final results will only be seen 40 days after healing.

13.3.2. EYELINER

Clients choose a graphic procedure like eyeliner for many different reasons. Applying pigment on the eye's x point creates the illusion of an eye that is vertically wider, if the eye is of the ascending type, or horizontally wider, if it is a positive eye type. Before drawing a graphic eyeliner it is important to understand its geometric structure.

If we were to draw eyeliner on a one-dimensional surface like a sheet of paper, the result would be an elongated triangle which could be wider or narrower, longer or more streamlined, or have softer or rounder shapes (Fig.1).

There are also different typologies that refer to the way the eyeliner is drawn. The end of the eyeliner, often called the tail, can be made thinner, more tapered, or thicker, or it can be in between a triangle and a rounder shape (Fig.2).

Once the shape of the eyeliner has been chosen, it is time to decide on its thickness: it is important to achieve the right balance between the morphology of the facial features, the professional's advice, and the client's own taste.

It is best to analyze the special aspects of the step-by-step instructions for correctly applying eyeliner.

FIG. 2 EYELINER SHAPE

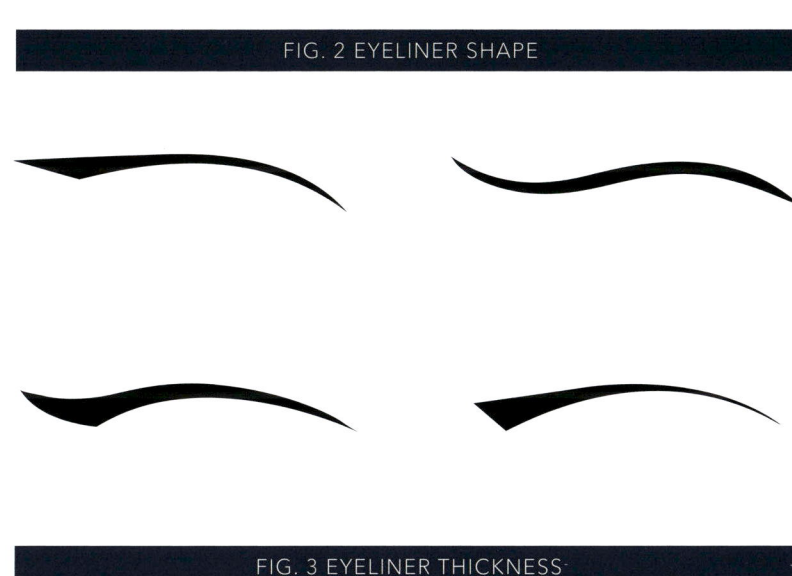

FIG. 1 EYELINER GEOMETRY

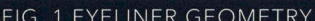

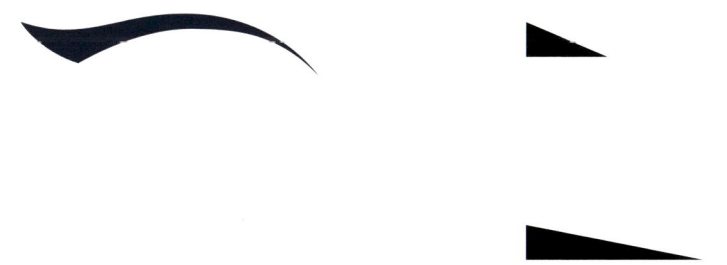

FIG. 3 EYELINER THICKNESS

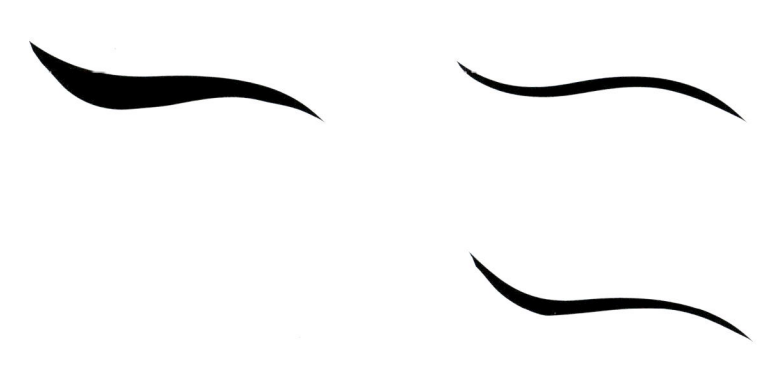

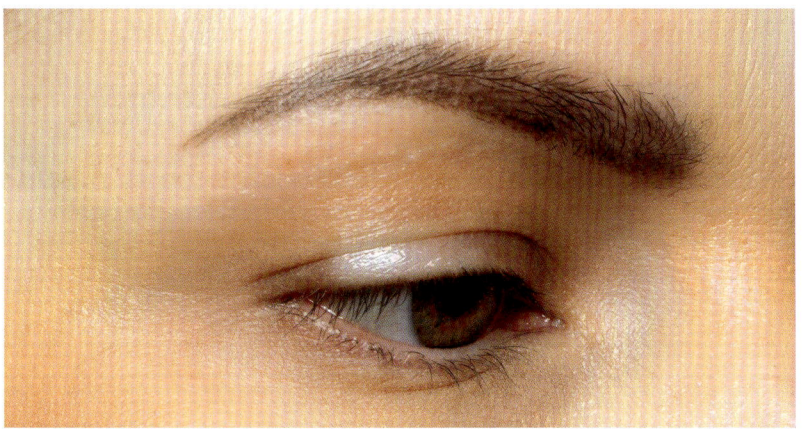

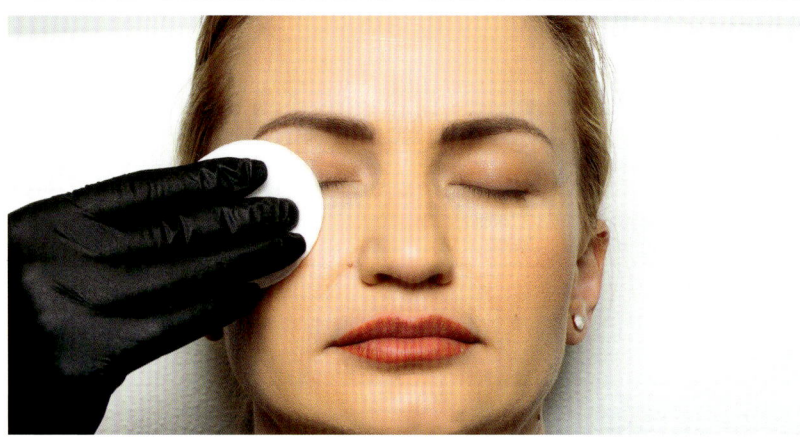

Before starting the eyelash enhancement procedure, it is advisable to ask your client how they draw their eyeliner in their daily makeup in order to discover the preferred color and thickness. At the same time, we analyze the shape and position of the eyes in our client's face, so we will be able to correct the shape and make the eyes' expression more balanced.

Before starting procedure, it is important to take into account all relevant hygienic aspects for the eye area. Remember that tissue between the lashes has a different morphology and sensibility than the eyebrow area, and it is more prone to inflammation, infections and other reactions. Therefore, it is of crucial importance to follow the highest safety and hygienic standards.

We proceed to gently clean the upper lid area with antiseptic liquid until makeup and other cosmetic products have been completely removed.

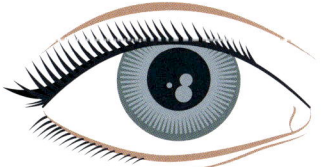

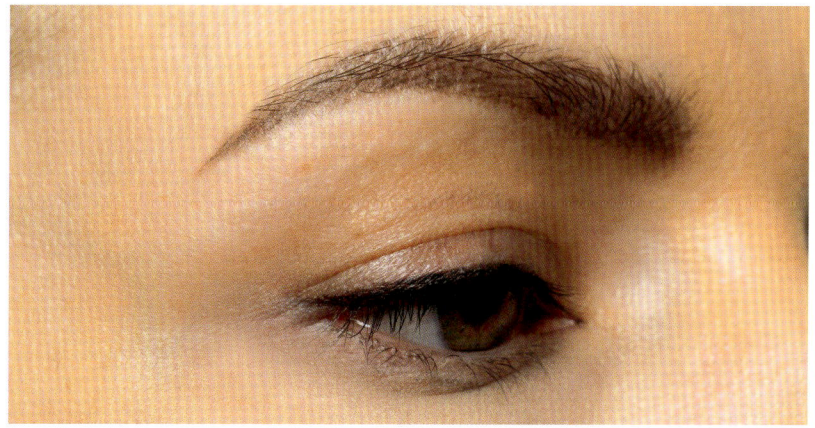

Proceed by sketching the design on the client. Use one marker in the desired color following the common visagistic rules for the eye area.

⚠ ATTENTION

In some countries only sterile, single-use markers are allowed for this purpose.

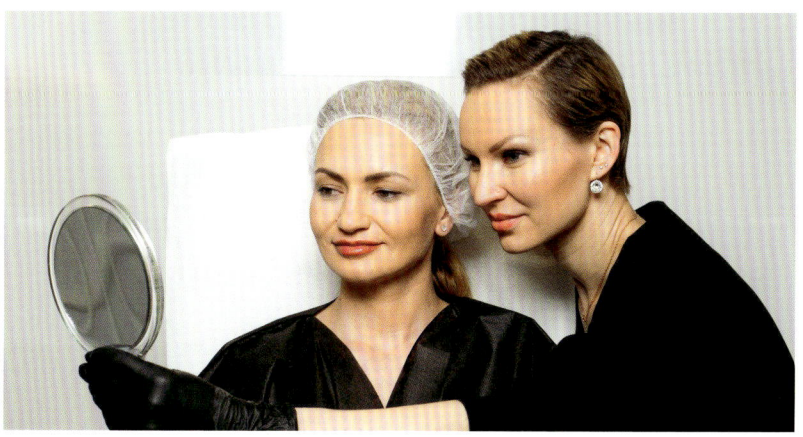

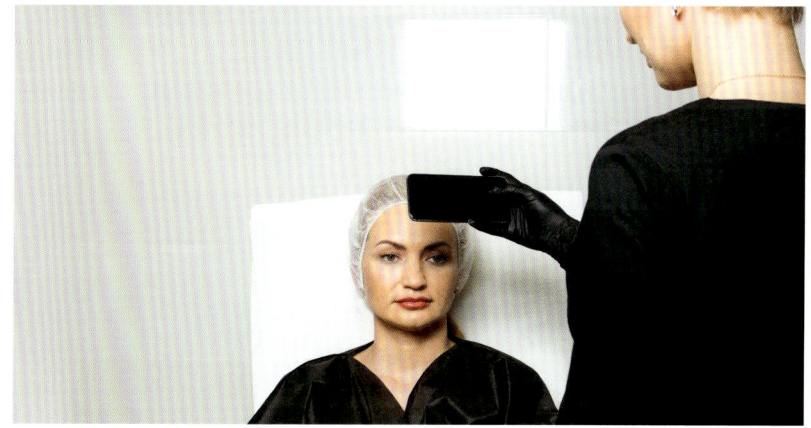

Once the sketch is ready, it is time to show the final design to the client and ask for approval. Two methods are recommended to help the client visualize the sketch. The first and more classic method is to view the sketch in a mirror from frontal and side angles. The second method consists of taking several pictures from different perspectives and showing them to the client. Take enough time to show the sketch to your clients, pointing out the improvements in terms of definition, balance, and symmetry. It will increase customer satisfaction once the procedure has been performed.

EYEBROWS

LIPS

EYES

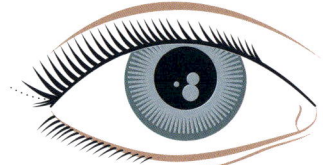

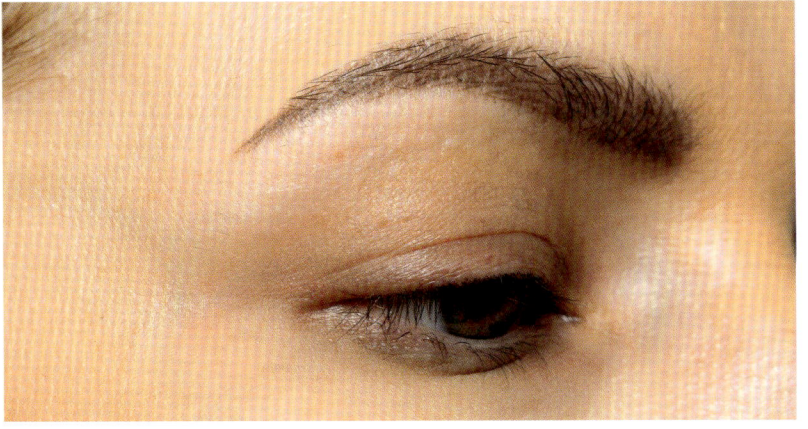

➡️ Bidirectional   ◢ 60°   🌡️ 3-Micro, 1-Liner

✋ Slow   ± 80/100   💧 Organic, Inorganic, Mix

Fix the design by drawing the lower line of the eyeliner and the external corner of the eye with the micropigmentation handpiece. Work very gently with low frequency (80–100 pps). It is important to fix the sketch prior to applying the numbing solution. Otherwise, the design will not be visible once we remove the solution.

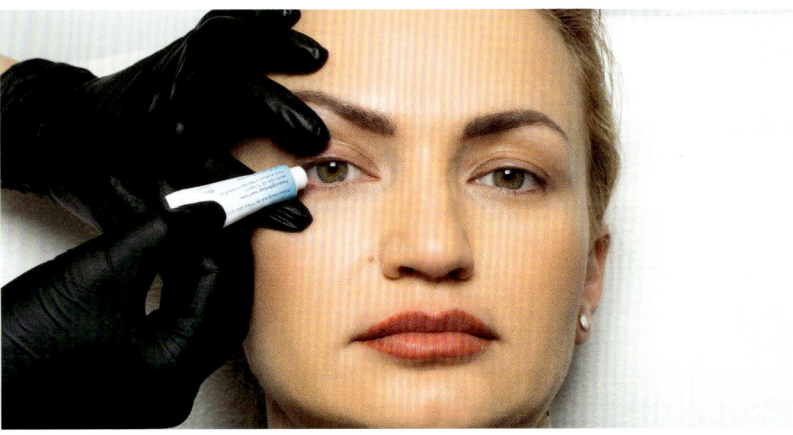

To avoid eye irritation from contact with pigments or other products, we will apply an ophthalmological cream which will create a sort of transparent, protective patina that will temporarily obstruct vision and disappear within a few minutes.

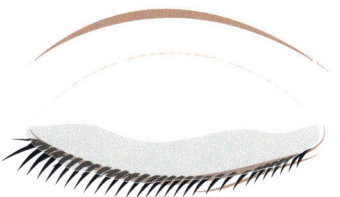

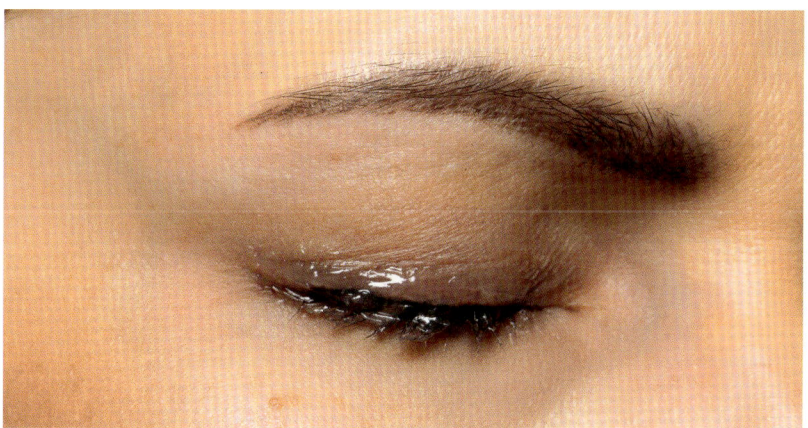

In countries that allow the use of topical numbing ointment, proceed by applying it to the external eye area, making sure not to let it come in contact with the eye itself.

Apply the numbing solution for 15 minutes then remove it with wet wipes.

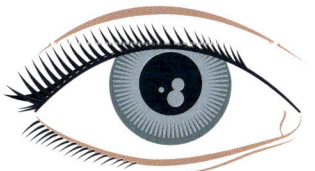

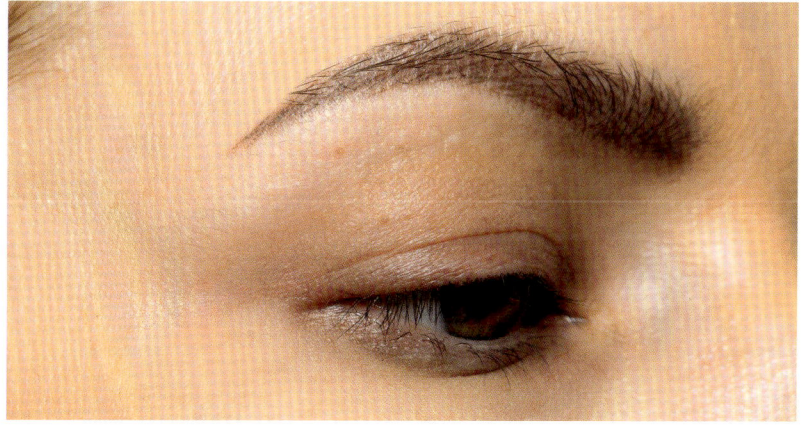

➡ Bidirectional ◢ 60°–90° ⬦ 3-Micro, 1-Liner

✋ Medium ± 100 💧 Organic, Inorganic, Mix

We start the first micropigmentation pass moving from the external corner of the eye towards the internal corner with short bidirectional zigzag movements that go back and forth. Then, proceed to draw a line in the area between the lashes following the same zigzag movements.

We recommend using the 3 point micro cartridge or 1-Liner with a working angle of 60° or 90°.

EYEBROWS

LIPS

EYES

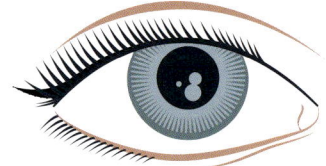

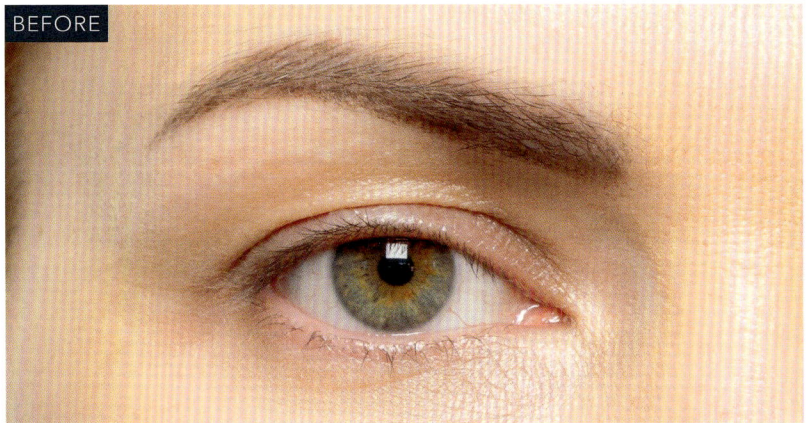

BEFORE

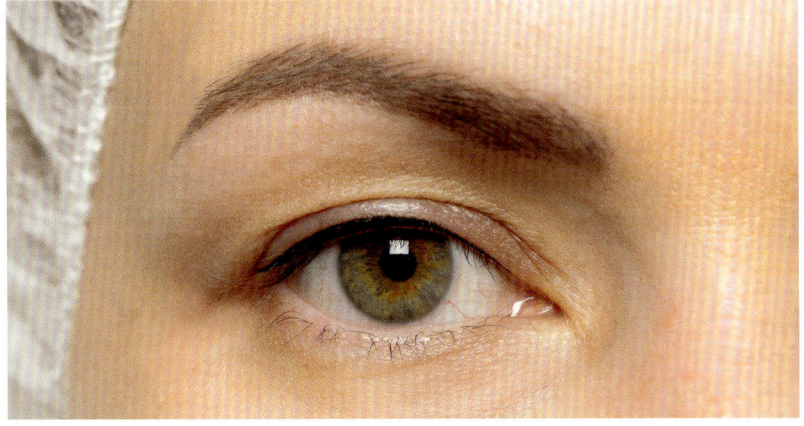

AFTER

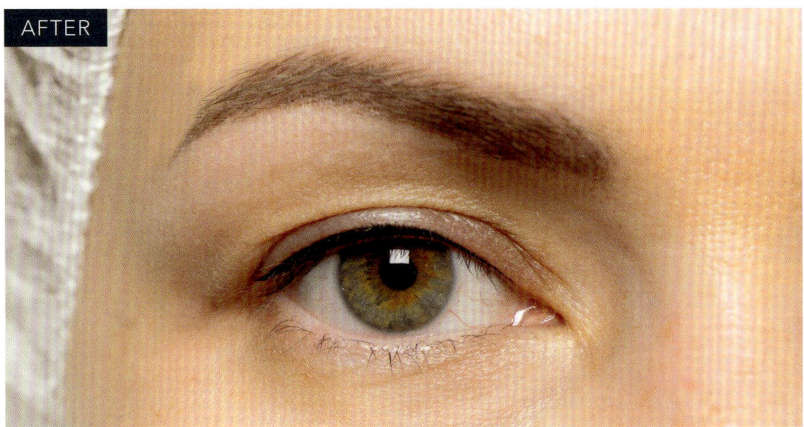

➡ Bidirectional ◪ 60°–90° ⬍ 3-Micro, 1-Liner

🖐 Medium ± 100 💧 Organic, Inorganic, Mix

Proceed to perform a second or even a third pass on the area between the lashes following same technique and movements until we achieve a very intensive and saturated fine line. Please do not perform more than three passes on the same area.

Next, start with the eyeliner micropigmentation, moving from the external corner of the eye towards internal corner according to the previous sketch. Make sure no empty space is left between lash line and external eyeliner.

Since procedures in the eye area deal with two different kinds of tissue, the skin and the conjunctiva, there is a risk of greater irritation compared to procedures for the eyebrows. As usual, the final results will only be seen 40 days after healing.

13.3.3. SHADING

1   INITIAL SITUATION

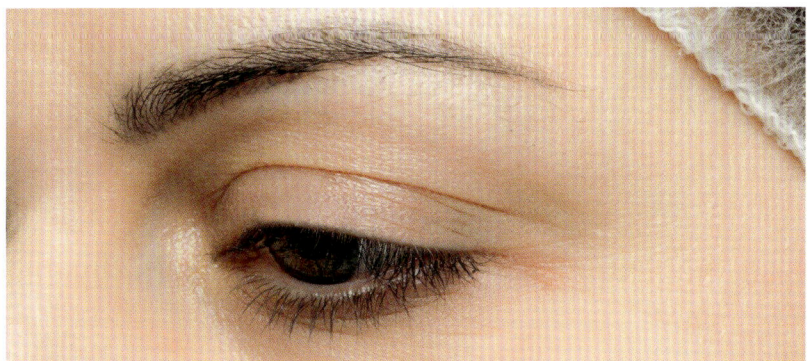

Before applying pigment between the lashes, take care of the hygiene of the area of application.

2   CLEANING

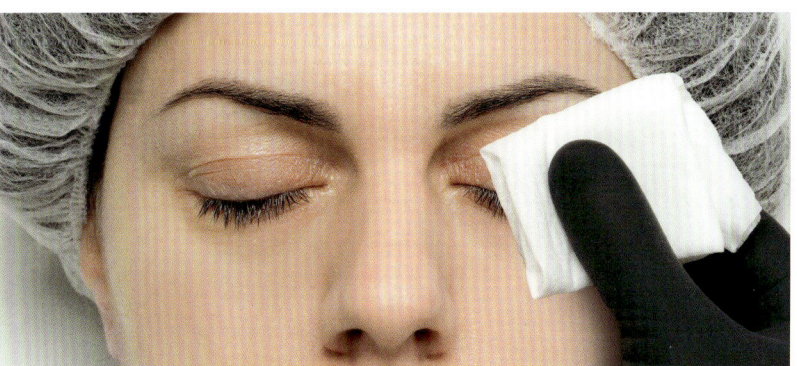

The first phase involves deep-cleaning the area to remove any previously applied makeup or cosmetic products, and to eliminate any potential non-pathogenic microorganisms.

3   APPLYING OPHTHALMOLOGICAL CREAM

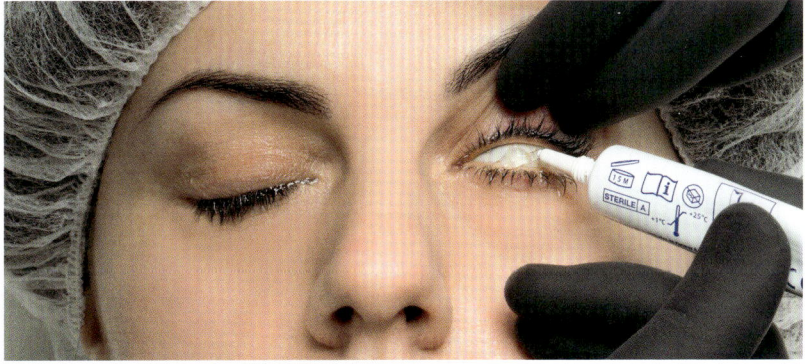

To avoid eye irritation from contact with pigments or other products, we will apply an ophthalmological cream which will create a sort of transparent, protective patina that will temporarily obstruct vision and disappear within a few minutes.

4   APPLYING 1ST NUMBING SOLUTION

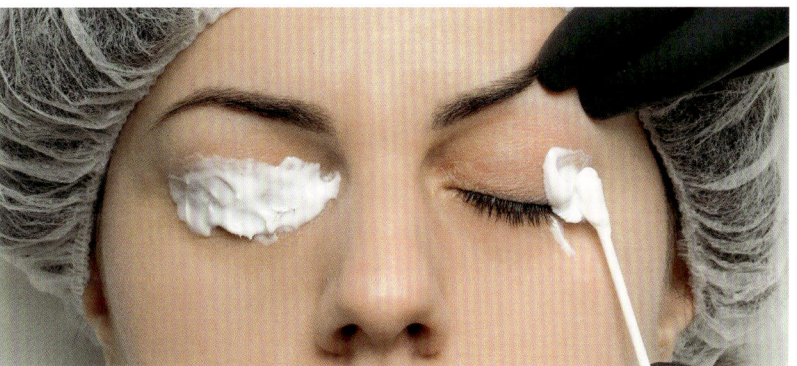

In countries that allow the use of topical numbing ointment, proceed by applying it to the external eye area, making sure not to let it come in contact with the eye itself.
Let the solution sit for around 15 minutes then remove it with the special wipes and plenty of water.

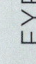

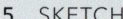

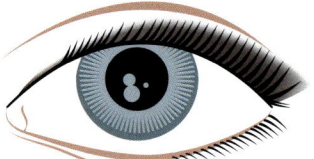

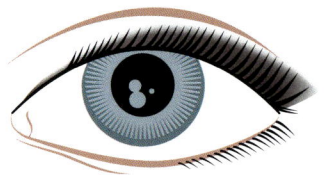

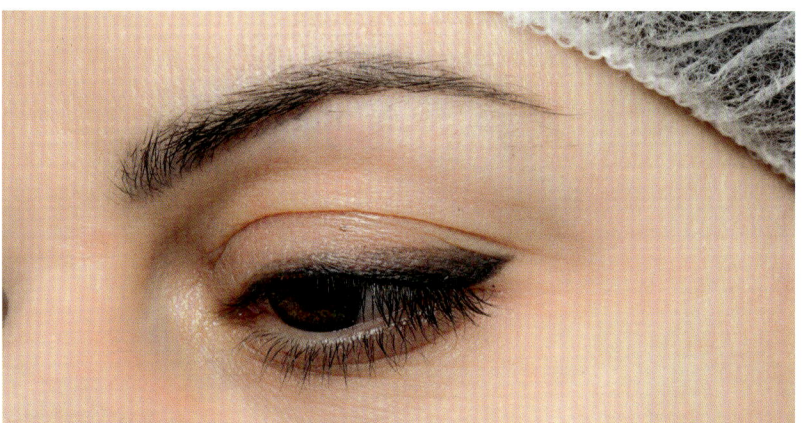

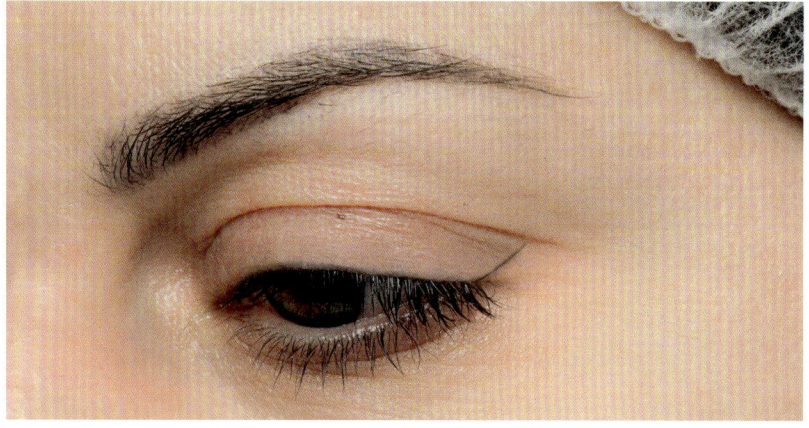

During the sketching phase, pigment will be applied on the eyeliner with an amiea mixing pen. With a sterile cotton tip you can shade the color upwards in order to show the final design to the client. This is a good method for reassuring the client about the final results. The extent of the shading depends not only on the client's taste and expectations, but especially on the anatomic structure of the eyelid. A wider eye with more space on the upper lash line can of course handle more blending and more intense colors.

➡ Bidirectional   ◢ 60°   🌡 3-Micro

✋ Slow   ± 80/100   💧 Organic, Inorganic, Mix

This involves creating just a light line along the outer corner of the eye to determine the orientation and height of the shading. By making small pricks along the inside of the lashes, the professional facilitates the opening of the skin and its absorption of the numbing solution.

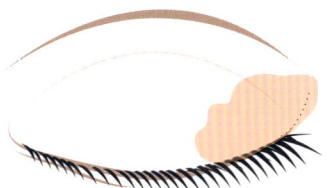

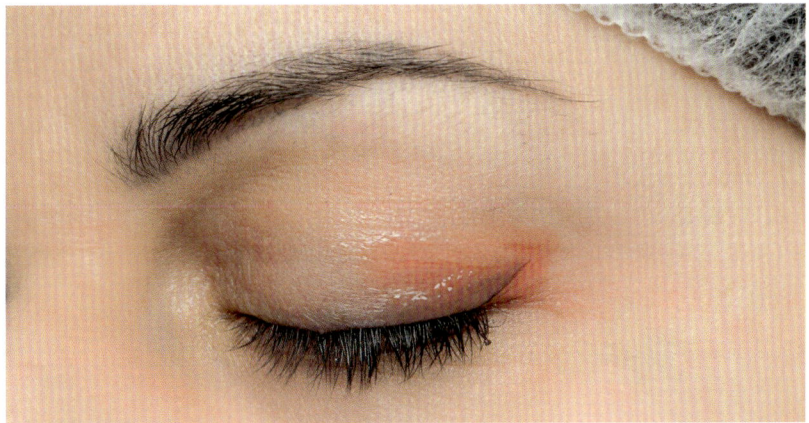

In countries where the law permits it, apply a numbing solution; this not only inhibits pain stimuli but also decongests the area, preventing bleeding which could dilute the color. Apply the second numbing solution.

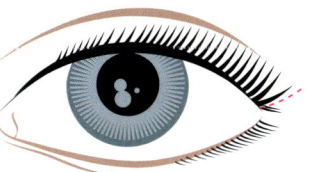

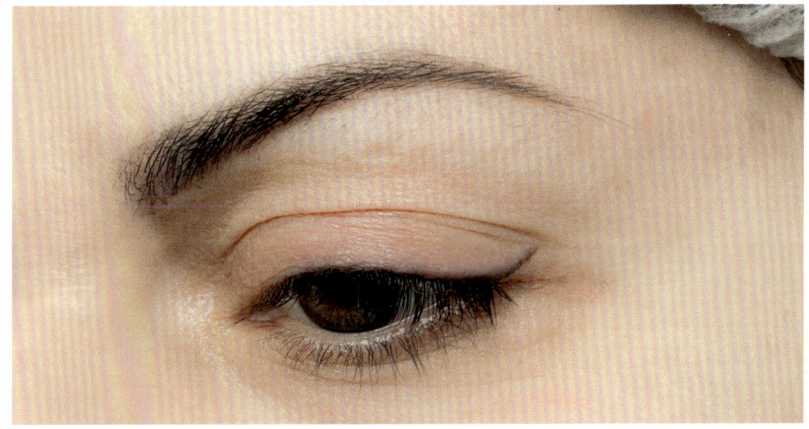

➡ Bidirectional	◢ 60°-90°	🌡 3-Micro
✋ Medium	± 100	💧 Organic, Inorganic, Mix

Protocol calls for inter-eyelash pigmentation to be done with a 3-point micro needle, at a 60°–90° angle with very slow, bidirectional movements, in order to achieve a thicker line and more intense color between the eyelashes.

EYEBROWS

LIPS

EYES

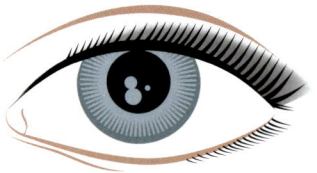

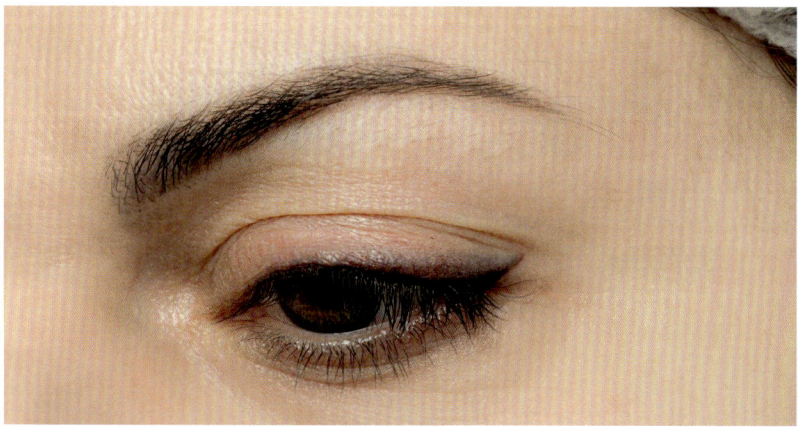

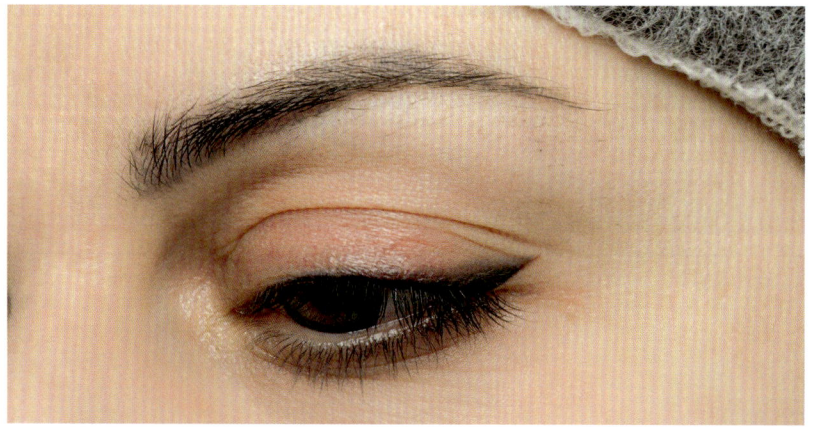

➡ Bidirectional	◿ 60°–90°	🌡 3-Micro, 3-Slope
✋ Medium	± 100	💧 Organic, Inorganic, Mix

Once the lash enhancement line is done, proceed to the first level of shading using a needle that corresponds to the thickness and extent of the blending intended. An initial level of color intensity is already visible in the eye.

➡ Bidirectional	◿ 60°–90°	🌡 3-Micro, 3-Slope
✋ Medium	± 120	💧 Organic, Inorganic, Mix

For the second level of shading, use bidirectional movements at a faster speed, at a 60°–90° angle, taking care not to apply color too opaquely. The motion should be quick to avoid true, opaque color.

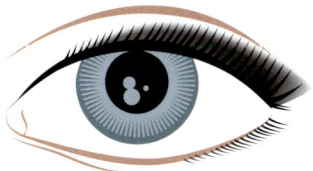

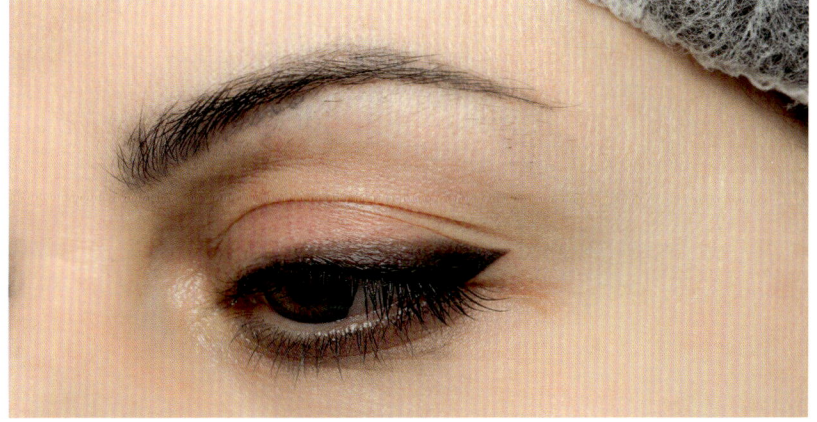

➡ Monodirectional   ◢ 60°   ◐ 3-Micro, 3-Slope

✋ Medium   ± 100   💧 Organic, Inorganic, Mix

It is also important for pressure to decrease as you move away from the deep dermis of the eyelashes, towards the medium dermis and the superficial dermis outside the lashline, finally reaching the epidermis. From here, use a monodirectional movement, but move from the eyelashes outward, at a 60° angle and moderate speed. This will feel like applying small brush strokes, allowing more control in creating a color gradient, which will be more or less obvious depending on the intended effect. The process involves at least three levels of shading.

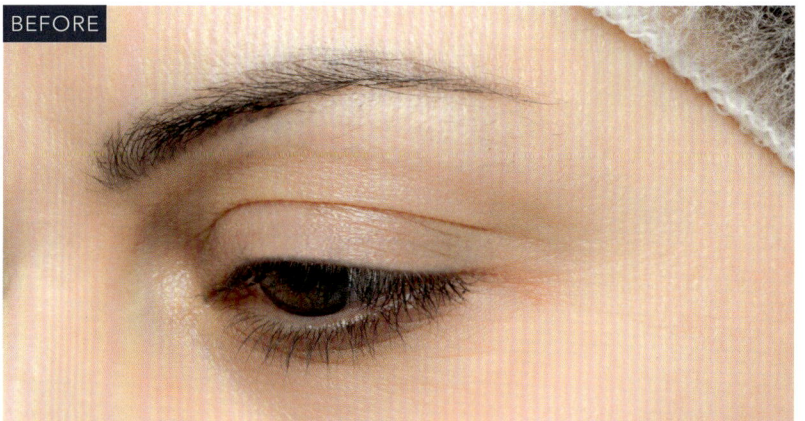

BEFORE

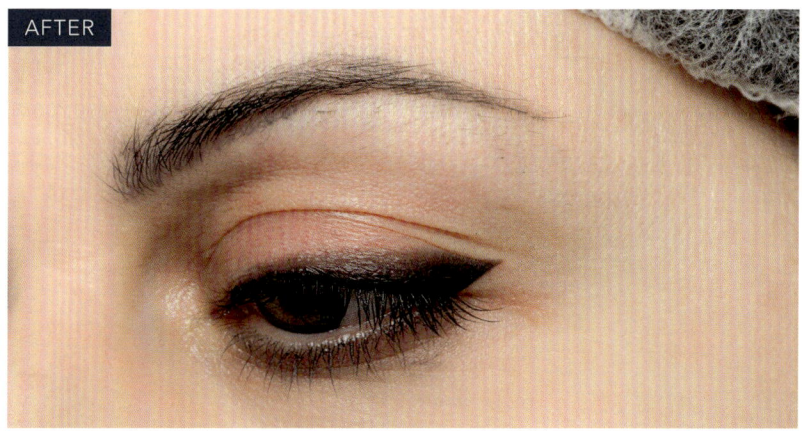

AFTER

Since procedures in the eye area deal with two different kinds of tissue, the skin and the conjunctiva, there is a risk of greater irritation compared to procedures for the eyebrows. As usual, the final results will only be seen 40 days after healing.

EYEBROWS

LIPS

EYES

SUGGESTIONS

After the end of a book or a training course, a crucial phase begins: practice. As with any sports, we prepare for the race by repeating the necessary movements until our performance meets our expectations.

The same holds for permanent makeup: before performing any procedure on a model, you must have put all of the information acquired here into practice, in terms of parameters, managing stress, and confidence with the equipment and facilities.

The first thing to do in order to achieve professional results is to go back over the entire course of study and try to find answers to any doubts or confusion you may find.

The next step is to practice over the next few months, using paper and pencil, in order to quickly memorize the way hair grows, develop excellent hand sensitivity, and perfect the lines that will form the basis of any application technique.

This requires consistency: by spending at least one hour a day on this phase, with the knowledge that the more time you put in now the faster you will grow as a professional.

After that step, it is time to practice on synthetic material and add more challenges to the previous phase: these include mastering the needle's vibration, managing the angles of application, and evaluating the depth and speed of hand movements.

At this point you will begin to simulate real procedures, along with their accompanying problems. Remember that technical defects will be more visible on latex and therefore you should not let various mistakes demoralize you.

The greatest professionals are those who never set aside this kind of practice even though they receive hundreds of clients; just like an Olympic champion never leaves the gym and continues to beat their own records each time.

Once you have acquired technical confidence, set aside emotional fears, and developed a memory of application techniques, you are ready for the next step which is performing procedures on models.

We recommend starting out by performing permanent makeup procedures on people close to you, such as family and friends, in order to feel calmer during the procedure, to better manage your emotions, and so that any small errors can be accepted more easily than would be the case with paying clients.

Continued theoretical study and constant practice strengthen any real dermopigmentation professional.

NOW IT'S YOUR TURN.

This is the opposite of a conclusion. The end lays the foundation for a new beginning. Any journey into a new world leaves visible signs behind. It would be great if these pages, full of practical advice, could above all serve to instill the kind of curiosity that is common among intelligent minds, those who are not satisfied with explanations.

The spread of beauty cannot be fulfilled in theory; it lives in reality. Without Dionysius, Apollo is confined, imprisoned in a perfect body, but devoid of life.

What I wish for you is that you become passionate about beauty, and feel that you have chosen a career that allows you to share your passion.

That is what happened to me, and that is why anywhere I travel in the world, I bring my own suitcase of knowledge and experience. Because sharing knowledge is the only thing that enriches both the giver and the recipient, defying any economic logic.

Released by MT.DERM GmbH,
Gustav-Krone-Straße 3, 14167 Berlin, Germany

© 2019 MT.DERM, Berlin

Publisher: Jan Hodok
Author: Toni Belfatto
In cooperation with Elena Nikora, Olga Kravchenko
and Sara Lopez
Layout: Alessio Papa, TRE BIT Communicazione
Layout Consultant: Wera Waleska Steiner
Project Management: Clemens Glade
Printing & binding: H. Heeneman GmbH & Co. KG,
Bessemerstraße 83, 12103 Berlin, Germany

ISBN 978-3-9819943-0-8